Anatomical terminology

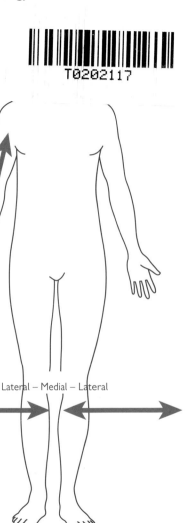

T0202117

Distal—Proximal

Lateral – Medial – Lateral

Coronal plane

Oxford Handbook of
Forensic Medicine

Published and forthcoming Oxford Handbooks

Oxford Handbook for the Foundation Programme 2e
Oxford Handbook of Acute Medicine 3e
Oxford Handbook of Anaesthesia 2e
Oxford Handbook of Applied Dental Sciences
Oxford Handbook of Cardiology
Oxford Handbook of Clinical and Laboratory Investigation 3e
Oxford Handbook of Clinical Dentistry 4e
Oxford Handbook of Clinical Diagnosis 2e
Oxford Handbook of Clinical Examination and Practical Skills
Oxford Handbook of Clinical Haematology 3e
Oxford Handbook of Clinical Immunology and Allergy 2e
Oxford Handbook of Clinical Medicine—Mini Edition 8e
Oxford Handbook of Clinical Medicine 8e
Oxford Handbook of Clinical Pharmacy
Oxford Handbook of Clinical Rehabilitation 2e
Oxford Handbook of Clinical Specialties 8e
Oxford Handbook of Clinical Surgery 3e
Oxford Handbook of Complementary Medicine
Oxford Handbook of Critical Care 3e
Oxford Handbook of Dental Patient Care 2e
Oxford Handbook of Dialysis 3e
Oxford Handbook of Emergency Medicine 3e
Oxford Handbook of Endocrinology and Diabetes 2e
Oxford Handbook of ENT and Head and Neck Surgery
Oxford Handbook of Expedition and Wilderness Medicine
Oxford Handbook of Gastroenterology & Hepatology
Oxford Handbook of General Practice 3e
Oxford Handbook of Genitourinary Medicine, HIV, and Sexual Health 2e
Oxford Handbook of Geriatric Medicine
Oxford Handbook of Infectious Diseases and Microbiology
Oxford Handbook of Key Clinical Evidence
Oxford Handbook of Medical Sciences
Oxford Handbook of Nephrology and Hypertension
Oxford Handbook of Neurology
Oxford Handbook of Nutrition and Dietetics
Oxford Handbook of Obstetrics and Gynaecology 2e
Oxford Handbook of Occupational Health
Oxford Handbook of Oncology 2e
Oxford Handbook of Ophthalmology
Oxford Handbook of Paediatrics
Oxford Handbook of Palliative Care 2e
Oxford Handbook of Practical Drug Therapy 2e
Oxford Handbook of Pre-Hospital Care
Oxford Handbook of Psychiatry 2e
Oxford Handbook of Public Health Practice 2e
Oxford Handbook of Reproductive Medicine & Family Planning
Oxford Handbook of Respiratory Medicine 2e
Oxford Handbook of Rheumatology 3e
Oxford Handbook of Sport and Exercise Medicine
Oxford Handbook of Tropical Medicine 3e
Oxford Handbook of Urology 2e

Oxford Handbook of
Forensic
Medicine

Jonathan Wyatt

Emergency Department Consultant and
Forensic Physician,
Royal Cornwall Hospital,
Cornwall, UK

Tim Squires

Developer, Global Health Academy,
School of Biomedical Sciences,
The University of Edinburgh, UK

Guy Norfolk

Founding President,
Faculty of Forensic and Legal Medicine,
Royal College of Physicians of London, UK

Jason Payne-James

Editor, Journal of Forensic and Legal Medicine
Director, Forensic Healthcare Services Ltd,
Vice-President (Forensic Medicine),
Faculty of Forensic and Legal Medicine,
Barts & The London School of Medicine & Dentistry,
London, UK

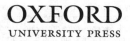

OXFORD
UNIVERSITY PRESS

OXFORD
UNIVERSITY PRESS

Great Clarendon Street, Oxford OX2 6DP.

Oxford University Press is a department of the University of Oxford.
It furthers the University's objective of excellence in research, scholarship,
and education by publishing worldwide in

Oxford New York

Auckland Cape Town Dar es Salaam Hong Kong Karachi
Kuala Lumpur Madrid Melbourne Mexico City Nairobi
New Delhi Shanghai Taipei Toronto

With offices in

Argentina Austria Brazil Chile Czech Republic France Greece
Guatemala Hungary Italy Japan Poland Portugal Singapore
South Korea Switzerland Thailand Turkey Ukraine Vietnam

Oxford is a registered trade mark of Oxford University Press
in the UK and in certain other countries

Published in the United States
by Oxford University Press Inc., New York

British Library Cataloguing in Publication Data
Data available

Library of Congress Cataloging-in-Publication-Data
Data available

Typeset by Glyph International, Bangalore, India
Printed in Italy
on acid-free paper through
L.E.G.O. S.p.A.

ISBN 978–0–19–922994–9

10 9 8 7 6

Oxford University Press makes no representation, express or implied, that the
drug dosages in this book are correct. Readers must therefore always check the
product information and clinical procedures with the most up-to-date published
product information and data sheets provided by the manufacturers and the most
recent codes of conduct and safety regulations. The authors and publishers do not
accept responsibility or legal liability for any errors in the text or for the misuse or
misapplication of material in this work. Except where otherwise stated, drug dosages
and recommendations are for the non-pregnant adult who is not breastfeeding.

Acknowledgements

We would like to acknowledge the help and advice in the preparation of this book received from the following individuals: IB, Leah Burgess, Ruth Creamer, Jenny Farrant, Zoe Ghosh, Rachel Goss, Sian Ireland, Hayley Johnson, Andy Lockyer, Richard Parry, Kim Picozzi, and Rob Taylor.

Contents

Contents

Detailed contents

15 Forensic science 495

Symbols and abbreviations

📖	cross-reference
>	greater than
<	less than
±	with or without
ACPO	Association of Chief Police Officers
ADD	accumulated degree days
ADH	accumulated degree hours
ADHD	attention deficit hyperactivity disorder
AF	atrial fibrillation
AIDS	acquired immune deficiency syndrome
AMHP	approved mental health professional
AP	anteroposterior *or* acid phosphatase
ARDS	adult respiratory distress syndrome
ATP	adenosine triphosphate
BAC	blood alcohol concentration
BMA	British Medical Association
BMG	bedside measurement of glucose
BMI	body mass index
BNF	*British National Formulary*
CAA	Civil Aviation Authority
CAGE	the 'cut-annoyed-guilty-eye' questionnaire to assess alcohol dependence.
CCTV	closed-circuit television
CIWA	Clinical Institute Withdrawal Assessment for Alcohol
CJD	Creutzfeldt–Jakob disease (most common human prion disease)
CNS	central nervous system
CO	carbon monoxide
CO_2	carbon dioxide
COHb	carboxyhaemoglobin
COPFS	Crown Office Procurator Fiscal Service (Scotland)
COPD	chronic obstructive pulmonary disease
CPS	Crown Prosecution Service
CSM	Crime Scene Manager
CT	computed tomography (scan)
DFMS	Diploma of Forensic Medical Sciences

DMJ	Diploma of Medical Jurisprudence (🕮 http://www.apothecaries.org)
DNA	deoxyribonucleic acid
DSH	deliberate self-harm
DSM	Diagnostic and Statistical Manual of Mental Disorders, American Psychiatric Association (revision V due in 2013)
DTTO	Drug Treatment and Testing Order
DVLA	Driver and Vehicle Licensing Agency
ECG	electrocardiogram
EEG	electroencephalogram
FEV_1	forced expiratory volume in 1s
FFLM	Faculty of Forensic and Legal Medicine (🕮 http://www.fflm.ac.uk)
FME	Forensic Medical Examiner
FP	Forensic Physician
FSS	Forensic Science Service
GAD	generalized anxiety disorder
GC–MS	gas chromatography–mass spectrometry
GCS	Glasgow coma score
GMC	General Medical Council
GP	General Practitioner
h	hour(s)
HEPA	high efficiency particulate air
HIV	human immunodeficiency virus
HOCM	hypertrophic cardiomyopathy
ICD-10	International Statistical Classification of Diseases and Related Health Problems (revision 11 planned for 2015)
ICV	Independent Custody Visitor
IEF	isoelectric focusing
IPCC	Independent Police Complaints Commission (🕮 http://www.ipcc.gov.uk)
IQ	intelligence quotient
ISS	Injury Severity Score (www.trauma.org)
LSD	lysergic acid diethylamide
m	metre/s
MAOI	monoamine oxidase inhibitor (antidepressant)
MAM	monoacetylmorphine
MB ChB	Bachelor of Medicine, Bachelor of Surgery
MCA	Mental Capacity Act
MDA	Misuse of Drugs Act
MFFLM	Member of the Faculty of Forensic and Legal Medicine
mg	milligram(s)

MHA	Mental Health Act
MI	myocardial infarction (AMI—acute MI)
min	minute(s)
MMSE	Mini-Mental State Examination
MRI	magnetic resonance imaging
MRCGP	Member of the Royal College of General Practitioners
NAI	non-accidental injury
NHS	National Health Service (UK)
NICE	National Institute for Health and Clinical Excellence
NMC	Nursing and Midwifery Council
NSAI(D)	non-steroidal anti-inflammatory (drug)
NSPIS	National Strategy for Police Information Systems
O_2	oxygen
PA	posteroanterior
PACE	Police and Criminal Evidence Act
PE	pulmonary embolism
PER	prisoner escort record
pCO_2	partial pressure of carbon dioxide
PCSO	Police Custody and Security Officer
PGDs	Patient Group Directions
PGM	phosphoglucomutase
PM	'postmortem' but often refers to an autopsy
PNC	police national computer
POM	prescription-only medicine
PF	Procurator Fiscal
PTSD	post-traumatic stress disorder
RCPCH	Royal College of Paediatrics and Child Health
RMO	Responsible Medical Officer
RSU	Regional Secure Unit
RTA	Road Traffic Act 1988 but also: road traffic accident (MVC motor vehicle collision)
s	second(s)
SADS	sudden adult death syndrome (also sudden arrhythmic death syndromes and seasonal affective disorders)
SaO_2	oxygen saturation
SARCs	Sexual Assault Referral Centres
SCIWORA	spinal cord injury without radiographic abnormality
SCT	supervised community treatment
SIDS	sudden infant death syndrome
SIO	Senior Investigating Officer
SOCO	Scene of Crime Officer

SOP	standard operating procedure
SSRI	selective serotonin reuptake inhibitor (antidepressant)
SUDI	sudden unexpected death in infancy
TB	tuberculosis
TCA	tricyclic antidepressant
THC	tetrahydrocannabinol (active ingredient in cannabis)
TIA	transient ischaemic attack—a temporary inadequacy of the circulation in the brain, usually resolving within 24h. Sometimes known as a 'mini stroke'. A TIA is a medical emergency.
V&G	'View and Grant' procedure
VES	victim examination suites
UK	United Kingdom
UV	ultraviolet
VF	ventricular fibrillation
VT	ventricular tachycardia

Anatomical terminology

The body is described in the anatomical position—upright, hands by the side with palms to the front.

The three planes of section of the body are at right angles to each other.

- Coronal—parallel with the front and back of the body.
- Sagittal—parallel with the sides of the body.
- Transverse—in a body in the anatomical position these horizontal planes are parallel with the ground.

The sagittal section which bisects the body is known as a *midline* section or *median* section. Planes parallel to this are known as *parasagittal* sections.

On a transverse plane, a point closer to the front is *anterior* or *ventral*—those closer to the back are *posterior* or *dorsal*.

Points closer to the head are described as being *superior* (or *cranial*) to those *inferior* (or *caudal*) points nearer the feet.

When referring to two points in the same coronal plane, the one nearer the midline is said to be *medial* and the one further away *lateral* with respect to one another.

When referring to two points on the same limb, the one nearer the trunk is said to be *proximal* and the one nearer the hands or feet *distal* with respect to one another.

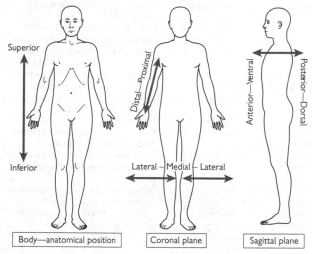

Fig. 1 Anatomical terminology.

Prefixes

Prepositional prefixes

Prefix	Meaning	Example
A- or An-	absence of	Anoxia—lacking oxygen
Ante-	before	Antemortem—before death
Anti-	against	Antiseptic—preventing infection
Circum-	around	Circumoral—round the mouth
Contra-	against or opposite	Contralateral—on the other side
De-	away from	Dehydrate—to remove water
Dia-	through	Dialyse—to pass through a membrane
Dis-	apart	Dissection—cutting to pieces
Dys-	abnormal	Dysfunction—abnormal function
En- or Endo-	within	Endometrium—inside lining of the womb
Epi-	on or upon	Epidermis—outer skin layer
Extra-	outside	Extracorporeal—outside the body
Exo-	outside	Exoskeleton—hard, protective outer material e.g. shell of crab
Hetero-	different	Heterogeneous—of mixed content
Homo-	same	Homosexual—attracted to same sex
Hyper-	excessive or increased	Hypertrophy—increase due to overgrowth
Hypo-	inadequate or underneath	Hypodermic—beneath the skin Hypotension—low blood pressure
Infra-	below	Infraorbital—below the eye socket
Inter-	between	Intercostal—between the ribs
Intra-	within	Intramuscular—within the muscle
Juxta-	alongside	Juxtaposition—lying alongside
Para-	close to or parallel to	Paravertebral—near the spine or Paramedian—parallel to midline
Per-	through	Percutaneous—through the skin
Poly-	many	Polymorphic—having many forms
Post-	after	Postmortem—after death
Pre-	in front of	Prepatellar—in front of the kneecap
Retro-	behind	Retrosternal—behind the breast-bone
Sub-	beneath	Subclavian—beneath the collarbone
Supra-	above	Supralabial—above the lips
Syn-	together	Syndactyl—fused or webbed fingers
Trans-	through or across	Transect—cutting across

Anatomical prefixes

Prefix	Meaning	Example
Abdomin(o)-	abdomen	Abdominal
Angio-	blood vessels	Angiogram—the X-ray picture of blood vessels produced by angiography
Arthro-	joints	Arthritis—inflammation of the joints
Cardio-	heart	Cardiomyopathy—disease of the heart muscle
Broncho-	small airways	Bronchopneumonia
Cerebr(o)-	brain	Cerebrovascular accident (stroke)
Chol(e)-	bile	Cholesterol—steroid essential to the formation of bile acids
Chondr(o)-	cartilage	Chondritis—inflammation of cartilage
Col(o)-	large bowel	Colostomy—artificial outlet of colon
Cost(o)-	ribs	Costochondral—rib cartilage
Encephal(o)-	Brain	Encephalogram—brain activity
Entero-	intestines	Enteritis—bowel inflammation
Gastro-	stomach	Gastroscope—instrument to examine the stomach
Haem(o)-	blood	Haemothorax—blood in the chest cavity
Hepat(o)-	liver	Hepatomegaly—enlarged liver
Myo-	muscle	Myocardium—muscle of the heart
Myel-	marrow	Poliomyelitis—inflammation of part of spinal cord
Nephr(o)-	kidney	Nephrectomy—surgical removal of kidney
Neur(o)-	nerve	Neurotoxic—poisonous to nerves
Ophthalm(o)-	eye	Ophthalmoscope—eye-viewing lens
Oste(o)-	bone	Osteomyelitis—inflammation of bone marrow or spinal cord
Pneum(o)-	air	Pneumothorax—air in the thorax
Splen(o)-	spleen	Splenomegaly—enlarged spleen

Suffixes

Prefix	Meaning	Example
-aemia	pertaining to blood	Anaemia—shortage of blood
-algia	pain	Neuralgia—pain along a nerve
-ectomy	cutting out	Appendicectomy—removal of appendix
-genic	producing	Pathogenic—causing disease
-itis	inflammation of	Laryngitis—inflammation of the throat
-lysis	destruction	Autolysis—enzymatic digestion of cells
-megaly	enlargement of	Acromegaly—big hands and feet
-oma	swelling or tumour	Carcinoma—cancer
-osis	non-inflammatory	Fibrosis—pathological scarring disorder
-pathy	disorder of function	Cardiomyopathy—heart muscle disorder
-plasia	growth	Hyperplasia—overgrowth of tissue due to increase of cells
-stomy	making a hole	Tracheostomy—surgical opening in windpipe

Glossary of medical terms

Medical language for the non-medic

To a non-medically trained individual, medical terminology can be quite bewildering. The following simple glossary is aimed at providing a brief explanation of those medical terms which appear relatively frequently in medical records, statements, and reports with a forensic context. Many of the terms listed here are considered in detail elsewhere in the book (see Index).

Abortion—termination of pregnancy (whether therapeutic or spontaneous).

Acetaminophen—alternative name for paracetamol.

Alveoli—air spaces in the lungs where gaseous exchange takes place.

Anaemia—deficiency of red blood cells in the blood.

Anaerobic—without O_2.

Analgesia—insensitivity to pain without any loss of consciousness. Also used to describe pain relief.

Anaphylactic (shock)—a severe (sometimes fatal) reaction subsequent to second exposure to an antigen following previous sensitization. A medical emergency requiring urgent attention.

Aneurysm—dilatation of blood vessel (especially an artery). Rupture is often a medical emergency and can be rapidly fatal.

Antidote—an agent which reverses the effect of a toxin or poison.

Apnoea—a transient cessation of respiration.

Arrhythmia—an abnormal heart beat rhythm.

Asymptomatic—not displaying the symptoms of a disease.

Ataxia—inability to coordinate voluntary muscle movement (e.g. when intoxicated due to alcohol or other substances).

Atheroma—the fatty degeneration or deposit in an artery.

Atrium—chamber of the heart receiving blood from the veins.

Atypical—a finding which is not usual or expected given other circumstances.

Auscultation—to listen to the sounds made by organs such as the lungs to assist diagnosis.

Avulsion—to tear away accidentally or surgically a part of the body.

Bradycardia—a relatively slower heart beat (<60/min in an adult).

Brainstem—part of the brain regulating basic life functions, composed of the midbrain, pons, and medulla oblongata and connecting to the spinal cord. Absence of brainstem activity is an important aspect of the definition of death.

Bronchopneumonia—an infection of the lung (including the bronchi) caused by bacteria, viruses, or other micro-organism.

Buccal—relating to the mouth or cheek.

Cardiovascular—pertaining to the heart and blood vessels.

Carotid (artery)—the two main arteries supplying blood to the head and brain, vulnerable to incised wounds of the neck.

Cerebellum—the part of the brain which maintains muscle coordination (two lateral lobes and one median lobe, situated behind the brainstem).

Cerebrovascular event (or 'accident')—rupture or obstruction of a blood vessel of the brain ('stroke').

Cirrhosis—generalized disruption of the liver caused by chronic conditions (e.g. hepatitis, alcohol misuse).

Coagulation—change from a liquid to a solid/semi-solid state by chemical reaction.

Colposcope—device to enable examination of the cervix, vagina, and vulva.

Comminuted (fracture)—a fracture in which the bone is shattered or crushed into more than two pieces.

Comorbidity—two or more coexisting conditions (e.g. substance dependency and depression).

Compliance—to comply with a treatment regimen.

Compound fracture—a fracture resulting in a breach of the skin and tissues through which bone may protrude.

Contraindicated—when circumstances render a treatment inadvisable.

Contusion—bruise (haematoma).

Convulsions—abnormal and involuntary contraction of the muscles (e.g. epilepsy or a withdrawal state).

Cranium—the skull.

Defibrillation—process of restoring the normal rhythm of the heart by electric shock.

Diastole—passive relaxation of the chambers of the heart permitting them to refill with blood.

Differential diagnosis—an alternative diagnosis which presents with the same or similar signs and symptoms (e.g. bruising and Mongolian blue spot).

Dilatation (dilation)—to expand or stretch or open (e.g. vasodilation).

Dissecting (aneurysm)—rupture of the vessel due to a weakness.

Ecchymosis—a subcutaneous haematoma (bruise).

Embolism—an obstruction in a blood vessel due to gas (e.g. nitrogen in the 'bends'), a blood clot or other foreign body (PE—pulmonary embolism blocking the pulmonary artery).

Emphysema—lung disease leading to rupture of the alveoli.

Encephalitis—inflammation of the brain.

Endocarditis—inflammation of the lining of the heart and valves.

Endocrine (system, gland)—hormonal secretions which are distributed by the blood stream.

Erythema—redness of the skin caused by dilation of the capillaries often as a result of inflammation or infection.

Evisceration—the process of removing the internal organs for dissection.

Exothermic—a reaction which produces heat.

Exsanguination—complete hypovolaemia (blood loss) ('bleeding to death')

Extravasation—the flow of fluid (e.g. blood) from a vessel into the surrounding tissue.

Fenestration—a natural or artificial opening in a surface (e.g. a surgical incision).

Fibrillation—irregular contraction of the myocardium resulting in a loss of pulse (see defibrillation).

Fibrosis—any increase in interstitial fibrous tissue.

Fissure—a natural cleft in an organ (e.g. brain, liver) or a split (injury) in any tissue.

Fetus—unborn child aged from the start of the 9th week following conception (embryo—before 9 weeks) until birth.

Foramen—natural opening usually through the tissues, especially bone (e.g. foramen magnum in the base of the skull, permitting connection of brain and spinal cord.)

Fulminant—rapid and severe (e.g. sudden onset of extreme pain).

Haematoma—a collection of blood (large bruise).

Haemodynamic—(study of) blood movement.

Haemolysis—the destruction or erythrocytes (red blood cells) resulting in anaemia.

Haemophilia—a hereditary condition inhibiting blood clotting resulting in excessive (and possibly fatal) bleeding.

Haemoptysis—to cough up blood (often a consequence of a severe respiratory infection, cancer or pulmonary embolism).

Haemothorax—an accumulation of blood in the pleural cavity.

Hypoxia—deficiency of O_2.

Idiopathic—arising from an unknown cause.

Idiosyncratic—observations peculiar to an individual or a group of individuals sharing common characteristics.

Impairment—reduction in normal function.

Infarction—localized death (narcosis) of tissue as a result of ischaemia (absence of oxygenated blood) (myocardial infarction = 'heart attack').

Infectious—communicable disease caused by an infectious agent (cf. 'contagious'—transmitted by contact).

Influenza—highly contagious respiratory disease (e.g. H5N1, 'Avian' or 'bird' flu, H1N1, 'swine' flu, H2N2, 'Asian' flu).

Interstitial—usually refers to fibrous tissue within, but not a component part of, an organ or other tissue.

Intoxicant—any substance capable of producing an abnormal state of intoxication ('poisoning').

Intoximeter—a device capable of measuring the concentration of a substance (e.g. alcohol) usually in the breath ('breathalyser'). 'Home' versions are available but are not necessarily accurate.

Intra-abdominal—within the abdomen.

Intra-articular—within the cavity of a (bone) joint.

Intracranial—within the skull.

Intradermal—within the skin (or between the layers of the skin).

Intramuscular—within a muscle.

Intranasal—within the nose.

Intrathoracic—within the chest (thorax).

Intrauterine—within the uterus (e.g. IUD or intrauterine device is a contraceptive known as a 'coil').

Intravaginal—within the vagina.

Intravascular—within a blood vessel.

Intravenous—into a vein (e.g. IV injection).

Ischaemia—reduced blood (and therefore O_2) supply to a tissue.

Lateral—situated away from the medial plane (e.g. the shoulders are lateral to the sternum).

Lesion—term referring to any abnormal tissue resulting from disease or trauma (injury or wound).

Lymphatic (system)—network of conduits permitting the flow of lymph fluid around the body. Has an important function in the immune process.

Myocardium—muscle of the heart (e.g. cardiomyopathy is a disease of the muscle of the heart which can result in sudden death prior to a diagnosis.)

Necrosis—cell or tissue death.

Neonate—a newborn within the first month of life.

Occlusion—blockage of a vessel.

Oedema—accumulation of fluid in or around cells often leading to swelling.

Opiate—a drug containing or derived from opium (e.g. diamorphine).

Opioid—drugs in the same class as opiates, including those of both natural and synthetic origin (e.g. pethidine).

Pericardial—located around the heart (e.g. the pericardial sac).

Petechiae—tiny 'pin-prick' haemorrhages associated with asphyxia.

Plasma: the fluid part of blood (water and dissolved constituents such as proteins).

Pneumonia—respiratory disease, inflammation of the lungs (excluding the bronchi—see bronchopneumonia) caused by bacteria, viruses or other micro-organisms.

Pneumothorax—accumulation of air in the pleural cavity frequently resulting in a collapsed lung. Often a result of trauma.

Posterior—back or 'dorsal' (anterior = front or 'ventral').

Proctoscope—instrument used to examine the anus and rectum.

Prophylactic—a preventative measure.

Psychosis—a psychiatric condition in which the person ('psychotic') experiences a distorted reality and exhibits severe personality changes. Psychoses are symptomatic of a range of psychiatric diseases rather than being a diagnostic of a particular illness. Can result from alcohol and/or drug misuse (especially associated with hallucinogenic drugs).

Pugilistic—typical 'pugilists' pose adopted by bodies in fires as a result of extreme flexion or muscle contraction (dehydration and protein denaturation).

Pulmonary—relating to the lungs.

Putrefaction—state of decomposition associated with foul-smelling odours.

Resuscitation—the procedure to revive or attempt to revive an unconscious and/or pulseless person.

Schizophrenia—a relatively common psychiatric condition associated with hearing voices and paranoia although the psychosis experienced by a schizophrenic may take various other forms.

Sclerosis—a pathological change resulting from increased growth of fibrous tissue (atherosclerosis) or interstitial tissue (multiple sclerosis).

Seizure—physical manifestation (e.g. fit/convulsion) resulting from abnormal electrical impulses in the brain (e.g. epilepsy).

Septicaemia—infection of the bloodstream ('blood poisoning').

Serum—the fluid part of blood (the plasma) which remains after clotting factors (e.g. fibrinogen) have been removed.

Speculum—instrument for examining body cavities (e.g. the vagina).

Stab—a penetrating wound inflicted by the thrust of a sharp instrument.

Stellate—a star-like appearance associated with gunshot injuries. A stellate fracture is one in which the break radiates away from a central point (usually the site of impact).

Stenosis—abnormal narrowing of a blood vessel (or other channel).

Stillbirth—the delivery of a fetus who has died during pregnancy, labour, or delivery.

Stroke—an ischaemic event (CVA, cerebrovascular accident) caused by an artery to the brain becoming blocked or ruptured.

Subarachnoid haemorrhage (SAH)—bleeding (as a result of head injury or cerebral aneurysm) into the subarachnoid space (i.e. between the arachnoid membrane and the pia mater). A SAH has a high mortality even following early treatment.

Subcutaneous—below the layers of the skin.

Subdural haemorrhage—bleeding (usually as a result of head injury) within the dura mater (membrane covering the brain).

Sublingual—beneath the tongue (as in the administration of buprenorphine).

Suffocation—a form of asphyxia in which a mechanical obstruction prevents breathing.

Suicide—a manner of death: the intentional taking by a person of his/her own life.

Superficial—e.g. a wound which affects only the surface layer. Often of little clinical significance, a superficial wound may contain a great deal of significant information in a forensic context (e.g. a patterned abrasion).

Supine—lying on the back, face up.

Syndrome—a group of signs of symptoms which characterize a disease, although in isolation none are diagnostic.

Systole—active contraction of the heart muscle which generates the pressure required for circulation.

Tachycardia—a relatively fast heart beat (>100/min in an adult).

Tamponade—compression of an organ (e.g. cardiac tamponade in which bleeding into the pericardial sac exerts pressure onto the heart).

Therapeutic—pertaining to treatment. In toxicology, contrasts with 'toxic' or 'fatal' and indicates that the measured concentration of a substance is within the normal or expected range given the standard therapeutic dose.

Thoracic—relating to the chest or thorax.

Thrombo-embolism—a detached fragment of blood clot which forms an emboli and potentially blocks an artery (DVT = 'deep vein thrombosis').

Thrombus—a blood clot in a vessel, often formed at a site of atheroma. If detached, a thrombus becomes a thromboembolism.

Torso—the body excluding the head and limbs.

TOXBASE—℘ http://www.toxbase.org. The primary clinical toxicology database of the National Poisons Information Service.

Trachea—('windpipe') part of the respiratory system connecting the larynx ('voicebox') to the bronchi.

Tranquillizer—drugs intended to relieve anxiety and insomnia (increasing levels of drowsiness occur as potency increases).

Triage—a protocol to assign priorities based on medical need, probability of survival and available resources. Used in Emergency Medicine (especially in major incidents and war).

Unconscious—a patient exhibiting significantly reduced capacity for sensory perception.

Unresponsive—a patient who fails to respond to external stimuli, but who is not unconscious.

Vagus nerve—(cranial nerve X) cranial nerve extending from the brainstem to the viscera. Regulates heart beat and breathing plus various other functions. Vagal stimulation can result in sudden death.

Vasoconstriction—narrowing of the blood vessels (particularly the arteries by the contraction of the muscular wall).

Vasodilatation—relaxation of the wall of the blood vessel resulting in increased lumen (opening).

Vasovagal (episode, attack, response)

Ventilate—procedure to assist breathing in an unconscious patient.

Vitreous humour—fluid of the eye filling the space between the lens and the retina. Anatomically isolated (unlike aqueous humour at the front of eye where the fluid is continuously replenished).

Chapter 1

Scope of forensic medicine

Introduction to forensic medicine

The appeal of forensic medicine

Forensic medicine is inherently fascinating. The extent to which forensic medicine subject matter features in popular novels, films, and television is a testimony to this!

The scope of forensic medicine

The term 'forensic medicine' means different things to different individuals. Most simply, forensic medicine may be defined as incorporating those areas of medicine which interact with the law or the legal process. Using this broad definition, it is clear that a large number of areas of medicine have potential forensic implications. The scope of forensic medicine is so broad that perhaps uniquely in medicine, no single practitioner can have any realistic hope of claiming to be an expert in all aspects of this diverse specialty.

Forensic practitioners

There is a wide range of practitioners who perform work which may be regarded as 'forensic in nature', as outlined here.

Forensic pathologists

These individuals are pathologists who have specialized within the field of forensic pathology. They are principally involved in assisting the legal process investigating deaths which may have legal implications (e.g. homicides, suicides, other 'suspicious deaths', industrial deaths). Their work involves analysis of crime scenes as well as performing autopsies and frequently takes them to court.

Clinical forensic practitioners

Doctors working in clinical forensic medicine have struggled to find a term which has stuck! The original term 'police surgeon' has been superseded by a variety of other terms, including forensic medical examiner ('FME') and forensic physician. The role is heavily based around the police custody unit, involving the examination, care, and gathering evidence of detainees.

Forensic nurses

Nurses are developing roles in police custody centres which have traditionally been the province of doctors. Many larger custody units in the UK have forensic nurses working within them. Being on site, they are quickly available to assess and treat detainees and are particularly adept at managing medication and chronic illness issues.

Forensic psychiatrists/psychologists

Doctors and nurses working within this branch of forensic medicine focus particularly on individuals with possible mental disorders who have committed crime (or are accused of having committed crime).

Forensic odontologists

Forensic dentists are experts in the analysis of bite injuries.

Forensic scientists
Forensic science is a rapidly expanding area, with numerous important subspecialty areas, particularly toxicology.

Other specialists who have important forensic roles
Many specialists whose principal role is other than forensic medicine nevertheless fulfil forensic roles. These include:
• Paediatricians
• Emergency physicians
• Entomologists
• Forensic anthropologists
• Forensic archaeologists
• Gynaecologists
• Genitourinary physicians
• General practitioners (GPs).

Forensic medicine understanding by other professionals

Lawyers and police officers have traditionally regarded forensic medicine as a mysterious area which is difficult to comprehend. The façade of mystery and complexity is compounded by potentially confusing terminology, which at times can make it appear that forensic specialists are speaking a completely different language. However, once the terminology is explained (see 📖 Glossary of medical terms, p.xxvii), it becomes obvious that most of the principles underpinning forensic medicine are remarkably straightforward. Lawyers and police officers who are brave enough to tackle the medical terminology will be rewarded by an understanding of the forensic issues.

History of forensic medicine

Forensic medicine and forensic pathology

In the past, many people considered forensic pathology to be synonymous with forensic medicine. In many countries, including the UK, high profile murder cases allowed some forensic pathologists to develop almost legendary status. Their word was 'law' in some courts and it is only in the last two or three decades that the all-knowing approach of the forensic pathologist has been questioned. Almost certainly, received wisdom is now exposed to more rigorous critical analysis than before.

Origins

The origins of forensic medicine go back many years, with terminology varying. Depending on the country and linguistic niceties, the terms forensic medicine, medical jurisprudence, juridical medicine, and forensic pathology have all been used to cover similar areas. A number of significant texts were published in the 19th century, the contents of which still have relevance today. In many respects, it could be argued that forensic medicine has changed little. Bodies still decompose in the same way, individuals remain violent towards each other in many ways. There are numerous previous references to the use of medical experts to assist legal processes in various jurisdictions. Such physicians were involved in criminal or civil cases, as well as public health, and are referred to frequently and rather confusingly in the 19th century as medical police.

A specialty unfolds

There is much dispute regarding the date when medical expertise in the determination of legal issues was first used. However, there is plenty of historical evidence showing that in pretty much all legal systems, 'medical men' advised or informed those creating law or dispensing justice.

Ancient China

In 1975, Chinese archaeologists discovered numerous bamboo pieces dating from approximately 220 BC (Qin dynasty) with rules and regulations for examining injuries inscribed on them.

Ancient Greece

Other historical examples of the link between medicine and the law exist throughout the world. Forensic medical principles were used in Athenian courts and other public bodies—the testimony of physicians in medical matters was given particular credence, although this use of physicians as expert witnesses was not particularly structured.

Roman times

The Roman Republic's constitution, *Lex Duodecim Tabularum*, had references to medicolegal matters, covering such topics as determining the length of gestation (to determine legitimacy), disposal of bodies, punishments dependent on the degree of injury caused by an assailant, and poisoning. Interestingly, in some jurisdictions nowadays the doctor is still asked to classify the degree of injury to determine punishment.

The Middle Ages

The *Constitutio Criminalis Carolina*, the code of law published and proclaimed in 1532 in Germany by Emperor Charles V, is considered to have originated legal medicine as a specialty: expert medical testimony became a requirement rather than an option in cases of murder, wounding, poisoning, hanging, drowning, infanticide, and abortion. Medicolegal autopsies were well documented in parts of Italy and Germany five centuries before the use of such procedures by English coroners. The use of such expertise was not limited to deaths or to mainland Europe. Cassar, for example, describes the earliest recorded Maltese medicolegal report (1542): medical evidence established that the male partner was incapable of sexual intercourse and this resulted in a marriage annulment. Fortunatus Fidelis has been identified as the earliest writer on medical jurisprudence, with his *De Relationibus Medicorum* being published in Palermo, Italy in 1602. The authors of this text hope they are continuing a noble tradition!

The last two centuries

From the late 1800s, substantial texts began to appear in the English language. In 1783, William Hunter published an essay entitled *On the Uncertainty of the Signs of Murder in the Case of Bastard Children* and this is often considered the first true forensic medicine publication from England. John Gordon Smith wrote in 1821 in the preface to his own book: 'The earliest production in this country, professing to treat of Medical Jurisprudence *generaliter*, was an abstract from a foreign work, comprised in a very small space. It bears the name of "Dr. Farr's Elements," and first appeared above 30 years ago [in 1788]'. George Male's *Epitome of Juridical or Forensic Medicine*, first published in 1816, was possibly the first major English language text. He was a physician at Birmingham General Hospital and is often considered the father of English medical jurisprudence. John Gordon Smith stated in *The Principles of Forensic Medicine Systematically Arranged and Applied to British Practice* (1821) that: 'It is but justice to mention that the American schools have outstripped us in attention to Forensic Medicine'—so there's nothing new there then and he may have been referring to the work of Theodric Romeyn Beck. It is instructive to read some of these texts which are now almost 200 years old. By the end of the 19th century, a framework of forensic medicine that persists today had been established in Europe, the UK, America, and related jurisdictions.

Developing clinical forensic medicine

A possible working definition is: 'Clinical forensic medicine includes all medical [healthcare] fields which may relate to legal, judicial, and police systems'. This embraces all aspects of clinical forensic medicine. Although for some practitioners it may mainly involve the healthcare and forensic assessment and management of individuals detained in custody, for many a much broader range of forensic contact may be achieved.

Scope

High profile issues (e.g. detention in Guantánamo Bay), have recently raised the profile of awareness of abuses of human rights and civil liberties. Coupled with assorted miscarriages of justice, management, and care of detained convicted prisoners, unconvicted prisoners and suspects of crime have become increasingly relevant to the proper legal process. Increasing recognition that these groups, as well as those who are complainants of, or victims, of crime should have appropriately competent doctors or other practitioners to assess them, has resulted in more emphasis being placed on skills, competence, and training.

Failure of basic rights

Examples of injustice and failure to observe basic human rights or rights enshrined in statute in which the input of medical professionals may be considered at least 'poor quality' and at worst 'criminally negligent' have occurred and continue to occur. The death of Steve Biko in South Africa, the conviction of Carole Richardson in England, and deaths of native Australians in prison are widely publicized instances. Reports from the European Committee for the Prevention of Torture and Inhuman and Degrading Treatment in the early 1990s drew attention to the lack of independence of some police doctors. Conflicting needs and duties of those involved in the judicial system are clear and it is sometimes believed that recognition of such conflicts is comparatively recent, which would be naïve and wrong. In England and Wales, the Human Rights Act 1998, whose purpose is to make it unlawful for any public authority to act in a manner incompatible with a right defined by the European Convention of Human Rights, reinforces the need for doctors to be aware of those human rights issues that touch on prisoners and that doctors can influence. It is worth noting that this law was enacted almost 50 years after publication of the *European Convention on Human Rights and Fundamental Freedoms*. There appears to be a future role for the forensic physician within bodies, such as the recently established International Criminal Court.

Potentially conflicting roles

The forensic physician may have several conflicting roles when assessing a prisoner or someone detained by the state or other statutory body. Three medical care facets that may conflict have been identified: the role of medicolegal expert for a law enforcement agency; the role of a treating doctor; and the examination and treatment of detainees who allege that they have been mistreated by the police during their arrest, interrogation, or the various stages of custody. The forensic physician must be mindful of these conflicts and his/her over-riding duty to the patient.

Structure in the UK

In the UK, The Metropolitan Police Surgeons Association was formed in 1888 with 156 members. In 1951, the association was reconstituted as a national body—the Association of Police Surgeons. The name was later changed to The Association of Forensic Physicians, to reflect the independence from the police. In an exciting development in 2006, the Faculty of Forensic and Legal Medicine was created as a new Faculty of the Royal College of Physicians (www.fflm.ac.uk), giving clear recognition of the specific need for, and role of, clinical forensic medicine and forensic physicians.

Forensic medicine around the world

Lack of global consensus

Unfortunately, unlike well-defined specialties such as cardiology, color-ectal surgery, or emergency medicine, there is no international consensus as to how forensic medicine should be delivered. Forensic pathology, clinical forensic medicine, and their related specialties (forensic science, toxicology, forensic anthropology, and forensic odontology) may be provided in entirely different ways in different countries.

Training, research, and funding

Often, forensic subjects are funded by justice ministries rather than health departments and so appear to be relatively underfunded. Some countries have a wealth of academic forensic units that embrace forensic research. Others, such as the UK, appear to undervalue the role of forensic medicine and the need for properly funded research. Similarly, training schemes are variable around the world, and globally (as compared with the UK) governments appear to have wider recognition of the inter-relationship of the different forensic subspecialties.

Delivery of the service

In many jurisdictions, both the clinical and the pathological aspects of forensic medicine are undertaken by the same individual or by groups of doctors working closely together. The use of GPs (primary care physicians) with a special interest in clinical forensic medicine is common: England, Wales, Northern Ireland, Scotland, Australasia, and the Netherlands still all remain heavily dependent on such doctors to provide a service.

The future of forensic medicine

Given the increasing focus on many aspects of forensic medicine, the specialty seems set to develop further. Forensic practitioners working in different aspects of the specialty and in different parts of the world will need to work together to carve out the best future.

Professional bodies and discipline

General Medical Council (🔊 http://www.gmc-uk.org)

The General Medical Council (GMC) is the organization which keeps a register of doctors in the UK and regulates them, as well as UK medical schools. The GMC was established by an Act of Parliament in 1858. It attempts to ensure proper standards in the practice of medicine. UK doctors need to be on the medical register in order to have a licence to practise.

The medical register

In order to practise medicine in the UK, doctors need to have a recognized medical qualification and be registered with the GMC. Registration may be provisional or full provisional registration is given to medical graduates who become first-year doctors ('Foundation year 1'). This provisional registration subsequently becomes full registration after satisfactory completion of the first year. The GMC sets standards for undergraduate, preregistration, and postgraduate medical education. It has the power to grant or remove registration from doctors, as outlined next.

Good Medical Practice

The publication entitled *Good Medical Practice* produced by the GMC (last updated in 2006) includes clear guidance on the standards, guidance, and principles which doctors are expected to adhere to.

Key sections in *Good Medical Practice* are:
• Duties of a doctor
• Good clinical care
• Maintaining good medical practice
• Teaching and training, appraising, and assessing
• Relationships with patients
• Working with colleagues
• Probity
• Health.

Fitness to practise procedures

Following a complaint, the GMC investigates and can take appropriate action. The GMC may decide to investigate a doctor's fitness to practise if there is evidence to suggest serious professional misconduct and/or seriously deficient performance. The panel convened by the GMC includes medical professionals and lay members. The GMC has the power to suspend a doctor or place conditions upon his/her registration.

The future of the GMC

The GMC has been criticized from several sides. Doctors note a high rate of suicide amongst those undergoing 'Fitness to Practise' procedures, whilst the GMC was heavily criticized after the inquiry into Dr Harold Shipman. The GMC has recently undergone considerable change, becoming more involved in revalidation and postgraduate education.

Nursing and Midwifery Council (⅍ http://www.nmc-uk.org)
The Nursing and Midwifery Council (NMC) was established in 2002. It performs a similar regulatory role for nurses and midwives in the UK as the GMC does for doctors. These functions include:
- Keeping a register of all nurses and midwives, ensuring that they are properly qualified and competent to work in the UK.
- Setting standards for education, training, and conduct that nurses and midwives need in order to deliver high quality healthcare consistently throughout their careers.
- Ensuring that nurses and midwives keep their knowledge and skills up to date.
- Investigating allegations relating to impaired fitness to practise.

Forensic organizations

Forensic organizations can be divided broadly into those which may be involved primarily in developing standards, training, and disseminating knowledge (e.g. the Faculty of Forensic and Legal Medicine ℘ http:// www.fflm.ac.uk) and those which focus on research and education (e.g. the American Academy of Forensic Sciences ℘ http://www.aafs.org). Both named organizations may have substantial other roles. The Forensic Science Society in the UK has been undergoing a transition as it moves towards being a professional body (℘ http://www.forensic-science-society.org.uk). Around the world, there is recognition that all forensic practitioners need appropriate theoretical and practical training and that once trained, continuing professional development is essential. In courts, particularly those of an adversarial nature, lack of basic training or failure to maintain a knowledge of current facts or trends in your area of practice can result in personal embarrassment and the risk of compromising justice. This may even result in sanctions from a professional body.

Consent

Introduction

Interactions between health professionals and patients in a legal setting (e.g. a police custody unit) are understandably overshadowed by the legal process. Equally, interactions in other settings (e.g. hospital) can have similar legal implications which are not always appreciated. The over-riding duty of a doctor, nurse, or other health professional is usually to try to provide first-class care for their patients. However, in some situations, additional responsibilities of the health professional in relation to the legal process can significantly reshape the relationship with the patient. This is particularly true of medicine within the custody unit, where the doctor/nurse often has a 'dual role' of treating the detainee and recording information which has the potential of being used against him/her in a legal sense. On some occasions, the patient may have no healthcare issues which he/she wishes to be addressed, so that the entire focus is upon gathering information for forensic/legal purposes. An example is the examination of a detainee suspected of rape when the doctor focuses upon recording injuries and gathering samples for DNA analysis. The potential tension between providing care and assisting the legal process needs to be appreciated by the forensic practitioner. An overview of issues of consent, capacity, and confidentiality is given in the following sections—these issues are considered in more detail in relation to custody medicine on pp.196–7.

Consent

Issues of consent in the custody setting are fully considered on pp.196–7. Considerations relating to consent in a forensic setting often include more than simply whether a patient agrees to receive a certain treatment. Indeed, the consent (or refusal) by an individual for a particular forensic intervention (e.g. examination, intimate search, taking of samples) can be of considerable importance to the individual. The implications of both giving and refusing consent need to be carefully explained to the patient. When considering the stated wishes of the patient, the doctor and/or nurse involved also need to consider whether or not the patient has (at that time) the capacity to make this decision (see Mental capacity, p.16).

Consent to treatment in children aged less than 16 years

The law relating to consent to treatment in children aged less than 16 years in England and Wales is based upon a (now famous) case involving Gillick heard by Lord Fraser in 1986—see boxed text. Children aged less than 16 years can be legally competent to give consent if they have sufficient understanding and maturity to understand fully what it proposes.

The Gillick case

In 1985, an activist and mother of 10 (Mrs Victoria Gillick) was involved in a high profile case (Gillick v West Norfolk and Wisbech Area Health Authority) which was considered by the House of Lords. Mrs Gillick was opposed to a health departmental circular which advised doctors that the prescription of contraceptives to children aged less than 16 years was a matter for the doctor's discretion and that contraceptives could be prescribed without consent of parents. The House of Lords focused on the issue of consent, rather than parental rights, finding that children could consent if they fully understood the proposed medical treatment.

Fraser guidelines

Lord Fraser set out the criteria for healthcare professionals to provide advice and treatment, as follows:
- The young person will understand the professional's advice.
- The young person cannot be persuaded to inform their parents.
- The young person is likely to begin, or to continue having, sexual intercourse with or without contraceptive treatment.
- Unless the young person receives contraceptive treatment, their physical or mental health, or both, are likely to suffer.
- The young person's best interests require them to receive contraceptive advice or treatment with or without parental consent.

Mental capacity

Mental Capacity Act 2005 (England and Wales)

The assessment of an individual's mental capacity to consent to (or refuse) an intervention can be difficult and is the focus of the Mental Capacity Act 2005. This Act applies to those aged over 16 years in England and Wales. It sets out the legal framework for acting and making decisions for those individuals who lack the capacity to make particular decisions for themselves. The five statutory principles set out in the Act are:

1 A person must be assumed to have capacity unless it is established that they lack capacity.
2 A person is not to be treated as unable to make a decision unless all practicable steps to help him to do so have been taken without success.
3 A person is not to be treated as unable to make a decision merely because he makes an unwise decision.
4 An act done, or decision made, under this Act for or on behalf of a person who lacks capacity must be done, or made, in his best interests.
5 Before the act is done, or the decision is made, regard must be had to whether the purpose for which it is needed can be as effectively achieved in a way that is less restrictive of the person's rights and freedom of action.

Assessment of competence

The Act is quite specific in stating that no one may be labelled as being incapable simply due to a particular medical condition or diagnosis. A person is competent if he/she:

• Is able to understand and retain the information pertinent to the decision about their care (i.e. the nature, purpose, and possible consequences of the proposed investigations or treatment, as well as the consequences of not having treatment).
• Is able to use this information to consider whether or not they should consent to the intervention offered.
• Is able to communicate their wishes.

Time-specific nature of the assessment of competence

An important feature of the Act is the way that it sets out that the assessment of an individual's capacity to make a decision is time specific (i.e. it acknowledges that it may change with time). So, for example, an individual who is heavily under the influence of drugs and/or alcohol may lack capacity until the time that the effects of the drugs and/or alcohol have worn off.

Confidentiality

Background

The basic ethical principle underlying any consultation between a doctor and/or nurse and a patient is that details of this consultation will remain confidential. This principle of secrecy is ancient, dating back to the Hippocratic oath. It is still considered to be very important by the GMC in the UK. Healthcare professionals need to take extreme care in protecting confidential information—this particularly applies to the safe and secure storing of medical records. It should also be noted that the ethical (if not legal) duty of confidentiality of a doctor or nurse extends beyond the death of a patient. It is worth acknowledging that medical information about a patient is frequently shared between healthcare professionals (e.g. GP and hospital specialist) acting in the best interests of their patient as part of routine practice with the implied consent of the patient.

Confidentiality in custody (see ℅ http://www.fflm.ac.uk)

Interactions between a doctor and/or nurse and detainee in custody take two principal forms: occasions when the detainee is a patient requiring treatment and occasions when the healthcare professional wishes to perform an intervention (e.g. taking of samples for DNA analysis) which will form part of the legal process. Both interactions require consent and whereas the former might be considered along standard lines as far as confidentiality is concerned, in the latter situation, the doctor/nurse will be recording information which may be shared with the investigating police officer—this needs to be clearly explained to the detainee (see 📖 p.197).

Disclosure of information

There are a number of instances where it is either deemed to be acceptable, desirable, or legally required to break patient confidentiality, with or without the patient's consent, as follows:
- When a court (legally) demands it (detainees need to be warned of this when they consult a doctor/nurse in custody).
- When there is suspicion of terrorist activity.
- The Road Traffic Act 1988 requires disclosure to the police of information leading to the identification of a driver involved in a traffic offence.
- GMC guidance is that gunshot wounds should be reported to the police (℅ http://www.gmc-uk.org).
- Disclosure in the public interest is ethically and legally permissible, but not mandatory. The GMC advises that this might include situations where someone might be exposed to death or serious injury (℅ http://www.gmc-uk.org).

Medical defence organizations can be an invaluable source of assistance to doctors who are faced with dilemmas and/or requests for disclosure of information.

Preparing a witness statement

As a forensic practitioner, you will frequently be required to prepare a witness statement in relation to criminal proceedings. The statement is a way of providing evidence in court that is as valid as if the evidence were given live and it is worth remembering that a well-constructed witness statement may well prevent an unnecessary attendance at court to give evidence in person.

When preparing a witness statement for court you are required to sign a declaration of truth and you need to be aware that any dishonesty in a signed statement amounts to perjury and may lead to prosecution.

The format of a witness statement

A sample statement can be found at 📖 Sample witness statement, p.20. Statements should generally be typed and to facilitate the process it is sensible to set up a template that contains the declaration of truth and all your personal details on your computer. When writing your statement, remember that it needs to be understood by lay people, so make sure that all medical terms are properly explained in terms that an average member of a jury can understand.

The header and footer

The header of the first page of a witness statement should include your full name, your date of birth (or a statement that you are aged over 18 years), and the following declaration of truth followed by your signature and the date:

'This statement (consisting of … pages each signed by me), is true to the best of my knowledge and belief and I make it knowing that, if it is tendered in evidence, I shall be liable to prosecution if I have wilfully stated in it anything which I know to be false or do not believe to be true.'

The header of subsequent pages only needs to read 'Continued statement of …' together with the page number. There should be space in the footer of all subsequent pages for your signature.

Introduction

An introductory section should include details of your qualifications, job title, and relevant experience. This provides you with the opportunity to demonstrate your level of expertise. If you have only been appointed recently it is appropriate to give details of the induction training that you have undertaken.

Basic information

The following should be provided:
• Details of who requested the statement
• Name of the examinee
• Date, time, duration, and place of the examination
• Reason for the examination
• Names of others present during the examination
• Form of consent.

Background

Details of the allegation/history of events should be included, making clear who provided the history (e.g. police officer who briefed you, examinee, etc.).

Past medical history

You should provide details of all relevant past medical and psychiatric history (as long as the examinee has consented to this), including details of medication taken and any history of substance misuse.

Examination findings

Present your examination findings in a logical manner, beginning with general comments and observations (e.g. demeanour and behaviour) and then listing in order the anatomical areas or body systems that were examined.

Injuries should be listed systematically, noting their nature, size, shape, colour, and position. Where there are multiple injuries, it is acceptable to append body maps to your statement and to refer to these when describing the injuries. The absence of abnormalities should be noted and you should ensure that you make clear which areas of the body have been examined (e.g. 'A full examination of all body surfaces together with an internal examination of the mouth revealed no evidence of injury').

Forensic samples

A list of any forensic samples taken during the course of the examination should be provided together with the unique reference number you used when labelling the sample. You should indicate when and to whom you handed the samples.

Treatment and advice

Your statement should record the details of any treatment provided and/or advice given.

Opinion

Whenever it is within your area of expertise, you should provide an opinion on your findings. However, you should bear in mind that you have probably only heard one side of the story (that of the examinee and his or her version of events) and this is likely to limit the scope of your opinion. Whilst it is acceptable to state that the injuries were consistent with the version of events provided, you should acknowledge that alternative mechanisms are possible unless the findings were so unique that cause and effect can be safely inferred. Where appropriate, you should indicate the limits of your expertise (e.g. 'It is outside my area of expertise to comment on the likely cause of these injuries').

Sample witness statement

Witness Statement

(Criminal Justice Act 1967 s.9; Magistrates' Courts Act 1980 s5A(3A) and 5B; Magistrates' Courts Rules 1981 r.70)

Statement of: Dr John Fagin
MBChB, MFFLM, MRCGP, DMJ

Age of witness: Over 18
Occupation of witness: Registered Medical Practitioner

This statement (consisting of 2 pages each signed by me) is true to the best of my knowledge and belief and I make it knowing that, if it is tendered in evidence, I shall be liable to prosecution if I have wilfully stated in it anything which I know to be false or do not believe to be true.

Dated the 10th February 2011

Signature: ....

Qualifications

My qualifications are MB ChB (Bachelor of Medicine, Bachelor of Surgery), MFFLM (Member of the Faculty of Forensic and Legal Medicine), MRCGP (Member of the Royal College of General Practitioners), and DMJ (Diploma in Medical Jurisprudence).

Experience

I am a registered medical practitioner and have been a forensic physician (police surgeon) working for the Metropolitan Police Service since 1988.

I have lectured on both induction and developmental training courses for forensic physicians and was a member of Council of the Association of Forensic Physicians from 2001 to 2004. I have published several articles in the field of clinical forensic medicine and I was also the coauthor of a chapter in a textbook of clinical forensic medicine.

Presentation

On 2nd February 2007, I attended Dock Green police station, where I was asked to examine Angry MAN (custody record number: DG/1190/11). I was informed by the police that MAN had been arrested on suspicion of possessing an offensive weapon. He had apparently been punching his cell door repeatedly throughout the night and I was asked to examine him and to note any injuries. My examination was conducted in the cell. It began at 03.52 hours and concluded at 04.07 hours.

This is a professional statement regarding my examination findings made at the request of Inspector Dixon.

Consent

MAN declined to provide written consent to my examination, but did consent verbally. He understood that I may have to produce a report based on the examination and that details of the examination may have to be revealed in court.

History

MAN refused to give me any medical history or other details. He said that he just wanted me to record that the police had been refusing to answer the bell in his cell so he had had to punch the cell door in order to get attention. He made no allegations regarding the circumstances of his arrest.

Examination

On examination I noted MAN's demeanour to be angry and agitated. He was fully conscious. His breath smelt of intoxicating liquor. There was no slurring of speech or evidence of incoordination. His pupils were of normal size (4.5mm) and he had a normal pulse (76 beats per minute) and blood pressure (120mmHg/74mmHg).

There was some erythema (redness) with slight swelling and tenderness over the 3rd, 4th, and 5th metacarpophalangeal (knuckle) joints of the right hand, where MAN indicated he had been punching the door.

At this point of my examination, MAN demanded to see the notes I had been writing. Despite reassurances to the contrary, he accused me of being biased towards the police and his behaviour became increasingly abusive and threatening. In view of this, I left the cell and terminated the examination.

Opinion

The minor injuries to MAN's right knuckles were consistent with his account that he had been punching his cell door with his right fist. No other injuries were noted, but the presence of additional injuries cannot be excluded because a full body surface examination was not conducted in view of MAN's behaviour.

Signed..

Appearing in court

Good preparation is the key to surviving court appearances. Do not be misled into thinking this is unnecessary when you are anticipating a brief appearance in a lower court or at a 'simple' inquest. Somebody wants you there for a reason—and that reason is unknown so preparation is always vital.

Technical preparation

- Agree fees in advance.
- Check your notes and documentation well beforehand.
- Think about what issues are likely to be relevant to the case.
- Try and anticipate the questions that you will be asked.
- Ensure that you have a reasonable knowledge of medical conditions that have a bearing on a case—there is nothing worse than giving the oath in the witness box while thinking 'I wish I had looked up the pharmacokinetics of cocaine before I came to court today'.
- Ask in advance to see any expert report prepared for the defence.

Practical preparation

- Ensure you know the location of the court and contact numbers.
- Make adequate transport arrangements. If driving, check that there is car parking available.
- Bring a spare clean copy of your report.
- Arrange with the usher for the right oath to be ready.
- Check the layout of the court.

Personal preparation

- Decide on how you want to come across.
- Practise your introduction.
- Dress appropriately.

How to address the presiding officer

- Coroner   'Sir/Madam'
- Magistrates Court:
  - Magistrates   'Sir/Madam' or 'Your Worship'
  - District Judge   'Sir/Madam'
- Crown court:
  - Circuit judge (His/Her Honour Judge…)   'Your Honour'
  - High Court judge (the Honourable Mr/Mrs Justice…) 'My Lord/Lady'
- High Court (the Honourable Mr/Mrs Justice…)   'My Lord/Lady'
- Court of Appeal (Lord/Lady Justice…)   'My Lord/Lady'

The pre-trial conference

This is a forum in which the advocate and doctor can ensure their mutual understanding of the facts. It is used too infrequently in criminal cases, but is important in ensuring that vital medical evidence is neither omitted nor misrepresented. So ask to see the advocate before you give evidence (this gives you the additional opportunity of finding out what your barrister's first questions will be).

Giving your evidence

What to take into the witness box
- Contemporaneous notes.
- A clean copy of your expert witness report (but not your witness statement).
- You may need to take copies of textbooks that you referred to—ask in advance.
- Props can be helpful (e.g. samples of instruments used in the examination, such as a vaginal speculum).
- A bundle of court documents will be provided for you where relevant—read sections carefully before answering questions on them.

Procedure in the witness box
- Walk slowly and purposefully to the witness box.
- Stand still in the witness box with your feet facing the judge—avoid fidgeting.
- Address the judge/jury—not the barrister.
- Speak clearly and with confidence in simple terms that lay people can understand.
- Avoid arguing with the barrister.

Evidence in practice
You will first be required to take the oath or affirmation. Your barrister will then ask you to tell the court your name, professional address, job description and/or qualifications, and experience before leading you through your evidence in chief, during which you will be taken through your witness statement. Following your evidence in chief, you will be cross-examined by the opposing barrister. Your barrister will then have the opportunity to re-examine you about points that were raised during cross-examination. Finally, the judge may ask you some questions.

Pitfalls in giving evidence
- Avoid partisanship.
- It is not your job to contend for a particular verdict or judgment.
- You are an advocate for your opinion only.
- Avoid overinterpretation.
- Confine your opinions to your own area of expertise.

Surviving cross-examination
- Remember it is not *you* that is on trial.
- Don't allow yourself to be led into areas outside your expertise.
- Don't be afraid to say 'I don't know'.
- Avoid humour.
- Try to anticipate the direction that the questions are taking you.
- Answer questions fully.
- If the barrister prevents you from answering fully then seek help from the judge.

Professional and expert medical evidence

When it comes to attending court there are essentially only two types of witness:

- A witness of fact.
- An expert witness.

A witness of fact is called to give evidence only about what they have seen or heard, whereas the expert witness is called to give opinion evidence—to interpret the facts using his or her expertise.

The professional medical witness

The waters are muddied because the Lord Chancellor's Department and Crown Prosecution Service recognize, for the purposes of fees, an intermediate class of witness known as a 'professional witness'. The professional medical witness is someone whose evidence is confined to matters of fact, but who is in possession of knowledge of those facts as a result of action taken in his or her professional capacity (i.e. they have treated the patient at some time). As a witness to fact, the professional witness can be summoned and compelled to give evidence.

Difficulties often occur when doctors come to court believing they have been called as professional witnesses of fact but find themselves being questioned on matters such as the causation and age of injuries they have observed. It is the judge's duty to step in when such questioning starts, to establish the witness' status and thus determine if he/she can give expert evidence. Unfortunately, not all judges intervene in this way—it is then up to the doctor to point out their lack of experience or knowledge and to seek the judge's protection. In order to avoid these difficulties, always enquire if you are being called as professional or expert witness whenever you are asked to attend court. If you consider that you are only able to give professional evidence of fact in relation to your involvement in the case, you should make this clear as soon as practicable so that an appropriate expert can be instructed.

Duties of an expert medical witness

Duty to the court

As an expert you owe a duty to exercise reasonable skill and care to those instructing you. However, when instructed to give or prepare evidence for court proceedings in England and Wales, your over-riding duty is to help the court on matters within your expertise. This duty over-rides any obligation to the person instructing or paying you.

Independence

As an expert, you should provide opinions that are truly independent, regardless of the pressures of litigation. In this context, a useful test of 'independence' is that you should satisfy yourself that you would express the same opinion if you had been instructed by the opposing party. Remember, it is not your job to promote the point of view of the party instructing you or to engage in the role of advocate.

Recognize the limits of your expertise

You should confine your opinions to matters which are material to the disputes between the parties and provide opinions only in relation to matters which lie within your expertise. You should indicate without delay where particular questions or issues fall outside your expertise.

Consider all relevant material

You should take into account all material facts before you at the time that you give your opinion and your report should set out those facts and any literature or any other material on which you have relied in forming your opinions.

Opinions

If you are not satisfied that an opinion can be expressed finally and without qualification, you must say so. For example, you should indicate if an opinion is provisional, or qualified, or if you consider that further information is required. If you are aware that there are other possible interpretations of the evidence you must say so and you should inform those instructing you without delay of any change in your opinions on any material matter and the reason for it.

Medical negligence

The civil law of negligence is designed to provide compensation when one individual has been injured by another's negligence. In order to successfully seek compensation for negligence a person has to establish:

• That the defendant owed him a duty of care
• That he was in breach of that duty; and
• That the harm of which he complains was caused by that breach in the duty of care.

It is important to appreciate that a plaintiff has to satisfy all three of these tests in order to succeed in a claim of negligence—it is not just sufficient to establish that there has been a breach in the duty of care. Thus, in *Barnett* v *Chelsea and Kensington HMC*,[1] a widow was able to establish that a hospital doctor was in breach of his duty of care by failing to attend Casualty to examine her husband. He was in a terrible state when eventually seen and died within a few hours of being admitted to hospital. The cause of death was arsenic poisoning. Despite the liability of the doctor, the widow failed to secure any compensation because the evidence was that her husband would still have died even if he had been properly attended.

Duty of care

Therapeutic examinations

Where a doctor–patient relationship exists, there is usually no difficulty establishing that a plaintiff was owed a duty of care. Thus, a GP accepting a patient on to his/her list undertakes a duty of care to that patient, as does a forensic physician providing therapeutic care to a detainee in police custody. So, if as a forensic physician you neglect to exercise proper care in your work and your patients are harmed as a result, you can expect to be criticized and may face claims for compensation arising out of alleged clinical negligence.

Forensic examinations

The situation regarding duty of care becomes far less clear in relation to purely forensic duties undertaken by doctors on behalf of the police. For example, the Court of Appeal ruled that a forensic physician who examined an alleged rape victim, owed the victim no duty of care to attend as a prosecution witness at the alleged rapist's trial, even if the failure to attend court resulted in the collapse of the trial and an exacerbation of the victim's psychiatric trauma.[2] In such circumstances, the court ruled, the doctor is carrying out an examination on behalf of the police and does not assume any responsibility for the victim's psychiatric welfare. The doctor's duty was simply to take care in the course of the examination not to make the patient's condition worse.

The medical standard of care

The second hurdle that a plaintiff has to overcome in order to successfully sue a doctor for negligence is that the doctor was careless. The onus of proof is on the plaintiff. The standard of care demanded of the doctor is the standard of a reasonably skilled and experienced practitioner of similar status acting with ordinary care in accordance with a reasonable body of medical opinion (the so-called 'Bolam test').

'Reasonable' in this context means that the body of medical opinion has to stand up to logical scrutiny ('the Bolitho test'). Thus, in defending a claim of negligence it is not enough for a defendant to simply call a number of doctors to say that what he had done was in accord with accepted clinical practice. The judge must consider the evidence and decide whether that clinical practice puts the patient unnecessarily at risk. Medical opinion can be rejected if the court is satisfied that the views held by a group of doctors are such as no reasonable body of doctors could hold.

Causation

The third, and final, hurdle that a successful plaintiff has to overcome is to establish causation—proving, on the balance of probabilities, that their injury, their worsened or unimproved condition, was caused by the doctor's negligence. In practice, this is often the most problematic aspect of a patient's claim.

Gross negligence manslaughter

A doctor may be criminally liable if a patient dies as a result of gross negligence, which is negligence that went *'beyond a mere matter of compensation between subjects, and showed such disregard for the life and safety of others as to amount to a crime against the State, and conduct deserving of punishment'*.

Three criteria must be fulfilled for a finding of gross negligence manslaughter:
• There must be a duty of care.
• The duty must have been breached and that breach caused death.
• The breach must have been so grossly negligent as to justify a criminal conviction.

In the case of *Adomako*, four states of mind are listed, any one of which may be grounds for a finding of gross negligence.[4] These are:
• Indifference to an obvious risk of injury to health.
• Actual foresight of the risk coupled with the determination none the less to run it.
• Appreciation of the risk coupled with an intention to avoid it but also coupled with such a high degree of negligence in the attempted avoidance as a jury may consider justifies conviction.
• Inattention or failure to advert to a serious risk which went beyond mere inadvertence in respect of an obvious and important matter which the defendant's duty demanded he/she should address.

References
1 HMC [1969] 1 QB 428.
2 N v Agrawal (1999) Times Law Report June 9.
3 R v Bateman (1925) 19 Cr. App. R 8.
4 R v Sullman, Prentice and Adomako. (1993) 15 BMLR 13 CA.

Forensic aspects of death

Definition and diagnosis of death

Death may be considered as the cessation of life at either the cellular level or the overall level of an organism. Traditionally, Bichat's triad has been used to define death of a person: 'failure of the body as an integrated system associated with the irreversible loss of *circulation*, *respiration*, and *innervation*'.

Cell death

Different tissues within the body vary considerably in the extent to which they can withstand hypoxic and other insults. Loss of aerobic respiration and cell death occurs relatively rapidly in brain cells after circulation of blood ceases and delivery of oxygen stops. In contrast, muscles, tendons, and other musculoskeletal tissues can survive hypoxic insults for relatively long periods.

Brainstem death

The death of an individual is traditionally characterized by a lack of any circulation or respiration. With advances in medical science, it has become possible to artificially maintain circulation and ventilation in some patients who would otherwise die and whose brain is no longer working normally. Functioning vital centres in the brainstem are required in order for spontaneous respiration to continue—failure of these centres results in 'brainstem death'. This is essentially a clinical diagnosis, and it is often of considerable legal and ethical significance, usually in an intensive care setting, and sometimes involving the possibility of organ transplantation.

Diagnosis of brainstem death

In order to diagnose brainstem death, the patient needs to be deeply unconscious, with no spontaneous respiration (i.e. on a ventilator), with no reversible metabolic condition (e.g. hypoglycaemia, electrolyte imbalance, acidosis), no drug intoxication, and no hypothermia. Once these conditions are satisfied, clinical tests are applied to establish the diagnosis. Tests differ slightly between countries, but the UK criteria are that a consultant (or their deputy, qualified for more than 5 years) and another doctor establish the following on two separate occasions:

- Both pupils are unresponsive and there is no corneal reflex.
- There is no vestibulo-ocular reflex (no eye movement on slow installation of ice cold water into each external auditory meatus).
- Stimulation within the cranial nerve distribution fails to elicit a motor response.
- There is no gag reflex or response to bronchial stimulation and there is no respiratory effort on stopping artificial ventilation, having allowed pCO_2 to rise above the normal range.

Vegetative state

A person is deemed to be in a 'vegetative state' when he/she is in a deep coma, with spontaneous breathing and stable circulation, but is unaware of his/her self and the environment. Spontaneous eye opening may occur.

Confirmation (and diagnosis) of death

Although there are many occasions when it is perfectly obvious even to a lay person that death has occurred (e.g. decapitation, decomposition), there have been a number of well-publicized instances when a person labelled as being dead, unexpectedly 'wakes up' in the mortuary. Sometimes the underlying condition is profound hypothermia. It is perhaps surprising, given its potential importance, that the medical profession has only relatively recently focused upon standardizing the diagnosis of death. The Academy of Medical Royal Colleges produced guidelines on diagnosing death after cardiorespiratory arrest when clear signs that are pathognomonic of death (e.g. hypostasis, rigor mortis) are absent (🕮 http://www.aomrc.org.uk). Key points are summarized as follows:

- There is simultaneous and irreversible onset of apnoea and unconsciousness in the absence of a circulation.
- Appropriate attempts at resuscitation have been made (and failed).
- The deceased person should be observed for a minimum of 5min using a combination of absent central pulse on palpation and absence of heart sounds on auscultation (and in hospital setting, asystole on ECG monitor).
- Any spontaneous return of cardiac or respiratory activity during this period of observation should prompt a further 5min of observation from the next point of cardiorespiratory arrest.
- After 5min of continued cardiorespiratory arrest, the absence of papillary responses to light, of the corneal reflexes, and of any motor response to supraorbital pressure should be confirmed.
- The time of death is recorded as the time at which these criteria are fulfilled.

Waking up after being certified dead

Instances of patients recovering having been declared dead by a doctor appear to be rare, but well-publicized. There are examples from both prehospital and hospital settings. In 1996, Mrs Maureen Jones was seen to move and then breathe spontaneously at her home in Thwing, East Yorkshire after a doctor had earlier declared death and left the house (🕮 http://news.bbc.co.uk/1/hi/uk/7419652.stm).

In Vietnam in August 2003, a man named Nguyen Van Quan (aged 73 years) was found alive after spending a night in a hospital mortuary, having previously been declared dead by doctors (🕮 http://news.bbc.co.uk/1/hi/world/asia-pacific/3173327.stm).

Some terminology

The 'mode of death' refers to the final pathophysiological process leading to death (e.g. coma, pulmonary oedema), whereas the 'manner of death' classifies death according to the preceding events (homicide, suicide, accident, natural causes).

Changes after death: lividity

An appreciation of the range of changes which occur to a body after death is crucial to enable accurate interpretation of postmortem findings, particularly in relation to estimating the timing of death (see 📖 p.37) and identifying the possibility of any foul play (before or after death).

Postmortem lividity

This is also known as (postmortem) hypostasis, livor stasis, or livor mortis. It refers to the changes in the appearance of the skin which occur after death due to movement of blood under the influence of gravity. Bluish-red discoloration of dependent areas starts to become apparent between 30min and 3h after death. Lividity typically continues to develop in the first 12h, during which time it blanches under digital pressure. Areas which are in direct contact with a firm surface (e.g. the sacrum) do not exhibit hypostasis. After about 18–24h, the lividity becomes fixed. Knowledge of this may allow recognition that a body has been moved more than 18h after death.

Colour of lividity

Lividity tends to have a bluish-red appearance and may change with time, although such colour changes are not entirely predictable. Deaths which are the result of carbon monoxide poisoning demonstrate characteristic 'cherry red' (or 'cherry pink') lividity, reflecting the presence of carboxy-haemoglobin.

Distinguishing lividity from bruising

This is rarely a problem in practice, especially in the early postmortem period when lividity exhibits blanching under pressure from a finger.

Lividity in internal organs

Internal organs may show changes of lividity at the same time as it becomes apparent in the skin and can occasionally cause confusion as to the cause of death. This is especially true of blood collections at the back of the neck which can be mistaken for being the result of manual strangulation.

Absence of lividity

Some individuals who were either profoundly anaemic or who had suffered exsanguination prior to death fail to show any evidence of lividity. Lividity may also be difficult to identify in individuals with highly pigmented skin.

Rigor mortis

The process whereby muscles stiffen after death is well known to both the specialist and lay person. As the amount of adenosine triphosphate (ATP) within muscle decreases after death, the actin and myosin fixes together to produce the characteristic stiffness of rigor mortis. With the passage of time, as the tissues start to break down, so rigor mortis disappears and flaccidity returns.

Typical progression of rigor mortis

Although the process occurs in all muscle groups, postmortem rigidity is first apparent in the smaller muscles (e.g. in jaw and eyelids) and then becomes evident in the remainder. Typically seen first in the face, it then progresses to the shoulders, and finally in the large muscle groups of the limbs (Nysten's rule), as follows:

- In the initial 30min after death, no rigidity is apparent (except possibly in the unusual instance of cadaveric spasm—see later in this section).
- Between 30min and 3h after death, the limbs remain flaccid, but there may be evidence of rigidity affecting the jaw and other muscles of the face.
- Rigidity becomes established in all muscle groups by the time of 6h and remains so until 24–36h after death.
- From the time of 24h onwards, rigidity starts to diminish, with the muscles becoming obviously flaccid again from the time of around 36h.

Assessing postmortem rigidity

The development and extent of rigor mortis can provide useful information when trying to make an assessment of the time since death (see 📖 p.37), but a number of factors can hasten or delay this process. The process is delayed by cold ambient temperature and/or preceding debilitating illness. It is hastened by higher ambient or body temperature and by physical exertion (or convulsions) immediately prior to death. The presence and extent of rigidity can be tested for by attempting to extend/move various joints. If sufficient force is applied, postmortem rigidity can be 'broken' and if already fully established, will not subsequently return.

Cadaveric spasm

There have been anecdotal reports of rigidity occurring almost instantly after death—this phenomenon has been termed 'cadaveric spasm'. It is a highly controversial area, with many experts questioning whether or not it really exists.

Changes after death: decomposition

Putrefaction

The typical destruction of a body after death by bacteria is termed putrefaction. Bacteria from the bowel (e.g. clostridia) and lungs thrive in the
anaerobic environment and spread around the body. The process is
understandably accelerated in patients who die from generalized sepsis
as bacteria have already gained a head start and the body temperature
tends to be elevated at the time of death, creating more favourable conditions for bacteria to multiply. Similarly, putrefaction occurs more rapidly
in bodies left in hot ambient conditions and in individuals with obesity.
Bacteria utilize the protein-rich content of the blood—putrefaction may
be delayed when there has been significant haemorrhage prior to death.

The putrefactive process

There is no fixed sequence of events as a body decomposes: considerable
variation occurs between individuals and according to the ambient temperature. As a result, analysis of the process is not usually helpful in trying
to make an accurate estimation of the time interval since death occurred.
Bodies which are left in below-freezing conditions may be preserved
into the long term without evidence of significant putrefaction. Bodies
which are left in water tend to decompose more slowly. The process of
decomposition tends to follow a characteristic pattern:

- At standard room temperatures, the first external evidence is usually
  greenish skin discoloration of the right iliac fossa, occurring within the
  first few days. This green discoloration becomes more prominent and
  spreads to involve the remainder of the anterior abdominal wall and
  other parts of the body during subsequent days.
- The abdominal wall, scrotum, and face become distended (sometimes
  grotesquely so) by gas (including methane and the offensive smelling
  hydrogen sulphide) produced by bacteria. There may be palpable
  crepitus. The tongue may also swell, the eyes protrude, and bloody
  fluid exude from the mouth and nostrils ('purging')—some of these
  features may be mistaken for injury involved in causing death.
- At about 1 week after death, bacteria spread through the venous
  system, resulting in characteristic *'marbling'* of the skin (reflecting
  intravascular haemolysis)—branching dark red (becoming green) lines.
- As time passes, the hair becomes loose and superficial fluid-filled skin
  blisters appear.
- As weeks pass, the skin discoloration changes to dark green.
  Fingerprint identification starts to become difficult. Maggots and
  rodents may play a significant role in the destructive process. Body fat
  may liquefy.

Adipocere

Under certain (particularly anaerobic) circumstances, body fat can be
hydrolysed by bacteria to a greasy waxy substance called 'adipocere' (also
known as 'corpse or grave wax'). This process requires several months
and tends to occur when bodies are buried or left submerged in water.

Mummification

Drying of a body after death can result in mummification of all or part of it. This process can occur in both hot and cold climates. As it dries out, the skin turns hard and leathery. The limbs may alter position as the muscles and tendons shrink.

Skeletalization

The process of decomposition whereby the soft tissues of a body gradually disappear after death to leave a skeleton takes place at various rates, depending upon the conditions. In warm conditions, skeletalization can occur within a matter of months, although in temperate climates the process usually takes about 2 years.

Body farm—Forensic Anthropology Center

The most famous of several 'body farms' in the US was started by Dr William Bass in the University of Tennessee, Knoxville, in 1971. Body farms study the decomposition of human bodies placed in different outdoor environments. Research involving the detailed recording and analysis of the condition of the bodies over time (including the activity of insects) provides insight into the process of decomposition. The results of work undertaken at body farms has obvious applications in crime scene investigation, in terms of the following:

• Identification of bodies in various stages of decomposition.
• Estimation of the time since death.
• Determining the manner of death.

Individuals can donate their bodies to body farms for the advancement of forensic anthropology and science.

Time interval since death

Attempting to estimate the time interval since death (and hence the time of death) can be crucial in the investigation of potentially suspicious deaths, particularly in relation to confirming and establishing alibis. The forensic physician attending the scene of death often plays a key role in the estimation of time of death. Unfortunately, there is no single forensic test which can be applied to provide a definite and exact answer. Combining analysis of temperature and extent of rigor mortis is most commonly employed.

Body temperature

As time passes after death, the temperature of the body reduces. The rate of cooling varies according to a number of factors, including the ambient temperature, the size of the body, clothing, air currents, and humidity. A variety of charts have been published which contain cooling curves, enabling extrapolation taking into account the measured core temperature and the other factors already outlined. Core temperature is measured by using a rectal thermometer, although there may be instances where this is inappropriate (e.g. alleged sexual assault).

Rough guide

As a rough guide, the lightly clothed torso of a body at room temperature will feel warm for approximately the first 8h.

Rigor mortis, lividity, and putrefactive changes

The presence and extent of rigor mortis and/or any putrefactive changes may provide a guide to the time interval since death, as outlined on 📖 Rigor mortis, p.33, Changes after death: lividity, p.32, and Changes after death: decomposition, p.34.

Gastric contents

Attempts have been made for many years to try to estimate the time of death. An average meal will usually have left the stomach by 4h. However, in general terms, the rate of gastric emptying is too variable for this to be relied upon. Also, unless death is sudden, the events leading up to death can significantly hasten or delay gastric emptying. Analysis of undigested gastric contents can, however, provide very important information about what was consumed shortly before death (e.g. undigested chips and curry sauce might help to indicate that an individual found dead in the street had visited the local chip shop since being seen leaving the public house).

Vitreous humour

Changes in the chemical composition of various fluids, particularly the vitreous humour (fluid in the back of the eyeball), appeared to hold promise in attempting to accurately identify the time of death. Potassium gradually rises within the vitreous humour after death, but unfortunately, the initial potassium level and the rate of subsequent rise are too unpredictable for this to be a truly useful method at the present time.

Summary—practical estimation of time since death

The following may assist as a approximate guide:

- No lividity or rigor mortis is apparent within the first 30min.
- Lividity and postmortem rigidity starts at between 30min and 3h after death, during which time the limbs remain flaccid, but rigidity may be apparent in the muscles of the jaw and face.
- The torso of a lightly clothed body in a warm room will feel warm to the touch for the first 8h.
- Lividity blanches until the time of about 12h.
- Rigidity is established by the time of 6h and remains so until about 36h.
- Lividity becomes fixed at around 18h.
- From 24h onwards, rigidity diminishes and the body becomes flaccid again from about 36h onwards.
- Green discoloration appears on the skin in the right iliac fossa after several days, gradually spreading thereafter.
- Marbling of the venous system occurs at about one week after death.

Death scene investigation

Resuscitation considerations

When a body is discovered, the first consideration is whether death has occurred. If a person is still alive, or possibly so, emergency resuscitation measures need to be commenced. Attempts to preserve life take precedence over concerns about preserving evidence. Except when there is evidence of rigor mortis and/or decomposition, it can be quite difficult for the person who finds a body to determine whether or not to commence resuscitation. This particularly applies to those situations where prolonged resuscitation might be successful (e.g. a body retrieved from cold water after a recent drowning episode). When death has clearly occurred, a doctor is called to confirm death and examine the scene.

Suspicious or not?

On finding a body, any suspicion that death was not due to a natural disease process will prompt initiation of a detailed investigative process. If there are no initial concerns, but concerns arise later, it is almost inevitable that the opportunity to gather some vital information and clues from examination of the scene will be lost. For this reason, the investigating police officers tend to adopt a low threshold for declaring a scene of death as 'suspicious', with the forensic physician often being called upon to assist with this initial analysis.

Protection of the scene

Preservation of the evidence and avoidance of contamination are two guiding principles for those tasked with protection for the scene of a suspicious death. This is achieved by:
- Identifying what constitutes the 'scene' at an early stage.
- Using cordons to secure the setting.
- Carefully considering the entry route to the scene (e.g. using a rear entrance to a house when a body is discovered in the hallway adjacent to the front door.
- Preserving evidence outdoors by use of a protective tent.
- Minimizing movement within the cordoned area and restricting access to only those who need to be there.
- Ensuring that all those who attend the scene wear a protective suit, gloves, and overshoes.
- Gathering evidence (e.g. photographing shoeprints) at an early stage, before it is lost due to movement of the investigating team.

Health hazards

There are many potential risks to the health of the investigating team, depending upon the nature of the scene. Bodies found in enclosed spaces can present a risk due to production of noxious gas. The aftermath of explosions and fires presents obvious dangers. Extreme risks at terrorist scenes include 'booby traps' and exposure to noxious chemicals and biological substances.

The investigating team

The exact composition of the individuals who attend a suspicious scene varies slightly according to different jurisdictions. However, there are similar basic themes. In addition to calling upon the services of relevant doctors, the investigating police officer will invariably call upon the specialist services of Scenes of Crime Officers ('SOCOs')—also known as Crime Scene Investigators. Specialist investigators will obtain photographs and/or videos of the scene, examine for evidence (e.g. look for, analyse, record, and swab bloodstains), and collect possible trace and other evidence.

Role of the doctor at the scene

In the UK, the first doctor called to a suspicious death is a forensic physician, often followed later by a forensic pathologist. The duties of the doctor include the following:

- To confirm that death has occurred.
- To examine the scene and the body for marks and injuries (including possible resuscitation injuries) and provide a preliminary opinion as to whether it might have been due to homicide, suicide, 'accident', or natural causes. The doctor will typically record handwritten information and diagrams detailing the position of the body, any obvious injuries, and other relevant nearby objects.
- To record that important information which cannot be gathered later. This includes: assessing/recording both ambient and body temperature, the presence and extent of lividity and rigor mortis. The decision as to whether it is appropriate to record rectal core temperatures is usually taken after discussion with the investigating team—this measurement is understandably avoided if there is any suspicion of sexual assault. Non-invasive alternatives for measuring temperature include using the tympanic route.

Management of the body

A full external inspection of the body at the scene provides useful and important information. However, care should be taken to move and handle it as little as possible and in particular, to avoid postmortem injury. Appropriate trace evidence can be collected from the body at the scene. All interventions (including taking samples, moving, etc.) need to be recorded in detail. Once all evidence (trace, photographs, etc.) have been taken, the body needs to be placed in a plastic body bag with complete zip and accompanied to the mortuary suite by a police officer (to confirm and preserve the chain of evidence).

The coroner system in England and Wales

Background

The coroner is an experienced (registered) lawyer or doctor (or both) who has a role in the investigation of sudden deaths. The coroner is an independent judicial officer who is tasked with trying to establish the following ('who, when, where, and how'):

- Who the person was who died.
- When the person died.
- Where the person died.
- How the person died (both the medical cause of death and the circumstances that led to the death).

Reporting deaths to the coroner

Most deaths which are not unexpected and which result from natural causes and where a doctor is prepared to issue a death certificate do not need to be referred to a coroner. Doctors will typically report deaths to be considered by a coroner under the following circumstances:

- When no doctor treated the deceased during his/her last illness.
- When no doctor has seen the deceased within the past 14 days.
- When death occurred under an anaesthetic and/or during or after an operation.
- When death was sudden and unexplained or accompanied by any suspicious circumstances.
- When death might be due to an industrial injury or disease.
- When death may be the result of an accident, suicide, homicide, violence, neglect, abortion, or poisoning.
- When death occurs in prison or police custody.

Investigation by the coroner

The coroner may investigate deaths of an individual whose body lies within his/her designated 'area'. So, for example, in addition to investigating those deaths which occur in their locality, the local coroner may also investigate deaths which occurred abroad when the body is returned (e.g. the Oxfordshire coroner investigated military deaths which occurred in Afghanistan in 2009 when the bodies were returned to RAF Brize Norton).

Autopsy

The coroner may instruct a pathologist to perform an autopsy in order to try to establish the cause of death. Note that whilst taking into account the wishes of the family in this respect, it is the coroner's decision as to whether or not an autopsy is required.

Coroner's officers

The coroner is assisted by a team of coroner's officers, who often have a police, nursing, or paramedic background. The coroner's officers gather information (including reports from police officers and doctors) which may help the coroner to decide whether or not to have an autopsy and hold an inquest.

History of the coroner

The office of coroner has a long history. Although it has changed somewhat over the years, it was established more than 800 years ago in early medieval England. The initial role of the coroner was to 'keep the pleas of the crown', hence the derivation of the term and Shakespeare's 'crowner'.

Coroner's inquest

When to hold an inquest
The coroner will hold an inquest if there is reason to suspect a person:
- Died in a violent or 'unnatural' fashion.
- Died suddenly and from an unknown cause.
- Died in prison or custody or in such circumstances to require an inquest under any relevant Act.

Purpose of an inquest
An inquest is intended to be a fact finding, not a fault finding, exercise and usually proceedings in the coroner's court are suspended until after the outcome of any criminal proceedings. Witnesses at an inquest are not required to answer questions which may incriminate them in relation to any crime—the coroner has a role to ensure that witnesses are aware of this.

Format
The inquest is typically held in public, often with members of the press present. Witnesses are called in an order which is decided by the coroner. The degree of formality of the coroner's court depends upon the coroner, but each witness will be asked to take an oath or affirm. In addition to the coroner, any party with a 'proper' (reasonable) interest may be able to question the witnesses, either directly or via a solicitor.

Jury
Under certain circumstances, a jury (comprised of 7–11 members from the crown court jury list) will be required. These circumstances include deaths which occur:
- In prison, police custody, or possibly caused by a police officer.
- In industrial accidents.
- In circumstances which may recur to prejudice public health/safety.

Verdict
Contrary to popular belief, the verdict includes all of the relevant information: who, when, where, and not just how. Understandably, the focus is usually upon 'how' a person died, where there are a large number of possible verdicts, which include: death by natural causes, misadventure/accidental death, industrial disease, dependence upon drugs, unlawful killing, and lawful killing (including self-defence). Most of the verdicts are based upon the 'balance of probabilities', but a verdict of suicide can only be recorded when the coroner believes that the evidence supports this 'beyond reasonable doubt'. An 'open verdict' may be given when the cause of death cannot be established. The coroner can also give a 'narrative verdict' if this most accurately explains the circumstances leading to death. The term 'neglect' may be used either as a verdict or, more usually, as an additional factor in other verdicts.

Recommendations by the coroner

Based upon the information derived from the investigations in the course of an inquest, a coroner may make specific recommendations. Such recommendations may focus upon preventing recurrence of a sequence of events which resulted in an individual's death.

Implications for other legal proceedings

The system is designed to prevent the verdict from determining any associated question of criminal or civil liability. However, the coroner's verdict is frequently relied upon in civil proceedings (and claims against insurance policies).

The professional witness at an inquest

Attending an inquest as a professional witness (typically doctor, nurse, police officer) can be a difficult experience, depending upon the circumstances. Here is the view of one doctor:

'I have attended High Courts, sheriff courts, Crown Courts, and magistrates' courts as a professional and expert witness in relation to a variety of alleged offences, including rape, murder, and child abuse. Interestingly, these experiences have never been as stressful as the occasions when I have attended the coroner court as a professional witness! Being directly questioned by relatives of the deceased in an emotional and sometimes threatening and inappropriate manner has proved to be much more tricky to handle than the cleverest barrister…'

Two principal distinctions between the coroner's court and other courts from the perspective of the professional witness are that witnesses can have questions put to them by any interested party and that the intention is to establish the facts and not to apportion blame. However, there is the obvious potential for the professional to be blamed in an open and emotional way by relatives for failing to prevent the death of their loved one. Herein lies the opportunity for the coroner to demonstrate his/her skill in sensitively handling relatives, yet ensuring witnesses are handled fairly, all whilst establishing the facts.

Fatal accident inquiry in Scotland

Background

In some ways, the fatal accident inquiry is a Scottish equivalent of the English coroner's inquest, although there are certain significant differences. As at an inquest, the fatal accident inquiry investigates the circumstances of some deaths which have occurred in Scotland, but unlike the inquest, the fatal accident inquiry is not able to investigate deaths which occurred outside Scotland.

Fatal Accidents and Sudden Deaths Inquiry Act 1976

Under this act, the procurator fiscal in the area that the person died investigates the circumstances of sudden, suspicious, accidental, unexpected, and unexplained deaths, and any deaths where circumstances might cause serious public concern. The procurator fiscal is legally qualified and (unlike the English coroner), is unlikely to be medically qualified.

The *procurator fiscal* in Scotland has a wider remit than the coroner has in England and Wales. The principal difference is that the procurator fiscal is also involved in organizing and pursuing criminal proceedings on behalf of the Lord Advocate. The first decision for the procurator fiscal faced with a sudden death is whether criminal proceedings are required or whether a fatal accident inquiry should be held. The procurator fiscal may instruct a forensic pathologist to perform an autopsy and/or other postmortem investigations, such as toxicological analyses of body fluids.

Fatal accident inquiries may be mandatory or discretionary:

- A mandatory fatal accident inquiry is required in all cases of death occurring in legal custody or during the course of employment (unless a previous criminal trial has already adequately established the circumstances of the death).
- A discretionary fatal accident inquiry may be held in a case of sudden, suspicious, or unexplained death if the Lord Advocate (as advised by the procurator fiscal) considers it to be in the public interest. The wishes of the relatives and any criminal proceedings are taken into account in making this decision.

Reporting deaths to the procurator fiscal

The criteria for deaths which should be reported to the procurator fiscal are very similar to those used for the coroner in England and Wales (see 📖 The coroner system in England and Wales, p.40). Approximately 25% of all deaths in Scotland are reported to the procurator fiscal, usually by a doctor, the police, or the Registrar General.

A fatal accident inquiry is advertised in the press at least 21 days before it is held in a sheriff court.

Procedure at a fatal accident inquiry

As with the equivalent south of the border, the fatal accident inquiry is intended to be inquisitorial in nature, rather than formally apportioning blame. The procurator fiscal presents evidence in the public interest. Other interested parties will be able to attend and also have the opportunity to be legally represented. The Sheriff (judge) sits (in a sheriff court) without a jury and makes a determination of the factual circumstances of the death (i.e. time and place) and the cause of the accident. The Sheriff reaches this decision on the 'balance of probabilities'. Recommendations may be made (and if so, they may be published on the Scottish courts website ℘ http://www.scotcourts.gov.uk). The determination made by the Sheriff cannot be used as evidence in any subsequent separate legal proceedings. Interestingly, this determination may now also be the subject of judicial review and so may not be the final word.

History of the fatal accident inquiry

The Fatal Accidents Inquiry (Scotland) Act 1895 first formally introduced the fatal accident inquiry into Scottish law, prior to which it was left to the procurator fiscal to determine. The latest relevant legislation is the Fatal Accidents and Sudden Deaths Inquiry (Scotland) Act 1976, although there was a review of the fatal accident inquiry system in 2008, with the report on the consultation paper published in 2009 (℘ http://www.scotland.gov.uk/Publications/2009/06/03102428/0).

Homicide

Definition

Homicide is defined as the killing of a human being by a human being. Although the lay person often equates 'homicide' with 'murder', the two are very different terms. Homicide includes murder, but also manslaughter and other types of death. Note that forensic pathologists and other experts may express an opinion that a death was a homicide, but it is usually a court/legal system that decides it is a murder.

Terminology

A variety of terms have been applied to homicide in different circumstances:

- Filicide—killing of a child (by a parent).
- Fratricide—killing of a brother/comrade.
- Genocide—killing of an ethnic, religious, or other large group.
- Infanticide—killing of an infant.
- Mariticide—killing of a husband (by wife).
- Uxoricide—killing of a wife (by husband).

When is homicide not a crime?

Homicide can be regarded as not being a crime in certain circumstances and in certain jurisdictions. Perhaps the ultimate examples are (state sanctioned) capital punishment and deaths inflicted by soldiers from one country on those from another when the countries are at war. In a civilian setting, individuals may also claim that they caused the death of others in self-defence. Similarly, police officers (e.g. marksmen) may act legally when they cause the deaths of individuals who are risking the lives of members of the public and/or police, although any death occurring in such a situation will inevitably incur intense public and media scrutiny, as well as a formal investigation.

Mens rea and actus reus

Traditionally, from a legal perspective, for a person to have committed a crime, there needs to be the combination of both a criminal act ('*actus reus*') with a guilty mind ('*mens rea*'). It is worth noting that some crimes involve failing to act in a reasonable fashion (negligence), with the most notable crime being manslaughter.

International comparisons

The number of cases initially classified by the police as being homicides in England and Wales is liable to be different from the number which appears in the final statistics. Official figures take into account court decisions (e.g. that a death was due to suicide not homicide) and typically include murder, manslaughter, and infanticide, but not death caused by dangerous or careless driving or deaths following aggravated vehicle taking. Even allowing for different definitions and reporting, there are remarkably varied rates of homicide in different countries (and even between cities within the same country). The reported homicide rate in 2004 in South Africa was more than 10x higher than that in the USA, which itself was 3x higher than that in England and Wales (see Table 2.1). As far as individual cities are concerned, the homicide rate in Washington DC is approximately 30x that in London.

Table 2.1 Homicide rates in 2004 per 100 000 population

Japan	0.5
Morocco	0.5
Hong Kong	0.5
Ireland	0.7
Denmark	0.8
Norway	0.8
France	0.8
Germany	1.0
Italy	1.2
Netherlands	1.2
Australia	1.3
New Zealand	1.4
Spain	1.4
England and Wales	1.6
Portugal	1.8
China	2.2
Sweden	2.4
Northern Ireland	2.4
Scotland	2.6
Switzerland	2.9
Pakistan	3.6
India	5.5
USA	5.9
Mexico	10.9
Brazil	26.2
Russia	29.7
Jamaica	33.7
South Africa	69.0

UN data: http://data.un.org

Serial killers

Definition and background

There are few news items that create as much publicity, speculation, and sheer sensation as the reporting of cases of serial killers. Media and public interest is always understandably intense. It is worth remembering, however, that serial killing is relatively uncommon. Although the term would instantly conjure up an image in most people's minds, exact definitions vary. Serial killers are distinguished from mass murderers in that they commit crimes intermittently over a period of time, rather than all at the same time. Most definitions require at least three murders being committed in separate incidents by the same individual in the same fashion.

Serial killings may be classified into those involving an apparent sexual motive and those without.

Serial sexual killing

Many serial murders involve a sexual element, often targeting individuals apparently almost at random without any obvious connection to the killer.

Non-sexual serial killing

Some serial murders do not reflect any obvious overt sexual motive, but instead target specific individuals and/or minority groups within society.

Characteristics

There are some recurrent features which characterize serial killings, although not all of these are present in every case. It is worth noting the following:

- Most murderers are male.
- The murders are typically premeditated and preplanned, following a similar ritualistic pattern, often including a fantasy element, involving domination and/or sadism.
- There may be a significant period of time between each killing, sometimes referred to as a 'cooling off' period.
- The means chosen to effect killing tends to be violent and repeated in the same fashion on each occasion. The body may be mutilated after death and left in the same (characteristic and/or degrading) position. Sometimes the killer may move the bodies after death and attempt to clean up the crime scene.
- The murderer may remove articles from the crime scene, for reasons which are sometimes obscure. These articles may be referred to as 'souvenirs' or 'trophies'.

Jack the Ripper

In 1888, there commenced a series of brutal murders in the Whitechapel district of London, attributed to an unidentified serial killer, dubbed 'Jack the Ripper'. The exact number of murders attributed to this serial killer has never been established for certain, but is generally agreed to be somewhere between 5 and 12. Five murders in 1888 share striking similarities, with prostitutes being targeted, their bodies being mutilated, slashed ('ripped') open, and some internal organs removed. The investigation into the Whitechapel murders has been subjected to intense scrutiny over the years. Similarly, there has been considerable speculation over the possible identity of the killer.

Almost a century later, another slashing serial killer emerged in England, this time in West Yorkshire. He targeted women, including prostitutes, mutilating many of them. *Peter Sutcliffe* ('the Yorkshire Ripper') was convicted in 1981 of 13 murders of women between 1975 and 1980. Although declared 'sane' at his trial, he was later diagnosed with schizophrenia and locked up in Broadmoor Hospital.

Suicide

Background

A leading cause of death worldwide, suicide rates do vary significantly between different countries. Russia, Ukraine, and some neighbouring countries have particularly high rates, possibly associated with alcohol-related problems. The complete background to many suicides remains uncertain, but there are common recurring themes and factors, some of which may overlap:

- Chronic (long-term) depression and other (especially psychotic) mental illness.
- Alcohol and/or drug abuse.
- Chronic debilitating physical illness.
- Impulsive act following relationship break-up.

Less commonly, a different motivation is at work (e.g. self-immolation has been used as a means of protest, some terrorists use suicide attacks—see 📖 p.161).

Methods

Similar to the rates of suicide, the methods used to complete suicide varies considerably both within and between different populations. This partly reflects the methods available: firearms are a particular feature in countries (e.g. the USA) and communities (e.g. farming) with access to them. More violent methods tend to be employed by those with underlying psychotic illness. Recent data from the UK indicates the following:

- Suicide rates are higher in men than women.
- Hanging/suffocation is the most common method used by men and the second most common used by women.
- Drug poisoning (especially paracetamol and antidepressants) is the most common method in women and second most common in men.
- Other important methods of suicide (in diminishing order) are: drowning, jumping/lying before a moving object, falling from a height, firearms and explosives, use of sharp objects.

Suicide or not?

Distinguishing suicides from homicides, 'accidents', or even natural causes can be difficult. This difficulty is compounded by deliberate attempts (for various reasons) by perpetrators, family, and others to conceal what really happened. The investigating team needs to keep an open mind and consider carefully all of the information available. On occasions, it is impossible to tell what happened. On others, the background and circumstances (e.g. suicide note) may lead to an obvious conclusion that death was the result of suicide. Autoerotic asphyxia may at first appear to be suicide (see 📖 Autoerotic asphyxia, p.110).

Uncertainty and some famous deaths

The lives of many famous individuals come under tremendous scrutiny and it should come as no surprise that their deaths do too.

Marilyn Monroe (1926–1962), a globally famous actress from California was found dead at home on 5 August 1962. Her officially recorded cause of death was 'acute barbiturate poisoning', which was perhaps controversially stated to be the result of an accidental overdose. There has been much subsequent speculation about her death, particularly as to whether it might have been suicide, and there are also a number of conspiracy theories that it might have been the result of homicide.

Kurt Cobain (1967–1994) was lead singer of US rock band Nirvana. He was found dead at home on 8 April 1994. There was a suicide note next to his body. Autopsy revealed significant levels of diamorphine ('heroin') in his body, together with a fatal gunshot wound to his head. Despite numerous conspiracy theories about his death, there has never been any real evidence to suggest that it was anything other than suicide.

Michael Hutchence (1960–1997) was lead singer of Australian rock band INXS. He was found dead in a room of the Ritz-Carlton hotel in Sydney on 22 November 1997. His death was attributed to suicide by hanging. However, many individuals (including girlfriend Paula Yates and members of his family) questioned this, noting that he was naked when found and that there was no suicide note, postulating instead that he died as a result of autoerotic asphyxia (see 📖 Autoerotic asphyxia, p.110).

Paula Yates (1959–2000), Welsh television presenter, girlfriend of Michael Hutchence, was found dead at her home in London. Death was attributed to an overdose of diamorphine ('heroin'), which the coroner judged to be an accident, rather than suicide.

Michael Jackson, world famous eccentric pop star, died at the age of 50 years on 25 June 2009, having suffered a cardiac arrest at home in California. In a frenzy of media speculation, attention focused upon the drugs which he was prescribed (particularly propofol) and the role that drugs might have played in causing his death.

Dyadic death

Definition
Dyadic death is the combination of death by homicide followed by suicide in the perpetrator (homicide–suicide). Exact definitions are difficult, particularly in relation to the time period between homicide and suicide.

Types of homicide–suicide
'Standard cases' involve individuals who are well known to each other. Often, one spouse (most often male) may kill the other then kill him/herself. Sometimes, a parent may kill one or more children and/or spouse before committing suicide. Determining the underlying reasons that lead to dyadic death is understandably not easy, but deterioration in relationships between spouses appears to be a crucial factor. A significant proportion of cases involve mothers who kill their children and then themselves—many of the perpetrators suffer from depression and choose relatively non-violent methods of death. This has led to the proposal that dyadic death in these instances reflect an extension of the act of suicide.

Homicide followed by delayed suicide perhaps stretches the accepted definition of dyadic death, especially when the time interval between the two events is quite long. This is particularly true when suicide follows arrest of the perpetrator and when the act of suicide did not appear to be part of the original plan.

Random strikes against strangers may be carried out by individuals who carry a weapon and target people who are not known to them, with the apparent aim of killing as many people as possible. Often these attacks are carried out by perpetrators who have a military interest.

Religious and/or politically motivated attacks are primarily intended to kill as many people of a different faith/background as possible. Usually, the suicide of the perpetrator is an integral part of the attack.

Christopher Foster and family

In August 2008, flames engulfed an impressive mansion in a sleepy corner of Shropshire to leave a small village community in a state of shock. Three family members (Christopher Foster, his wife, and daughter) were missing, but such was the difficulty in investigating the devastated scene that it was several days before the bodies were all recovered. Forensic investigation, including analysis of closed-circuit television, gradually enabled a picture to be constructed of events leading up to the deaths. Although from the outside he appeared to be a successful businessman, 50-year-old Christopher Foster was actually facing financial ruin and the resultant transformation of his lifestyle and that of his family. It is believed that he shot his wife and daughter before setting fire to their house and killing himself.

Distinguishing dyadic death from double suicide

On occasions, it can be difficult to determine whether deaths may be the result of a double suicide rather than dyadic death. The same issue can face investigators of incidents when there are survivors.

Sudden death from natural causes

Background
Sudden unexpected death from natural causes can occur at any age and will inevitably be reported to the coroner (or procurator fiscal in Scotland) for investigation. This investigation will usually include the following:
- A report from a police officer and/or other individuals about the events leading up to death.
- A summary of known previous medical problems (usually obtained from the GP).
- Autopsy and/or toxicological and other analyses of body fluids (a small but significant proportion of individuals who at first appear to have died from natural causes turn out to have died from poisoning).

Sudden death in infancy is considered on p.88. Sudden death at other ages has a variety of underlying causes, sometimes relating to previously known disease and sometimes not. Not infrequently, despite thorough investigation, the cause of death remains unclear—a situation which is understandably frustrating and considered to be unsatisfactory for relatives.

Causes
The underlying causes of sudden unexpected death include the following:
- *Cardiac*—ischaemic heart disease, cardiomyopathy, congenital coronary artery anomalies, valve disease, coronary artery dissection, Wolff–Parkinson–White syndrome, Brugada syndrome, and other ion channel disorders.
- *Other cardiovascular disorders*—aortic dissection and rupture, pulmonary embolism.
- *Central nervous system (CNS) causes*—subarachnoid and other intracranial haemorrhage, epilepsy.
- *Infection*—meningitis, encephalitis, pneumonia, myocarditis, endocarditis.
- *Other*—asthma, gastrointestinal haemorrhage, metabolic collapse.

Death during sport/exercise
Sudden unexpected death during sport/exercise understandably generates alarm and often also interest from the press. Cardiomyopathy, congenital coronary artery anomalies, valve disease, and acquired ischaemic heart disease may cause sudden death during sport/exercise and are considered on p.62.

Brugada syndrome
This syndrome has been increasingly recognized as a cardiac cause of sudden death. It has a genetic component and is characterized by ventricular arrhythmias and sudden death, with electrocardiographic findings of ST segment elevation in V1–3 and right bundle branch block.

Other ion channel disorders

These include inherited disorders causing long QT interval on an ECG, which predispose to ventricular tachyarrhythmias (particularly torsade de pointes) and sudden death.

Aortic dissection and rupture

A tear in the intimal layer of the aorta can rupture externally into the pleural cavity or retroperitoneally (causing exsanguination) or into the pericardial cavity (causing cardiac tamponade). Certain groups (e.g. those with Marfan syndrome) are at particular risk, but it can occur spontaneously without any known risk factors.

Pulmonary embolism

Pulmonary thromboembolism commonly occurs in individuals with a variety of serious illnesses, when it can be the principal cause of death or simply contributory. Fatal pulmonary emboli also cause sudden death in individuals who are apparently fit and healthy.

Intracranial haemorrhage

Bleeding inside the skull can be rapidly devastating and can occur with little in the way of warning. Haemorrhage can take several forms, as follows:
- *Subarachnoid haemorrhage* occurring spontaneously usually results from rupture of a 'berry aneurysm', due to a congenital defect in the circle of Willis, or less commonly, due to an arteriovenous malformation.
- *Subdural haematoma* typically follows trauma, although the history may be lacking (see 📖 p.148).
- *Haemorrhage into the brain* may affect the cerebral hemispheres, cerebellum or brainstem, with the last being particularly poorly tolerated.

Infections

A variety of infections can cause sudden death, with symptoms being disregarded by the patient. Most notable infections include meningitis, encephalitis, and pneumonia. Microbiological tests at autopsy (especially postmortem blood cultures) can prove to be particularly useful.

Gastrointestinal haemorrhage

Brisk bleeding within the gut can occur in patients with known pre-existing disease (e.g. liver failure and oesophageal varices) or without (e.g. previously unrecognized peptic ulceration).

Metabolic disorders

The most frequently implicated metabolic problems causing unexpected sudden death are diabetic ketoacidosis, non-ketotic hyperosmolar diabetic hyperglycaemia, and adrenocortical insufficiency.

Accidents as a cause of death

Terminology

There is now disapproval of the use of the term 'accident' amongst certain professionals, although the law still uses it (e.g. 'accidental death', 'fatal accident inquiry'). Injury prevention experts argue strongly that accidents are defined as 'unforeseen, unpredictable events', whereas analysis of most injuries reveals inherent predictability and preventability.

What constitutes an accident?

Definitions vary, but an easy starting point is to consider an accident to include all traumatic deaths which are not due to homicide or suicide. Traumatic deaths are then classified into three easily identifiable categories with legal connotations, but unfortunately, it is not always easy to distinguish between these. There is relatively often particular difficulty distinguishing between death resulting from an 'accident' and that occurring due to 'suicide'. Note that some definitions of accidents include inadvertent ('accidental') poisoning, which is not strictly 'traumatic'.

Deaths from trauma

Trauma is a major cause of death at all ages, but exerts a relatively heavy toll on children and young adults. The majority of trauma deaths are 'accidents'—a detailed study from Scotland in 1995 revealed that there were 1305 deaths, of which 876 (67%) were accidents, 324 (25%) suicides, and 105 (8%) homicides.

Road traffic deaths (see 🕮 p.308)

Road traffic collisions have consistently contributed most to the number of deaths from trauma in the UK for many decades. Despite welcome significant reductions in the death toll in recent years, there were still 2538 UK road deaths in 2008. Travel by motorcycle is associated with the highest rate of death (see Table 2.2). Driver error (including excessive

Table 2.2 Relative fatality rates per hour travelled (car = 1)

Motorcycle	44
Pedal cycle	4
Pedestrians	2
Car	1
Van	0.3
Rail	0.2
Bus or coach	0.1
Water	0.1
Air travel	0.0

Source: 🕮 http://www.dft.gov.uk

speed, failing to look properly, and loss of control) are frequently cited contributory factors in all forms of collisions. Alcohol is a significant factor in a proportion of deaths, especially amongst pedestrians.

Falls
These are usually classified into 'high falls' (of 2m or more) and 'low falls' (from standing height or less). Background causes, patterns of injury, and potential for prevention is quite different for the two groups. High falls can result in immediately fatal (catastrophic) injury to the head, neck, thoracic aorta, as well as potentially fatal injuries (vertical shear pelvic fractures, liver and splenic injuries). Individuals who succumb after low falls include those who are at risk of intracranial (especially subdural) haemorrhage from head injury (e.g. alcoholics and those taking warfarin therapy) and the elderly who suffer osteoporosis related hip fractures.

Fire deaths (see 📖 p.158)
Significant contributory factors involved in fatal fires are cigarette smoking and alcohol consumption. Death more commonly results from the effects of smoke rather than burns. Detailed consideration of fire is covered on 📖 p.540.

Drowning (see 📖 p.112)
Deaths from drowning include those which occur in the home, swimming pools, the sea, and other environments. Epileptics are particularly at risk of drowning in the bath, whilst toddlers and young children may succumb in garden ponds and uncovered domestic swimming pools. The forensic and pathological aspects of drowning are considered in more detail on 📖 p.112.

Hanging (see 📖 p.106)
Most hanging deaths have underlying suicidal intent, but 'accidental' hanging can occur, particularly in children.

Environmental causes of death

The power of the environment is never far from view. Despite complex homeostatic mechanisms, humans are only able to tolerate relatively minor deviations from normal environmental conditions.

Heat illness

Exposure to high ambient temperatures can result in heat-related illness. Heat illness is a spectrum, ranging from relatively minor heat cramps and exhaustion, through to the life-threatening heat stroke. The very young and the elderly are at particular risk. Exertional heat stroke occurs in individuals who exercise vigorously in a very hot environment (e.g. army recruits). Drugs (especially chlorpromazine, haloperidol, and lithium) may induce heat illness in the form of *malignant neuroleptic syndrome*.

Heat stroke is characterized by a temperature of >40.6°C and altered conscious level. The usual homeostatic mechanisms fail, widespread cell damage occurs, and rhabdomyolysis, multiorgan failure, and disseminated intravascular coagulation may result in death. At autopsy, there may be relatively few specific findings.

Hypothermia

Hypothermia is defined as core body temperature of <35°C. An obvious hazard for winter climbers and skiers, hypothermia also affects middle aged (often alcoholics) outdoors, and individuals (especially the elderly) in residential environments, where the onset and progression may be more insidious. As body temperature drops, shivering occurs and conscious level drops. A well-known manifestation in some individuals (especially mountaineers) is paradoxical undressing—the result of deteriorating brain function. The pulse rate slows as body temperature drops, such that it can become difficult to tell if there are signs of life. Normal sinus rhythm becomes sinus bradycardia, slow atrial fibrillation, and other slow heart rhythms (e.g. heart block), before asystole ensues. Acute pancreatitis is a classic, if unusual effect of hypothermia. *Frostbite* can develop as a result of freezing of the extremities. At autopsy, evidence of direct cold damage to the extremities may be apparent, as may acute pancreatitis and/or acute gastric erosions.

Lightning

A lightning strike causes a very high-voltage direct current shock, albeit of short duration. Sudden vaporization of sweat and/or rain water by lightning may explode shoes and clothes off the victim and rupture ear drums. There may be deep muscle damage, coma from direct brain injury, and asystolic (almost flat-line electrical trace) cardiac arrest. Both survivors and those who die may have entry and exit wounds. Lightning causes characteristic superficial, feathered, or fern-like patterned burns. It is worth noting that prolonged cardiopulmonary resuscitation may be successful in the event of cardiac arrest.

Avalanches

Mountaineers and skiers (especially those off-piste) are at particular risk from avalanches, although there are occasional instances of roads, houses, and even villages being devastated. Injury and/or death may result from:
- Burial and asphyxia
- Blunt trauma from a fall
- Hypothermia.

Earthquakes

There are few unpredictable natural events which can wreak as much damage as earthquakes. Mass casualties can result from collapsing buildings and/or drowning from associated tidal waves (tsunamis). Significant health effects may follow the displacement of thousands of individuals. Survival of individuals trapped in collapsed buildings for many days is possible, focusing the attention of international rescue teams.

Floods

Severe flooding has affected many different parts of the world, but is seen in most dramatic form as a result of the monsoon rains in India and Bangladesh. Health risks include: drowning, loss of housing, loss of food supply, contamination of water, spread of infection.

Hurricanes

Also known as 'tropical storms', hurricanes are revolving seasonal low-pressure systems, which create violent storms. Strong winds and flooding typically cause dramatic damage to property.

Tornadoes

These powerful spiralling vortices of air occur on a relatively small scale, causing localized damage. Although they most frequently occur in North America, they have been reported in many parts of the world, including in the UK.

Volcanoes

Volcanic eruptions pose risks by explosions, noxious gases, pyroclastic and mud flows. Large eruptions are hard to predict.

Wild fires

Although these can occur naturally, in recent times, many fires which have devastated large areas in Australia and the USA are believed to have been started deliberately.

Deaths during sport

Background

The modern world embraces the concept that it is healthy to play sport. Health benefits, particularly relating to obesity and heart disease, are well recognized. It is ironic that taking part in activities designed to improve health actually result in death. There are two principal categories of sporting deaths: those related to vigorous exercise (mainly cardiovascular collapse) and those specific to the individual sport (specific injury).

Sporting deaths in history

Medieval hunting

Many deaths have occurred during sport, but few have changed the course of a country's history. One which did was the death of the English *King William II* ('William Rufus') in 1100. The third son of William the Conqueror was killed by an arrow through his chest whilst hunting in the New Forest.

Mountaineering

In more recent times, one fatal sporting incident to have really shocked a nation was the disaster on the Italian–Swiss border in 1865. Caught up in the fervour of the Golden Age of Alpinism, a team comprising English aristocrats and Swiss guides claimed the first ascent of the *Matterhorn in 1865*, but on the descent, a slip followed by a rope breaking, took the lives of four brave mountaineers, who fell >1000m to their deaths down the mountain's steep north face. The body of one climber, Lord Douglas, has still never been recovered and presumably remains buried in the Matterhorn's glacier. Such was the uproar about the deaths that they were discussed by Queen Victoria and politicians in the Houses of Parliament in London, where there were calls for the 'sport' of mountaineering to be banned.

Motor racing

The weekend of the 1994 San Marino Grand Prix at Imola saw the deaths of two motor racing stars. 31-year-old Roland Ratzenberger died during a crash in qualifying, followed the next day by the death of 34-year-old Ayrton Senna. The Brazilian world champion crashed into a concrete barrier at 135mph after six laps of the race. He sustained massive head injuries and was declared dead at hospital. The exact circumstances which resulted in Ayrton Senna's death have never been completely established, although his (Williams–Renault) team was cleared of manslaughter in an Italian court. These deaths did provoke a review of safety in motor racing, with subsequent significant improvements, particularly in relation to safety barriers.

Specific sport related deaths

Taking part in most sports does not pose a significant danger to life. Certain sports, however, are notoriously more dangerous than others. Different sports are associated with different specific injuries.

Adventure sports

- *Mountaineering, ice climbing, skiing, and snowboarding* carry risks of hypothermia, altitude sickness (including both cerebral and pulmonary oedema), falls, causing head and/or multiple injuries, as well as asphyxia and crush injuries in avalanches.
- *Parachuting and BASE jumping* (acronym: Building, Antenna, Span, Earth) may result in serious injury when a parachute fails to open or the individual fails to make it to the safe landing site.
- *Diving* carries risks of drowning and barotraumas.
- *Cave diving* is considered to be one of the most dangerous sports. The usual risks of diving are compounded by poor visibility and strong currents in caves, with the inability to escape in an emergency.
- *Sailing, canoeing, windsurfing, surfing, and swimming* are all associated with risks of drowning.
- *Hot air ballooning* results in serious injury when the balloon crashes into the ground or a power line, often due to pilot error or incapacitation.

Vehicle-related sports

Motor car racing, motorcycle racing, and mountain biking are all associated with injuries in the event of a crash. The same principle applies to *flying and gliding*.

Ball sports

- *Rugby* is known for serious injuries to the cervical spine, although the incidence of this appears to have fallen with changes in the rules and the way that the game is played.
- *Cricket* is played with a hard ball which can cause serious head injuries, particularly in batsmen not wearing helmets. Another unusual injury which is shared with some other sports (e.g. *baseball, ice hockey, karate*) is 'commotio cordis'—sudden death following a sharp blow to the chest, causing fatal ventricular arrhythmias despite a normal heart (see 📖 p.62).
- *Golf* is associated with occasional serious head injury (from both golfclub and ball) and lightning.

Other sports

- *Boxing* has well-documented risks of both short- and long-term head injuries (see 📖 p.151).
- *Horse riding/racing* has known risks of cervical spine and (trampling) multiple injuries.
- *Marathon running* is associated with heat-related illness.
- Even *fishing* can be dangerous, particularly in the context of sea fishing from the shore adjacent to strong tides.

Cardiovascular collapse during exercise

Sudden death during sport and/or vigorous exercise in young, apparently healthy, individuals does occur occasionally and usually reflects a cardiovascular event. Many involve previously undiagnosed cardiac problems.

Hypertrophic cardiomyopathy ('HOCM')

This is the most common cause of cardiovascular death in young athletes. Although hypertrophic cardiomyopathy has a genetic component, it often first presents as sudden death during exercise, possibly the result of a ventricular arrhythmia. Screening using ECGs and echocardiography has been used to try to identify sports players who have hypertrophic cardiomyopathy, in an attempt to prevent them from placing themselves at risk by vigorously exercising. The abnormalities (left ventricular hypertrophy and reduced left ventricle size) need to be distinguished from natural cardiac adaptations seen in some athletes (bradycardia, increase in thickness of left ventricular muscle, with increased left ventricular cavity size).

Congenital coronary artery anomalies

A variety of congenital anomalies of the coronary arteries occur. Although they are relatively common, they only cause problems infrequently. The problems which can result depend upon the nature of the anomaly. Blood flow can be reduced through abnormal coronary arteries either being kinked or compressed (e.g. when an artery runs through a 'tunnel' of myocardium, caused by an overlying 'bridge' of tissue) or by a 'steal' phenomenon (seen in abnormal arteriovenous fistulas).

Acquired coronary artery disease

Typically occurring from early middle age onwards, coronary artery atheroma can result in collapse due to arrhythmias and/or myocardial infarction.

Commotio cordis

A blunt force applied to the front of the chest (e.g. by a baseball, cricket ball, hockey puck, or opponent's hand/foot during contact sports) may result in fatal ventricular fibrillation. It is acknowledged that mechanical force applied to the chest may be 'translated' into electrical energy—indeed, this is the basis of the therapeutic 'precordial thump' used as immediate treatment of patients who are witnessed to develop ventricular fibrillation on a cardiac monitor. In the context of commotio cordis, there is believed to be a short vulnerable period of time for the development of ventricular fibrillation, immediately following the 'T' wave on the ECG.

Other causes

These include myocarditis, aortic stenosis, and heat illness.

Trauma scoring

Background

Trying to make an assessment of the extent of an individual's injuries is required in a number of different situations, including:

- A court attempting to classify the extent of injuries inflicted (and often to make an associated guess at the amount of force involved).
- A pathologist attempting to judge the likelihood of survival.
- Trauma team specialists focused upon improving treatment of patients with major trauma.
- Epidemiologists and researchers interested in analysing patterns of injury and/or comparing outcomes between various trauma systems.

The forensic pathologist's perspective

The forensic pathologist is often asked to comment upon the nature, extent, and survivability of injuries of individuals who have succumbed to trauma. Sometimes, particularly when injuries result from interpersonal violence, lawyers may attempt to imply that an individual's death was really the result of medical negligence, rather than due to overwhelming injury. It is worth bearing in mind the following points in relation to this:

- Relatively minor injury can result in death, particularly if the individual is unable to protect him/herself, possibly due to the concomitant effect of alcohol and/or drugs. An example would be the heavily intoxicated alcoholic who falls on his wine glass, causing deep buttock wounds, involving the gluteal vessels, from which he exsanguinates due to an inability to apply usual first aid measures or seek medical attention.
- Some individuals with significant pre-existing chronic illness (e.g. chronic obstructive pulmonary disease, COPD) may have such a limited reserve that they are unable to survive minor trauma in a way that a 'normal' person would. Similarly, individuals who have a bleeding disorder (either due to a congenital disease such as haemophilia, or acquired due to warfarin or other anticoagulant therapy) may suffer uncontrolled (fatal) haemorrhage from an injury which would ordinarily not cause death.
- Forensic pathologists obviously only perform autopsies on those who have died following trauma. They may therefore not be familiar with how some individuals with serious injuries can survive and are not necessarily in a good position to judge survivability.
- Trauma scoring can assist in identifying those injuries which are generally agreed to be unsurvivable.

Injury Severity Score

The most widely used score of anatomical injuries is the Injury Severity Score (ISS). The score is derived by first scoring each individual injury according to the Abbreviated Injury Scale (AIS), which attributes a score of between 1 and 6 to each injury as follows:

- AIS 1 = 'minor' injury (e.g. superficial skin abrasions).
- AIS 2 = 'moderate' injury (e.g. closed linear temporal skull fracture).
- AIS 3 = 'serious' injury.
- AIS 4 = 'severe' injury (e.g. bilateral pulmonary contusions).
- AIS 5 = 'critical' injury (e.g. massive splenic rupture with hilar disruption).
- AIS 6 = 'unsurvivable' injury (e.g. liver avulsion).

In order to calculate the ISS from the list of AIS scores for a patient, the three highest scores in different body 'regions' are squared, then added together. The Injury severity Score considers the body to have six different regions:

- Head/neck
- Face
- Chest
- Abdomen
- Extremities
- External (skin).

Possible ISS scores range from 1–75. The scoring system is non-linear and certain numbers (e.g. 15) are impossible. One traditionally accepted definition of major trauma is an ISS of >15.

Revised Trauma Score

The Revised Trauma Score (RTS) for a patient is an indication of the extent of physiological derangement caused by the injury. The score is calculated from knowing the Glasgow Coma Scale (GCS) score, systolic blood pressure, and respiratory rate. Each of these parameters is assigned a value to which a weighting factor is applied. The three resultant scores are added together to give the RTS, which can range from 0 (worst possible) to 7.84 (best).

TRISS methodology

Combining the anatomical injury score (ISS) with the extent of physiological derangement (RTS), within the context of the age of the patient and the nature of the injury, allows an estimate of the likelihood of survival for an individual patient ('TRISS methodology'). Patients who die with a probability of survival of >50% are 'unexpected deaths' and those who survive with probability of survival of <50% are classed as 'unexpected survivors', although individual results need to be interpreted with caution. TRISS methodology is used to compare the 'performances' of different hospitals and trauma systems.

Forensic autopsy

The autopsy: terminology and definitions

Autopsy

A postmortem examination which includes the removal and a full or partial dissection of the internal organs. Traditionally, it has been regarded as the 'gold standard' for the medicolegal investigation of death.

The word 'autopsy' is derived from the Greek '*autopsia*' meaning 'to see for oneself'. Sometimes the term 'necropsy' is used as an alternative, although this is more usually applied to a veterinary autopsy.

Postmortem examination

This term is used for any examination of the body after death—this is a wider term than 'autopsy' and includes, for example, the examination made by a GP or hospital clinician when certifying death, and techniques using radiology, computed tomography (CT), or magnetic resonance imaging (MRI) scans.

Although in common parlance an 'autopsy' is often referred to as a 'pm', it should be obvious that this term can lead to some confusion and is best avoided in official documentation or reporting.

View and grant

This is a procedure used in Scotland in which a doctor (who may or not be a forensic pathologist) *views* the body (an external examination) and *grants* the death certificate.

Whether the 'View & Grant' (V&G) has a role in modern forensic investigation is a matter of some controversy—although it is quick and can confirm the absence of external signs of trauma or violence, the lack of internal dissection means that an accurate and precise cause of death is less probable (the V&G has also been known as the '*view and guess*').

The extent to which it is necessary to determine an accurate and precise cause of death in all 'natural' cases referred to the legal authorities is an issue to be debated elsewhere, but here it suffices to note that the most important characteristic of a forensic procedure must be its ability to distinguish between a natural and an unnatural (accidental, suicidal, homicidal) death and to collect evidence for use in any subsequent criminal proceedings.

Diener

Derived from German ('servant'), rarely used in the UK, this term is applied to an Anatomical Pathology Technologist.

Prosector

The name given to a person who dissects a body.

The purpose of this chapter is not to give instruction on how to conduct an autopsy. Rather, it is intended to emphasize those aspects of the examination which contribute most to or, if performed poorly, detract from, a forensic investigation. The Royal College of Pathologists publishes autopsy guidelines with specific advice in a number of scenarios (🔗 http://www.rcpath.org).

Further reading

Home Office Police Advisory Board for Forensic Pathology and Royal College of Pathologists (2004). *Code of Practice and Performance Standards for Forensic Pathologists*. London: Home Office and The Royal College of Pathologists.

The Royal College of Pathologists (2002). *Guidelines on Autopsy Practice*. Report of a working group of the Royal College of Pathologists. London: The Royal College of Pathologists.

Scottish Government, COPFS, and The Royal College of Pathologists (2007). *Code of Practice and Performance Standards for Forensic Pathologists dealing with suspicious deaths in Scotland*. London: The Royal College of Pathologists.

Homepages of the professional bodies

Association of Anatomical Pathology Technologists (AAPTUK): 🔗 http://www.aaptuk.org
National Association of Medical Examiners: 🔗 http://www.thename.org
The Royal College of Pathologists: 🔗 http://www.rcpath.org
The Royal Society of Public Health: 🔗 http://www.rsph.org

Historical perspective

Ancient times

One of the earliest recorded examples of a postmortem examination relates to one of history's most notorious murders, namely that of Julius Caesar in 44 BC (see 📖 p.131). In Suetonius' account of the death, he states 'and of so many wounds none turned out to be mortal, in the opinion of the physician Antistius, except the second one in the breast'. The lawyer's question, oft asked of the forensic pathologist, 'which wound was fatal?' remains as relevant today as it was of interest then.

Although the ancient Egyptians practised a form of dissection (and retention of organs in Canopic jars) as part of a complex religious ritual, this was not related to a desire to investigate anatomy nor to understand disease or injury. Systematic 'scientific' postmortem investigation was undertaken by Galen (129–216) who dissected animals—his understanding of the rete mirabile makes it unlikely that he dissected humans. This had the unfortunate result of paralysing medical science for the next 1400 years because, for Galen, it 'proved' Hippocrates' theory relating disease to the four circulating humours (yellow bile, black bile, blood, and phlegm). As the 'four humour' doctrine became established within medical orthodoxy, there was little desire for further empirical experiment or investigation until the 13th century and the development of the centres of medical learning in Italy. The influence of the law faculty at Bologna was such that they used dissection to aid criminal inquiry—some of the earliest autopsies were, indeed, medicolegal cases. In 1410, the Catholic Church instructed an autopsy on the body of Pope Alexander V following a suspicion that he might have been poisoned. The findings were negative—of course, in today's practice this might not be surprising and is indeed an early testament to the wisdom of requiring toxicological analysis in such cases. Comparison should be made with the more recent case of Harold Shipman (see 📖 p.486).

Later Middle Ages

By the 16th century, the ecclesiastical authorities generally accepted that postmortem dissection was a legitimate investigative technique. This opened the way for the systematic study of human pathology and anatomy. Vesalius (1514–1564), Pauw (1564–1617), Harvey (1578–1657), Lancisi (1654–1720), and Boerhaave (1668–1738), amongst others, all made significant advances and in 1769 the Italian Giovanni Batista Morgagni (1682–1771) published *De Sedibus et Causis Morborum per Anotomen Indagatis* (On the Seats and Causes of Disease Investigated by Anatomy), often regarded as the first textbook of pathology. His observations established the link between pathological findings and clinical diagnosis, thus confirming the autopsy as a significant tool in medical investigation.

18th century

In addition to Morgagni, notable figures of the 18th century included Percivall Pott (1714–1788), who carried out an autopsy in England on the instructions of a coroner and Xavier-Bichet (1771–1802). Dubbed the 'Father of Histology', Xavier-Bichet focused on the tissues, rather than the organs themselves as the key to understanding disease. He may also have been one of the first to contract tuberculosis from a postmortem examination, dying of the disease at the age of only 30, thus unwittingly highlighting the Health and Safety aspects of mortuary practice. The growing interest in anatomy and dissection also gave rise to the so-called 'resurrectionists' who supplied corpses for dissection—the most famous being Burke (1792–1829) and Hare (1792–1870) in Edinburgh.

19th century

By the 19th century, the intellectual home of the autopsy had shifted north to Vienna. Karl Rokitansky (1804–1878) headed the Pathology Institute and is reported to have carried out in excess of 30 000 autopsies. He emphasized the need to carry out the same systematic examination in all cases, although his reluctance to use the microscope limited his scientific advancements. In Berlin, Rudolph Virchow (1821–1902) proposed that cellular pathology was the basis of disease and finally disproved the humoural theory of Hippocrates and Galen.

20th century

Doctors and medical students from around the world studied at Berlin, including one of the most notable of North American physicians William Osler (1849–1919). In 1905, he was appointed to the Regius Chair of Medicine at Oxford where he maintained a keen interest in observing and even carrying out postmortem dissection, telling his friend, Archibald Mallock: 'I've been watching this case for 2 months and I'm sorry I shall not see the postmortem'. The case was Osler himself.

The 19th century was perhaps the zenith of the autopsy as a medical research tool. In the 20th century, the clinical or hospital autopsy rate declined. It is probable that the decline is as much due to individual doctor's and more generally, the medical profession's changing perception of the role and value of the autopsy as it is to the scandals and controversy associated with, for example, the Alder Hey Children's Hospital. Recent research has tended to indicate that relatives *are* willing to consent to organ retention and research—the important factors appear to be that they are made aware of the reasons for the donation, the uses of the tissue, and the potential benefits of the research.[1]

More recently, within the forensic field, doctors and medical scientists are beginning to question the assumption that an autopsy is indeed, the 'gold standard' postmortem examination.

Reference

1 Millar T, Walker R, Arango J-C, *et al*. (2007). Tissue and organ donation for research in forensic pathology: the MRC Sudden Death Brain and Tissue Bank. *J Pathol* **213**:369–75.

Forensic or medicolegal autopsy

Autopsy or not?

Whether or not an autopsy is carried out on a body referred (in the UK) to the coroner/procurator fiscal (PF) is a decision made by the legal authority. In England and Wales, the coroner may request a home office pathologist to perform an autopsy in some suspicious deaths. In Scotland, the PF will also decide whether this should be a single or 'double-doctor' autopsy in accordance with the (legal) evidential requirements for corroboration. The second pathologist may be a specialist in a particular area (e.g. a paediatric pathologist).

Family consent

Once the coroner has ordered an autopsy, it is important to note that the consent of the family or relatives of the deceased is not required. In certain circumstances—usually when the death is not suspicious—the wishes of the family (particularly with regard to religious beliefs and practices) will be taken into account, although the thoroughness of the investigation should never be compromised.

Medicolegal autopsy

The purpose of the medicolegal autopsy is to investigate the manner of death. 'Medicolegal autopsies' may be divided into two types: those which investigate apparently non-criminal deaths and those ('forensic autopsies') which investigate suspicious or frankly criminal deaths.

Autopsies for apparently non-criminal deaths

This category includes deaths which appear to have resulted from accidents, suicides, and sudden deaths from natural causes. Many of these autopsies will be performed by 'general pathologists', others by forensic pathologists (depending upon local protocols and resources).

Forensic autopsies

These are performed by forensic pathologists on suspicious or frankly criminal deaths. The forensic autopsy is not a training or research tool and appropriate consent (or at least, advice) should be obtained from the relevant legal authority prior to embarking on any such activities.

Clinical autopsy

The clinical autopsy is primarily a treatment or diagnostic audit. It is a useful way of determining whether the clinical team's understanding of the disease and/or treatment process was correct—this, when used effectively, contributes to improved standards of care for patients presenting under similar circumstances. Other roles of the clinical autopsy include teaching and/or training, audit of death certification, and research. Relatives may give consent for a limited autopsy (e.g. leaving the head intact, with no removal of the brain).

The clinical (or 'hospital') autopsy requires:
- The consent of the deceased's family, and
- That the medical cause of the death is known, sufficient for a death certificate to be issued.

On no account should any doctor use the threat of referring a case to the coroner/PF as a way of obtaining consent to carry out a clinical autopsy.

If, during a hospital autopsy, there is any evidence of suspicious circumstances, the procedure should be halted immediately and the death referred to the legal authority.

Forensic autopsy procedure: summary

Developing a routine
All forensic autopsies follow the same procedure, which should be derived both from national guidelines and local practice. The basic outline of the procedure is:
- Examination of the scene of death where appropriate.
- Examination of clothing and property.
- Eliciting the history of the case.
- Identification of the body (to ensure that the body is that for which the pathologist has authorization to do an autopsy).
- X-ray examination, where indicated by the circumstances (e.g. gunshot injuries, fires, explosions, deaths of children).
- External examination.
- Internal dissection.
- Collection of routine tissue samples for histology.
- Collection of routine samples for toxicology.
- Forensic photography.
- Return of all tissues (with the exception of the above) to the body.
- Restoration of the body and preparation for collection by undertaker (usually the role of the anatomical pathology technologist).
- Recording of all findings (in writing or dictated and preferably *during* or *immediately* afterwards—on no account should writing up autopsy findings be left until after a number of cases have been completed).
- Statement of the cause of death (and comment as to the manner of death if required).
- Report of the examination (usually prepared by secretarial or administrative staff from recorded tapes or notes—it is essential that the report is carefully read and checked prior to being signed).

Guidelines
Adherence to Royal College of Pathologists' and local guidelines (such as the use of standardized autopsy report protocols and Standard Operating Procedures) is important. Note that the autopsy is not merely intended to ascertain *a* possible cause of death but, rather, to determine *the* cause of death. The investigation should, therefore be comprehensive, standardized (according to regulatory, local, and personal practice), and thorough.

Examination of internal organs
When examining internal organs consider:
- Weight, size, and shape (note that organ weights can vary significantly).
- Colour.
- Consistency (of external surface and internal cut surfaces).
- Lesions.

Although the macroscopic examination is important (and in many cases is sufficient to establish a cause of death), histology can reveal abnormalities not apparent during naked-eye observation.

Attitude and approach

The autopsy should be performed with appropriate dignity and respect for the deceased and on no account should unnecessary invasive or destructive procedures be carried out.

Although there is no single 'correct' way of doing an autopsy there may be several wrong ones. A pathologist should always be prepared to defend his or her chosen technique or method to colleagues and, ultimately, to the criminal justice system.

It is appropriate to be prepared to adapt a technique to the circumstances of the case, but a suspicious death is unlikely to be the right occasion to 'try out' a technique for the first time.

The autopsy report

Outline contents

The autopsy report should include the following information:

- Legal authority for the autopsy.
- Name and identifying details of the deceased.
- Name, appointment, and qualifications of the pathologist(s).
- Date of the examination.
- Place of the examination.
- External examination.
- Internal dissection (evidence of natural disease and injuries).
- List of all samples taken for histology (or 'routine samples').
- Toxicology samples taken.
- Any other tissues or organs retained (e.g. brain for preservation and later examination).
- Statement of the cause of death.
- Opinion as to the manner of death.
- Commentary/summary (which should justify conclusions and explain why alternative explanations were dismissed).

Details not required

It is not usually necessary to include a comprehensive description of the circumstances of the death, as this information is present in the police report. Similarly, a detailed medical history is not required, as this is available in the deceased's medical notes. However, the pathologist should comment on recent medical intervention, particularly if this arises from or contributes to, the event causing death.

Body diagrams

Body diagrams can be very useful and should be used in conjunction with the report to illustrate injuries and wounds, etc.

Negative findings

The autopsy report should include negative findings. It can then be assumed that the lack of a comment implies it was not specifically examined—this can be useful when referring to a report months or years later. It is helpful to use the term 'unremarkable' to describe a negative finding and limit use of the word 'normal' to those situations where there is a defined, standard, and objective state (e.g. the tricuspid valve having three flaps), which does not change with age. It is worth remembering that what is normal for a 19-year-old is not necessarily so for an 89-year-old.

Relatives

The autopsy report is a medical document and should not be shown to relatives, but it may be appropriate for the pathologist to speak to relatives about autopsy findings. The commentary section may be written in language which can be understood by non-medical people (e.g. lawyers and scientists), although it should retain detail and medical accuracy.

External examination

Prior to any incisions being made in the body, the pathologist should carry out a thorough external examination. The body must be turned over to permit an inspection of all aspects.

The following should be observed and noted

- Clothing, jewellery, etc. (if present in non-suspicious cases, these are often removed prior to the examination).
- Body length and weight (recorded in metric, but with an awareness of imperial conversions).
- Ethnic group.
- Skin pigmentation.
- State of decomposition.
- Rigor mortis (neck, extremities—the extent of refrigeration should also be noted).
- Livor mortis (see ☐ p.32).
- Congestion and oedema.
- Eyes (papillary size and symmetry have limited value at postmortem time).
- Teeth and gums.
- Ears.
- Fingernails.
- Genitalia.
- Breasts.
- Body hair.
- Hair.
- Tattoos and other deliberately inflicted markings.
- Personal hygiene and apparent nutritional state.
- Evidence of old injury (scars, including surgical interventions).
- Evidence of recent injury (bruises can be examined with localized incisions, if required).
- Marks of medical intervention.
- Needle puncture sites (old and recent, evidence of intravenous drug use).
- Presence of insects and trace evidence (e.g. glass, fibres, soil)—these should be collected by an appropriate expert or in accordance with guidelines. The pathologist should advise the senior investigating officer (SIO) if he/she requires the assistance of an appropriate specialist (such as an entomologist) and make a record of this in his/her notes.
- Other obvious features or characteristics of the body irrespective of whether these are related to the apparent cause of death (e.g. amputations, pugilistic posture in fire deaths).
- All injuries and marks of trauma need to be recorded (and photographed).

Forensic autopsy: evisceration

The evisceration of the body may be carried out by a technician or the pathologist. If carried out by an anatomical pathology technologist, the pathologist should be available to observe and comment on anything unusual or potentially significant (e.g. bruising under the skin in the neck area). Care must be taken not to mistake artefacts of evisceration as internal injuries—experience is an invaluable guide in this respect.

Procedure

Usually, a 'Y'-shaped incision (from the pubic bone to just below the suprasternal notch of the sternum and branching out to the shoulders) is made, enabling the skin to be reflected laterally. Using either bone-shears or a saw, the rib cage is cut, thereby enabling access to the internal organs. The ribs should be examined at this stage for any evidence of fractures (which may be a result of medical or bystander resuscitation or other trauma).

In addition to being an effective method of gaining access to the internal organs, the 'Y'-shaped incision is preferable to a straight incision, as it is less visible after the autopsy. This is a significant factor for the relatives of the deceased who may wish to view the body—ideally, there should be no signs that an autopsy has been carried out once a body has been prepared for presentation by an undertaker.

Approach to internal organs

Rokitansky's method indicates examination of the internal organs *in situ*. Techniques exist for the removal of all the organs en masse (following Letulle) or en bloc (following Ghon—four separate 'plucks': thoracic, coeliac, intestinal, and urogenital). Virchow's technique removes the organs individually. All techniques can be adapted according to the circumstances of the case and the personal preference of the pathologist.

Organs should be placed on a dissection block, which is either taken to a designated area or rests on the deceased's legs. It is important to ensure that there is an adequate water supply nearby.

The scalp is incised coronally, the flaps being reflected forwards and backwards. The skull is opened using an oscillating saw, usually by a technician under the supervision of a pathologist. Guidelines recommend that the pathologist removes the brain itself, although technologists often do this in non-suspicious cases. The interior of the skull should be examined by the pathologist.

Dissection: cardiovascular system

The forensic autopsy should examine and report the following (this is not an exhaustive list):

- Heart (weight—emptied of clot): including a comment on shape and size.
- Pericardial sac: quantity and colour of fluid.
- Atria: noting the presence of any thrombus.
- Right ventricle: noting the configuration and thickness and any evidence of old or recent ischaemic changes.
- Left ventricle: noting configuration and thickness and any evidence of old or recent ischaemic changes.
- Valves: noting configuration and any abnormality.
- Coronary arteries: noting their distribution and whether there is dominance of the left or right side. The extent of atheroma and presence of thrombus in individual arteries should be recorded.
- Aorta: recording the extent of any atheroma and/or thrombus.
- Carotid arteries: noting the extent of any atheroma and/or thrombus.
- Venae cavae: including the extent of any thrombus.
- Renal arteries: noting the extent of any atheroma and/or thrombus.
- Pulmonary vessels: noting in particular any thrombo-emboli.
- Other vessels: recording the extent of any atheroma and/or thrombus.
- Mediastinum: noting any abnormalities.

Limitations

The autopsy is unable to detect non-morphological causes of death, such as conduction system abnormalities (long QT syndrome, Brugada syndrome) or idiopathic ventricular fibrillation.

Myocardial infarction only becomes apparent macroscopically if the individual survives for > 24h afterwards, but microscopic changes of coagulative necrosis with inflammatory inflitrates and contraction bands may be apparent at 12h.

Dissection of the heart

There are several techniques for dissecting the heart. One of the usual methods (Prausnitz, following Virchow) dissects following the blood flow from the venae cavae to the aorta in the following sequence:

- Venae cavae
- Lateral margin of the right ventricle
- Pulmonary cone
- Pulmonary artery
- Left atrial veins
- Left atrium
- Left ventricular margin
- Aorta.

The technique itself is less important than the pathologist's ability to recognize significant morphological change (taking histology samples where necessary and/or required by a standard protocol). Coronary arteries should be sectioned at 3-mm intervals to assess the degree of atherosclerosis (opening the vessels longitudinally using scissors should be avoided as it becomes difficult to quantify any occlusion of the lumen). The whole heart should be sliced at 10-mm intervals parallel to the atrioventricular groove. Other structures (e.g. valves) can then easily be examined.

Assessment of coronary artery atheroma

It is difficult to make a precise assessment of the degree of occlusion to a coronary artery. Multiple transverse cuts along the arteries may indicate the minimum luminal diameter. It is worth considering using a chart to assess the cross-section of the artery.[1] For reporting purposes, an estimate of the percentage occlusion ('approximately 30%', '>70%') and a subjective description ('moderate', 'severe') is usually sufficient.

Categorization of sudden cardiac deaths[2]

1 Coronary atheroma and clear evidence of coronary thombosis and/ or acute myocardial infarction: very high probability of causing sudden death.

2 Coronary atheroma with at least one coronary artery <1mm diameter and evidence of old myocardial infarction: moderate to high probability of causing sudden death.

3 Coronary atheroma with at least one coronary artery <1mm diameter, but no evidence of old myocardial infarction: questionable probability of causing sudden death—depends on circumstances of death.

4 No evidence of ischaemic heart disease but evidence of congestive cardiac failure or significant left or right ventricular hypertrophy and/or dilation: moderate probability of causing sudden death (cardiomyopathy must be excluded).

5 No significant cardiac pathology/unexplained sudden cardiac death (sudden arrhythmic death syndrome, SADS): histology and toxicology essential if SADS is to be considered.

If there is a diagnosis of cardiomyopathy or SADS, the family should be referred family to an appropriate support group (e.g. The Sudden Adult Death Trust, ℘ http://www.sadsuk.org).

References

1 Champ CS and Coghill SB (1989). Visual aid for quick assessment of coronary artery stenosis at necropsy. *J Clin Pathol* **42**:887–8.

2 Davies MJ (1999). The investigation of sudden cardiac death. *Histopathology* **34**:93–8.

Dissection: respiratory system

The forensic autopsy should examine and report the following:

- Soft tissues of the neck: layer by layer dissection of the musculature, noting any bruising and/or damage to the thyroid.
- Hyoid and laryngeal cartilages: a fractured hyoid is associated with, but is not diagnostic of, deliberate neck trauma (e.g. strangulation). However, it can be damaged postmortem by careless handling.
- Larynx, trachea, and main bronchi: the presence of soot and products of combustion in a fire-related death is evidence that the person was alive and breathing at the time the fire started. Histology may also assist with this (see 'Fire deaths' later in this section).
- Pleural cavities: checking for adhesions and/or free fluid.
- Lungs (right and left weights): macroscopic findings are not always easy to interpret, but abnormalities and areas of bruising, infection, or infarction should be noted.
- Hilar lymph nodes.

Bronchopneumonia

This may be indicated by expressing pus from the lungs, but infection should be confirmed histologically. A focus on general pathological diagnosis rather than organism-specific diagnoses is a potential obstacle in improving public health monitoring of new and emerging infectious disease. Although organism-specific diagnostic testing is available, it is infrequently used, primarily because of contamination, cost, and in the forensic context, infection is caused by multiple organisms in an individual with increased susceptibility (as a result of aspiration or viral infection).

Pneumothorax

This should be considered prior to any incision. A simple test for a pneumothorax is to reflect laterally the chest skin and subcutaneous fat to form a 'bowl' which can be filled with water. Puncturing the intercostal space allows any air to escape—seen as bubbles in the water.

Drowning

Histological examination may reveal emphysema aquosum, interstitial congestion, and alveolar haemorrhage. Examination for diatoms may help.

Fire deaths

Histological analysis can help to determine if an individual died before or after a fire started: necrosis of bronchial epithelium and/or soot in the bronchial tree or alveoli indicate that the person was alive during the fire.

Dissection: endocrine system

The forensic autopsy should examine and report on the following:
• Parathyroids and thyroid
• Adrenals
• Pituitary.

Dissection: digestive system

The forensic autopsy should examine and report on the following:
• Tongue: note the classical sign of a bitten tongue.
• Mouth, tonsils, pharynx, oesophagus.
• Peritoneal cavity: noting the quantity/nature of fluid and the presence of adhesions.
• Stomach and its contents: noting residues or remains of tablets, foreign bodies, or other non-foodstuffs. A sample of stomach contents should be taken for toxicology in suspected poisoning.
• Duodenum and small intestine, large intestine, appendix, and rectum—together with contents of the bowel.
• Liver (weight): although liver damage as a result of an overdose of paracetamol, alcohol, or other drugs should be confirmed histologically (and with toxicological analysis), macroscopic examination of the liver is quite a good indicator of abnormality. Frequent findings include 'fatty' liver (related to alcohol), chronic passive congestion ('nutmeg' as it resembles the cut surface of a nutmeg), and cirrhosis.
• Gall bladder and bile ducts.
• Pancreas: this is often the first organ to autolyse.

Drug packages

If there is a raised index of suspicion, the digestive system should be thoroughly checked for drug packages and 'body-packing'. This is not routinely performed in all forensic autopsies.

Dissection: lymphatic system

The forensic autopsy should examine and report the following:
- Spleen (weight): external and sectioned.
- Cervical lymph nodes, mediastinal lymph nodes, mesenteric lymph nodes, para-aortic lymph nodes, and peripheral lymph nodes.
- Thymus: usually not recognizable.
- Vertebral bone marrow: rarely examined.

Dissection: musculoskeletal system

The forensic autopsy should examine and report the following:
- Spinal column: looking for fractures.
- Limb girdles: looking for fractures.
- Long-limb bones: searching for fractures externally or on palpation.
- Hands and feet: look for fractures externally or on palpation.
- Ribs/sternum: looking for fractures (prior to evisceration).
- General condition of skeleton: stating the condition for age.
- Muscles: only noted where exposed during routine dissection.

Dissection: cranium and nervous system

The forensic autopsy should examine and report on the following:
- Scalp: looking for obvious injury (but distinguishing and noting postmortem artefacts).
- Skull: searching for fractures and paying careful attention during the removal of the brain (it is important that an anatomical pathology technician is trained in this area).
- Middle ears and air sinuses: usually not opened.
- Meninges: looking for extradural (epidural), subdural, or subarachnoid haemorrhages.
- Cranial vessels: commenting on anatomical distribution, evidence of atheroma, and any apparent aneurysmal dilatation.
- Brain (weight): looking for haemorrhage, contusions, uncal or tonsillar herniation. Serial coronal sections of the cerebral hemispheres are made at 1-cm intervals. The cerebellum and brainstem need to be carefully examined.
- Spinal cord: not examined, unless there is a specific indication.
- Peripheral nerves: noted where exposed during routine dissection.

The brain

Approach

This is an area of potential controversy. It is usual in medicolegal cases to dissect the brain fresh (although non-forensic textbooks will often advise strongly against this). However, when indicated or as part of a local protocol, consider retaining the brain for preservation and later examination by a neuropathologist.

Fixation

The brain is usually fixed whole in formalin solution for 4 weeks. Subsequent histology is tailored to the individual circumstances. In the context of head (brain) injury, beta-amyloid precursor protein antibody is in widely used to indicate axonal injury.

Dissection: genitourinary system

The forensic autopsy should examine and report on the following:
- Kidneys (right and left weights): strip the capsules. Comment on the cortical ribbon, the corticomedullary junction, medulla, and the collecting system.
- Ureters and bladder: recording the amount of urine in the latter and collecting a sample for toxicological analysis.
- Internal genitalia and gonads.
- External genitalia: tattoos and piercings can be important aids to identification.

If the deceased is female, evidence relating to pregnancy should be documented.

Autopsy samples: legal issues

History

Following the adverse publicity relating to the activities of the pathologist van Velzen at Alder Hey Children's Hospital in Liverpool and similar incidents at other hospitals, including Bristol Royal Infirmary and Birmingham Children's Hospital, legislation was introduced to govern the retention and use of material obtained at postmortem examination.

Legislation

Although relatives' consent is not required for a coroner's autopsy (or PF in Scotland), the scope of what is permitted is limited by legislation. Guidance is published by the Human Tissue Authority.

England and Wales

In England and Wales, the pathologist can take tissue samples which are deemed necessary to establish the cause of death, or to carry out any other investigation as instructed by the coroner. On completion of these investigations, it is not lawful to retain the tissue without consent.

The family of the deceased are able to:
- Ask for the tissue to be disposed of; or
- Ask for the tissue to be returned to them; or
- Consent to further use of the tissue.

Scotland

In Scotland, the pathologist is also able to take tissue samples as deemed necessary to establish cause of death or to carry out other investigations as instructed by the PF. On completion of these investigations, tissue samples are retained as part of the medical record.

Tissues retained for research and other purposes

Tissues required for research, audit, teaching, or other purpose require authorization (Scotland) or consent (England and Wales). Consent must be informed and can be withdrawn at any time.

Although an investigation requiring retention of some human tissue might seem perfectly reasonable and justified to the detached scientific mind of a pathologist, this does not mean it is justified in terms of the legislation (nor indeed, from the bereaved relatives' perspective). If there is doubt about the legality of a proposed action, it is imperative to contact the appropriate legal authority and seek guidance. In Edinburgh, the Medical Research Council Sudden Death Brain and Tissue Bank retains brain and other tissue for research purposes—research use of tissue samples was authorized by 96% of bereaved relatives (ℬ http://www.edinburghbrainbanks.ed.ac.uk).

Further reading

The Human Tissue Act 2004; The Human Tissue (Scotland) Act 2006. Available at ℬ http://www.hta.gov.uk
The Report of the Royal Liverpool Children's Inquiry (Redfern Report, 2001). London: The Stationery Office. Available at ℬ http://www.rlcinquiry.org.uk

Autopsy samples: histology and toxicology

Bearing in mind the legal aspects (see 📖 p.86), samples for histology and toxicology can be taken during an autopsy if they are necessary for the determination of the cause of death or other postmortem investigation instructed by the appropriate legal authority.

Histology

A standardized range of tissue samples should be taken according to local protocol and embedded in paraffin blocks. It is necessary to decide what samples to section and stain depending upon the circumstances of the case. It is unlikely that all samples will be examined histologically in all cases as this is not scientifically justified and it is expensive and time-consuming. Histology should always be carried out in cases in which the macroscopic examination is not diagnostic of the cause of death and there is no other apparent cause (e.g. toxicology is negative).

Where relevant, samples taken from right and left organs should be cut differently to enable later identification and it is sensible to place them in separate containers. The autopsy report should always state what samples were collected (or refer to 'routine samples' if these are listed elsewhere). It may be worth considering referring 'difficult cases' to a colleague with relevant expertise in histopathology.

Toxicology

Routine collection of forensic samples should be considered during all forensic autopsies:
- Blood (from a peripheral vein)
- Urine (if present).

Other samples (vitreous humour, liver, stomach contents, hair, etc.) should be taken according to the circumstances of the death. Samples not required can easily be disposed of. There is no justification for not taking samples only to realize at a later date that they are required to determine a cause of death.

Forensic toxicology samples are considered in detail on 📖 p.456.

The paediatric forensic autopsy

Overview
The procedure for a forensic autopsy involving a child should be regarded as essentially the same as that for an adult. The purpose is to ascertain the cause of death and if relevant, provide a comprehensive statement of the findings for possible use as evidence in subsequent legal proceedings.

Special considerations
- A paediatric forensic autopsy should always be carried out by a forensic pathologist and a paediatric pathologist or if circumstances necessitate otherwise, by those with experience of and expertise in paediatric cases.
- Although deaths of children due to non-accidental injury are rare, it is wise to maintain a high index of suspicion when carrying out the examination. This should never be considered a justification to make unfounded allegations against individuals.
- The importance of a comprehensive and methodical approach cannot be overstated and all findings at autopsy should be carefully evaluated in the light of all the available evidence.
- In a case of sudden unexpected death in infancy (SUDI, SIDS) the autopsy will *by definition* not determine the cause of death. In order to make such a diagnosis of exclusion, it is imperative that all feasible investigative routes are followed.
- Body weights and lengths should be compared against standard published (centile) charts published for boys and girls.
- X-rays in the form of a skeletal survey may be appropriate in the detection of occult fractures resulting from child abuse and may play a role in helping to provide an opinion as to whether a newborn baby was a live birth or stillbirth. This works on the principle that in the case of the former, there will be evidence of gas within the lungs, gastrointestinal tract, and body cavities.
- There may be special microbiological considerations, involving swabs for culture from the middle ears and cerebrospinal fluid.
- The possibility of unusual, undiagnosed metabolic disorders may be investigated by a variety of tests on body fluids and tissues.

Exhumation

Definition

Exhumation is the legal removal of a body from the grave. It needs to be distinguished from unauthorized removal of a body (which can occur for a variety of reasons, including theft of items buried alongside the body). The term is usually not applied to the excavation of a mass grave.

Purposes

There are occasions when a grave may be opened and the body removed in order to rebury it elsewhere, or at the request of family (perhaps to retrieve a particular item). However, the term is most linked with the need to examine the remains in a search for new information. This may include one or more of the following:

- Ascertaining the identity of the person buried.
- Trying to confirm/establish the cause of death.
- A search for other forensic evidence.

Sometimes exhumation is performed if results of a previous autopsy are questioned and/or if a new suspicion arises about possible foul play (e.g. there is a suspicion that someone may have been poisoned).

Prior considerations

The most important prior consideration is to ensure that there is appropriate legal authority to proceed with the exhumation. Having gained appropriate authority/consent, the following information needs to be established:

- The exact location of the body. This should be identified with certainty (in order to be absolutely certain that the correct grave is opened).
- The nature of the casket used. Caskets are made of a variety of materials (e.g. wood, metal, plastic).
- Whether the body was embalmed and if so, what was used for this (see 'Embalming' section).

Embalming

Embalming aims to prevent natural decay, preventing infection, thereby protecting those who work with/handle the body. Embalming also makes the body much more presentable for the family to view. Arsenic was used traditionally as an embalming agent, subsequently replaced by formaldehyde and more recently by modern combinations of chemicals.

Exhumation process—key features

- The procedure must be carefully documented.
- Soil samples should be taken from the earth above/around the casket and retained for potential toxicological analysis.
- The remains may be removed for careful analysis.
- Identification of the body may use one or more of: fingerprints, dental record comparisons, DNA, and X-rays.
- Photographs may be taken, as appropriate.

Mass graves and war crimes

Approach

From a medical and scientific perspective, carrying out autopsies on suspected victims of war crimes and individuals located in mass graves is no different from performing medicolegal autopsies on any other deceased person. The function of the autopsy is to provide evidence for the purposes of identification, determining the cause of death, and, potentially, for use in any subsequent criminal proceedings. There are numerous war zones and areas of conflict in the world, a proportion of which arouse concerns relating to possible war crimes. The investigation of suspected war crimes is associated with significant challenges.

Logistical issues

The difficulties are more likely to arise from the logistics of the situation:
- Inadequate mortuary facilities (water, electricity, storage, ventilation).
- Availability of appropriately trained staff.
- Health and safety issues.
- Security concerns.
- Increased infectious agents and other hazards.
- Limited information technology/recording/reporting and administrative support.

Safety

On no account should a pathologist (or other expert working in the field) proceed until they are satisfied that the working environment is safe and conducive to appropriate professional standards of investigation. In addition, it needs to be emphasized that all staff (including professionals present for specific roles and local workers) must be informed about and adhere to the strictest and highest code of scientific ethics.

Team approach

Team work is just as crucial in the investigation of a mass grave in a conflict-country as it is in a murder investigation in the UK. However, as experienced and trained staff are less likely to be available, it is important that the professional experts facilitate and support a disciplined, integrated team approach. Evidence recovered from excavations needs to be considered within the context of all of the available information.

Health and safety issues

Mortuary hazards

The mortuary environment contains several hazards which can be grouped by type: biological (infectious agents), chemical (formalin, cyanide and organophosphates), radiation (radionuclides, implants), and 'industrial'. Workplace risks are controlled according to the ALARP principle ('as low as reasonably practicable', originating in the *Health and Safety at Work Act* 1974)—all personnel who enter a mortuary or autopsy suite should be familiar with the implications of this. The Royal College of Pathologists' guidelines make it clear that the forensic pathologist has a duty to inform the legal authority or the police if the mortuary provision is deemed inadequate or unsuitable.

'Industrial' type hazards include:

- Electricity
- Water
- Manual handling (e.g. bodies >100kg), weights, and associated machinery
- Sharp implements (scalpels, saws, etc.).

Risk reduction in the mortuary

All risks associated with the mortuary and autopsies can be substantially mitigated by proper and appropriate

- Assessment
- Personal protective equipment
- Autopsy procedures
- Facility design
- Equipment
- Standard operating procedures (SOPs)
- Implementation of legislation, regulations, and guidelines
- Safe working practices by all personnel.

Viewing facilities

Adequate viewing facilities for training purposes and to facilitate police and legal observers if and when required. In addition to providing a facility for the benefit of those who need to attend, a viewing gallery has the effect of taking non-key personnel out of the high-risk areas.

Definitions

- A *hazard* is something (e.g. an object or event) which has the potential to cause an adverse effect.
- A *risk* is the likelihood of that happening *and* a measure of the effect.

High-risk autopsy

Definition

The 'high-risk' autopsy may be defined as a postmortem examination of a deceased individual who has had, or is likely to have had, a serious infectious disease that has the potential to be transmitted to those present at the autopsy, thereby causing serious illness and/or death.

Identification of high-risk individuals

Cases considered to be 'high risk' include those involving:

- Individuals who have previously been tested positive for HIV and/or hepatitis.
- Individuals known to be intravenous drug users.
- Individuals known to have a perceived 'high-risk' life style—as well as intravenous drug users, this includes those with unprotected sexual contacts (both homosexual and heterosexual) and/or a history of travel to (and particularly living and working in) areas of the world acknowledged to have a high prevalence of HIV (e.g. many parts of Africa).

No body can be assumed to be 'no risk'

It is worth stating that unless every deceased person is tested and found to be negative, it must never be assumed that a body is not 'high risk'. Individuals who come to autopsy have higher rates of HIV and hepatitis than in the general population. Appropriate care and attention to safe working practices must always be a priority.

Risk reduction

The principal way to try to reduce the risk in a high-risk autopsy is to limit the personnel present in the autopsy suite to the absolute minimum required for legal and health and safety purposes (e.g. two pathologists if needed for the purposes of corroboration).

The 'high-risk' autopsy is not appropriate for use as a teaching/training autopsy and trainees (and others) are usually excluded from the autopsy suite.

Infection risks of autopsy

There are five routes to acquire infection in a mortuary:
- Percutaneous inoculation
- Inhalation
- Ingestion
- Skin contamination (in the absence of inoculation)
- Contamination of mucosal surfaces.

Blood-borne viruses and inhaled virulent pathogens are the main concerns. The Advisory Committee on Dangerous Pathogens (ℬ http://www.dh.gov. uk/ab/ACDP) categorizes infectious agents into four hazard groups.

Blood-borne agents are usually easier to control, because transmission requires an adverse event. These can be minimized by adopting safe working practices and adhering to agreed SOPs. Pathologists and other mortuary staff should take particular care when working in unfamiliar mortuaries with different SOPs. The splash risk remains localized.

Unless a self-contained breathing apparatus is worn (similar to a SCUBA unit), the risk of exposure to inhaled agents is ever-present. The risk from aerosol may be minimized by avoiding splash and where possible, by reducing dissection.

Hazard group 4
- Viral haemorrhagic fevers (e.g. Ebola, Lassa, Marburg, Congo–Crimean)—there is no natural reservoir or vector in the UK, but there is a risk of imported infection)—no autopsy should be carried out.
- Dengue—high-risk autopsy.
- Yellow fever—high-risk autopsy.
- Hendra and Nipah virus—an autopsy on a person suspected or known to have died from these conditions is an unwarranted risk and should not be done (in suspicious cases, advice should be obtained from the legal authority and medical specialists).
- Falciparum malaria—standard autopsy conditions.
- Leptospirosis—standard autopsy conditions.

Hazard group 3
HIV-1 and HIV-2
- Low infection risk.
- Sharps injuries should be avoided by safe working practices and wearing cut-resistant gloves (e.g. chain mail).
- Viable infection is known to survive for >2 weeks, so delaying an autopsy for a few days is not justified.
- It is not essential to use a separate 'high-risk' autopsy facility.
- There is a documented case of autopsy-acquired infection.[1]

Hepatitis B/C virus (HBV, HCV)
- Barrier protection to avoid sharps injuries.

Tuberculosis (TB)
- There are documented cases of pathologists contracting TB during autopsy (occupation risk to autopsy staff is approximately 100–200× that of the general public).
- Risk from aerosol—use recycling HEPA (high efficiency particulate air) filters and respirator hoods.
- Ventilation—downdraft tables help to keep aerosol away from the face.
- The risk is difficult to control—lungs can be perfused with 10% formalin before dissection, but this is not practical in most cases.

TB of the skin (tuberculosis verrucosa cutis) is a rare disease first described by Laennec. It has been called 'prosector's wart', as the lesions were often acquired in the autopsy suite, including the 'Father of modern medical education', Sir William Osler (1849–1919).

Creutzfeldt–Jakob disease (CJD)
- Low infection risk.

Hazard group 2
As the primary method of infection of the Hazard group 2 agents is by hand-to-mouth, standard hygiene procedures will minimize spread. Hazard group 2 agents have greater significance in a clinical setting.

Pathologists and all other personnel who may be required to attend an autopsy should be familiar with guidelines published by the Royal College of Pathologists: ℘ http://www.rcpath.org/resources/pdf/main_document.pdf

Although these guidelines refer to 'known' or 'suspected' cases, this does not mean that apparent 'low-risk' cadavers are free from infections. To minimize the hazard and risk it is imperative that all staff remain vigilant at all times and adhere to accepted SOPs and safe working practice.

Reference
1 Johnson MD, Schaffner W, Atkinson J, et al. (1997). Autopsy risk and acquisition of human immunodeficiency virus infection: a case report and reappraisal. Arch Pathol Lab Med **121**:64–6.

Further reading
The Royal College of Pathologists (2002). Guidelines on Autopsy Practice. Report of a working group of The Royal College of Pathologists. London: The Royal College of Pathologists.
—Appendix 1: Hazard Group 3 pathogens. ℘ http://www.rcpath.org/resources/pdf/appendix_1.pdf
—Appendix 2: Guidelines of assessing presence of Hazard Group 4 pathogens in a cadaver. ℘ http://www.rcpath.org/resources/pdf/appendix_2.pdf
—Appendix 3: Protocols for performing postmortem examinations on known or suspect 'high-risk' infected cadavers: Hazard Group 3 infections HIV, hepatitis C, tuberculosis, Creutzfeldt–Jakob disease. ℘ http://www.rcpath.org/resources/pdf/appendix_3.pdf
The Royal College of Pathologists (2009). Advice for pathologists and anatomical pathology technologists for autopsy of cadavers with known or suspected new/virulent strains of influenza A, 2nd edn. London: The Royal College of Pathologists.

Death certification

The death certificate should be a comprehensive, yet concise statement of the medical cause of death. The certificate is signed to the 'best of my knowledge and belief' and is not a legally binding document. The stated cause of death can be amended and challenged in a court.

Format of the death certificate

Part I

Ia   The immediate cause of death
(due to or as a consequence of)
Ib,c,d   The underlying cause of death

Part II

Other significant conditions contributing to the death but not relating to the disease or condition causing it.

In deaths due to external causes (i.e. non-natural deaths), the sequence might be:

Ia Intra-abdominal haemorrhage (i.e. fatally disrupted normal physiology).
Ib Transection of the aorta *(i.e. the primary injury)*.
Ic Stab wound to the abdomen *(i.e. the external event)*.

Note that speculation about, or over-confidence in, a specific immediate cause is unnecessary and potentially confusing. The option of choice is sometimes simply:

Ia Multiple injuries

There is some controversy about the use of probabilistic terms or, at the extreme of uncertainty, undetermined causes of death:

Ia Unascertained, presumed natural

On no account should this be interpreted as implying a lack of skill on the part of the medical examiner—indeed, there are circumstances, in which this is the most precise (and certainly the most honest) death certificate which can be written. It should not be used when it is difficult to choose between several possible causes of death, but limited to those circumstances in which no definite cause can be ascribed.

Causes of death which are reached by exclusion include SIDS (but not SUDI) and, arguably, drowning. Whereas SIDS is *by definition* associated with no known cause (indeed, if a cause is found at autopsy or other investigation then the death is not a SIDS death), drowning has a known cause, but there is often no evidence for this at autopsy (the presence of diatoms remains controversial).

Advice on completing death certificates

- The words 'suicide' (and words which imply that a death was deliberately self-inflicted) and 'accident' should be avoided. The death certificate is not intended to be a statement of the manner of death. So, for example, it is appropriate to write 'motor vehicle collision', but not 'road traffic accident'.
- Descriptions of terminal mechanistic events such as 'cardiac arrest' or 'respiratory arrest' should be avoided. These are prima facie evident and reveal nothing about what caused death.

The need for referral of deaths to a coroner or PF is considered on 📖 p.40 and p.44.

Further reading

Further information relating to death certification can be found at: Office for National Statistics (𝄞 http://www.ons.gov.uk)

General Register Office for Scotland (𝄞 http://www.gro-scotland.gov.uk)

It is noted that the Office for National Statistics and the General Register Office both publish comprehensive annual reports relating to mortality in England & Wales and Scotland respectively. All deaths are coded to ICD10 and include natural and unnatural (accident, suicide and homicide) deaths—so what doctors write affects national statistics!

An online guide to writing death certificates can be found at the National Association of Medical Examiners web site (𝄞 http://www.thename.org)

Asphyxia

Definitions and historical perspective

Definition

The term asphyxia causes much confusion, in particular in relation to its classification and definition. All textbooks emphasize that the term is derived from the Greek 'absence or lack of pulsation' but then go on to explain why this does not embrace its subtleties and complexities. Many textbooks describe the etymology of asphyxia and then assign different classifications for it. In fairness, much of the literature originates from forensic pathology where the term has to be used in determining a range of possible causes of death. In many ways, the concept of asphyxia is simple, like the concept of bruising—both can be medicalized and complicated in unnecessary and unhelpful ways. In the clinical setting, such distinctions are perhaps less relevant, because the assessment, documentation, and management of asphyxia survivors (from whatever cause) has different priorities.

A simple (but not completely accepted) view is to consider asphyxia to be a lack of oxygen by any means and that is the approach that is taken here. It is helpful to undertake some attempt at classification—broadly, asphyxia can be split into three groups: mechanical, non-mechanical, and miscellaneous forms.

Examples within each group are listed here:

Mechanical
- Strangulation
- Hanging
- Choking
- Compression asphyxia
- Smothering.

Non-mechanical
- Carbon monoxide poisoning
- Cyanide poisoning.

Miscellaneous
- Drowning.

This classification is similar to that of *external* (all forms of mechanical obstruction of the respiratory process) and *internal* (interruption of transport of oxygen at a cellular level). Clearly, non-mechanical forms of asphyxia, such as carbon monoxide and cyanide poisoning, also come within the realms of toxicology and poisoning and are considered on 📖 p.453. These different examples show the range of possible means by which asphyxia may occur.

Suffocation is a further term used, often interchangeably with asphyxia, although some authors have attempted to separate the two. In all cases of asphyxia/suffocation the possible outcomes are death or survival. The nature of the insult, its degree, and its length of time, will determine the clinical outcome in a survivor. Some may suffer no long-term effects; others may be left in a permanent vegetative state. If a person dies, then a forensic autopsy can help identify signs that would otherwise remain hidden (e.g. bruising to the neck muscles). The role of a clinician is to maximize documentation of forensically useful evidence in survivors of asphyxial insults in order to optimize management and, secondarily, to assist subsequent legal proceedings. It is best to avoid becoming too embroiled in the subtleties of definitions and classifications.

Phases of asphyxia

The following general sequence has been described as phases which take place as uninterrupted asphyxia progresses:

Dyspnoea phase

Expiratory dyspnoea with raised respiratory rate, cyanosis, and tachycardia—may last for a minute or more.

Convulsive phase

Loss of consciousness, reduced respiratory movements, facial congestion, bradycardia, hypertension, fits—may last for a couple of minutes

Pre-terminal respiratory phase

No respiratory action, failure of respiratory and circulatory centres, tachycardia, hypertension—may last a couple of minutes.

Gasping for breath

Respiratory reflexes.

Terminal

Loss of movement, areflexia, pupillary dilatation.

   This sequence of events may be altered, phases missed, and times changed, dependent on the asphyxia/suffocation mode and whether or not it is continuous or interrupted. The sequence may be interrupted at any point up until the terminal event. The possibility of resuscitation will depend on the circumstances—appropriate resuscitation efforts should be attempted if there appears to be any chance of a successful outcome.

Clinical features of asphyxia

In historical pathological terms, the 'classic signs of asphyxia' were: petechial haemorrhages, congestion, and oedema; cyanosis; right heart congestion; and abnormal fluidity of the blood. However, Knight suggested 'descriptions of an abnormal fluidity of the blood seen at autopsy in asphyxial deaths are part of forensic mythology and can be dismissed with little discussion', as postmortem clotting may also be seen after fatal suffocation. All signs are non-specific and thus must be considered clearly in the light of history and full examination. In clinical terms, petechiae, congestion/oedema, and cyanosis may be seen or described in living survivors of asphyxial insults. If venous return is occluded by compression, yet arterial flow persists, it may be expected that this will exacerbate physical signs and symptoms (e.g. oedema and petechiae).

Management of survivors

Careful examination is crucial in both survivors and deceased individuals. In the survivor, if there is visible neck swelling, local tenderness of hyoid, larynx, or other cartilages, MRI or other imaging may be required. Soft tissue or bony injury may be documented and identified. Consideration may also be given (particularly if there is stridor or a hoarse voice) to undertaking flexible laryngoscopy, taking images of any abnormality.

Autopsy findings

Evidence of asphyxia at autopsy includes those findings which are apparent in survivors (listed in the next section), together with one or more of the following:

- Intracranial bleed—haemorrhages may be present within the brain.
- Cerebral oedema, although not specific to asphyxial death, is commonly seen.
- Pulmonary oedema may suggest that the asphyxial/suffocation episode was relatively prolonged.
- Tardieu described haemorrhagic areas under the serosa of the thoracic cavity and related to the heart and great vessels. This is more commonly associated with mechanical asphyxia and includes an element of chest compression.
- Serosal haemorrhages may also be seen in other organs (e.g. serosa of bowel, thymus, epicardium).
- Right heart congestion may be noted and is probably simply a mechanical effect of compression of the chest.
- It has been suggested that hepatic congestion occurs in asphyxial deaths as a result of release of catecholamines.

Evidence of asphyxia in the living

Symptoms and signs that may be evident in the living following an asphyxia/suffocation incident include:

- Pain and tenderness around the neck.
- Damage to the larynx and associated cartilages.
- Damage to the hyoid bone.
- Dried saliva around the mouth.

- Cyanosis may be seen if the survivor is found shortly after the insult. Clearly, if the insult is removed, then cyanosis will disappear as adequate oxygen is received (e.g. by removal of a bolus after a Heimlich manoeuvre).
- Congestion and oedema may be seen, either as a generalized swelling of the entire face above the level of any compression, or with oedema and congestion in the most lax tissues, such as those around the eyes. This is caused by extravasation of fluid out of blood vessels into soft tissues. Such changes may remain for several hours or days and then resolve. In addition, substantial colour change may occur, which appears to relate to congestion of vessels without leakage of blood, but which also persists for longer than might be expected.
- Petechiae—small bruises (generally <2mm in diameter, but often much smaller and better seen on magnification) are caused by leakage of blood from thin-walled blood vessels due to raised intravenous pressure. This is exacerbated by continued inflow of blood from arterioles, endothelial damage caused by hypoxia, and a degree of acute rise in blood pressure. Petechiae may appear in any part of the body above the level of the compressive force that has caused the asphyxia. There is no predictor for the number and precise location of petechiae, which underlines the importance of a detailed external examination with good light. The scalp should be examined underneath the hair, as should the ears, mouth, and nose and all accessible mucosa. Petechiae may disappear after a few hours, but a well chosen photograph may capture a fleeting but forensically important sign. Note that petechiae can coalesce, forming much larger apparent bruises.
- Haemorrhage from body orifices may occur. Compressive forces can result in bleeding from orifices (mouth, nose, and ears). The mechanism is damage to small venules, in a similar manner to petechiae, but with blood leaking through mucosal or skin surfaces. Such bleeding is generally minor.
- Evacuation of bodily fluids may occur. Faeces and urine may be observed in both survivors and non-survivors. The mechanism is probably multifactorial with physical (compression) as well as emotional (e.g. fear) factors. Fatal cases may also have engorgement of the penis with leakage of semen.

Strangulation

Particular modes of asphyxia may have additional features that if sought can assist in determining the events. Strangulation can take many forms and may be done using ligatures or garrottes, or a hand/hands. It can happen accidentally (e.g. children with necklaces or other objects encircling the neck, catching on other items). The term *'throttling'* may also be used to describe pressure applied to the neck and is a technique unfortunately used not uncommonly in the security industry. Pressure may also be applied (dangerously) to the neck by application of the arm and forearm in an arm lock. Each of these methods may leave specific symptoms or signs, in addition to general signs of asphyxia, which need to be specifically looked for. In survivors where compression has been applied a number of effects may be apparent including:

• General signs of blunt force contact, including reddening, bruises, fingernail scratches—from both assailant and victim.
• Sore throat, pain on swallowing.
• Hoarseness, stridor.
• Neck, back and head pain.

These may be present alone or in combination. The end result of unresisted or uncontrolled strangulation or throttling can be death. Causes of death are multifactorial. Simple occlusion of the airway may cause loss of consciousness or even death by lack of oxygen. Pressure on the neck can cause occlusion of the first part of the vertebral arteries and the carotid arteries, stopping the flow of blood to the brain. In such eventualities death may be rapid. It is possible to occlude a single carotid artery with no adverse outcome. Pressure above the laryngeal cartilage can cause the base of the tongue to be elevated, occluding the nasopharynx. Stimulation of the vagus nerve and stimulation of the carotid sinus reflex may each play a part causing brady- or tachyarrhythmias. Direct damage to the larynx may result in soft tissue or blood occlusion of the larynx. Direct pressure below the larynx can occlude the trachea. There may be visible signs of pressure on the skin at the site of application of force and other signs, remote from the site of application. It is not possible to say how long pressure would have to be exerted on the neck for such an outcome, but that loss of oxygenated blood flow to the brain for 3min can be fatal.

Garrotting describes the use of an encircling band (often of metal) which could be tightened either quickly or slowly. It was originally used as means of controlled asphyxial death, and could be modified to include devices that would simultaneously destroy the spinal cord and cause dislocation of the upper cervical vertebra.

Accidental neck compression can occur in a number of ways. For example, there have been a number of deaths in children who have become entrapped in electric car windows that have closed whilst they are looking out of windows.

Factors affecting nature of injuries

The exact nature of injuries depends upon a number of issues including the type of object or implement causing the compression or occlusion (e.g. hands, arms, elbows, ligatures):

- Relative size of hands to neck.
- Force of compression, length of time of compression, and whether compression is consistent or intermittent.
- Whether compression was equal around the neck.
- Whether there was anything (e.g. clothes intervening) between assailant's hands and victim's neck.

Range of potential injuries

Injuries may appear alone or in combination and there is a wide range:

- No injury seen.
- Pain/tenderness at site of application of force with no visible injury.
- Reddening which may pass off after a few hours.
- Bruising or abrasions at point of compression (e.g. finger/thumb or line of a ligature)—this may appear early or late and persist for days.
- Petechiae above the site of compression in skin, eyes, and mucous membranes (e.g. lining of mouth)—such bruises may become confluent and enlarged.
- Damage to larynx/thyroid cartilage and/or hyoid, including fracture.
- Scratches to neck—from assailant and victim (as victim tries to pull away assailant's hands).
- Damage to mucosa of mouth and tongue due to direct pressure on teeth internally.
- Bleeding from mucosa where venous pressure increased (e.g. nose).

All areas of eyes, skin and mucosa (including in the mouth, eyelids, palate and uvula, scalp skin) above the level of compression need to be examined with a good light to identify any localized petechiae. Petechiae need to be identified early, as they fade and disappear within 24h or so. Petechiae may be caused by direct pressure. In manual strangulation or neck compression, petechiae may be florid and can coalesce to form larger bruises. In general, the longer and more powerful the force applied, the more likely that visual evidence of compressive force will be apparent. It is not possible to state when (in terms of timing) certain features may become present, as in many cases physical evidence of such asphyxiation or attack may simply not be present. It is not possible to state what force or what length of application of force is safe.

Ligatures

Neck ligatures can show additional signs depending on the type of ligature and how it was applied. If the ligature is broad and smooth surfaced there may be no visible mark. A thinner rough-surfaced ligature may leave abrasions in the living, or 'parchmented' areas in the deceased—valuable forensic information. There may be no ligature mark, but there may be residual evidence of a 'tide mark'—a level at which the ligature was applied and above which there may be congestion and swelling and petechiae. Patterns may give clues as to how the ligature was applied.

Hanging

Background

Unintentional ('accidental') or suicidal hanging involves the use of some form of ligature used to suspend the body by the neck. Any material capable of forming a ligature can potentially be used for hanging. Hanging is a relatively common method of suicide.

Suspension

Suspension of the body may be *complete* or *partial* (i.e. with the feet or some other part of the body remaining on the ground). A drop may or may not be employed. Most suicidal hangings are partial suspensions (e.g. over a door) and do not involve any drop.

Mode of death

A number of mechanisms may act alone or together to cause death. The mode of death is generally related to the means of suspension and any drop. When there is a full encircling ligature with the highest point of the noose situated posteriorly and the body suspended by its own weight, immediate compression of the arteries to the brain may occur, causing rapid death. If the point of suspension lies to one side, then other factors (e.g. laryngeal disruption and airway obstruction) may be more important in causing death.

Mechanisms which may be responsible for causing death

- Obstruction of arterial flow to the brain.
- Airway obstruction.
- Obstruction of venous return.
- Vagal stimulation in the neck.
- Brainstem/spinal cord injury resulting from neck fracture (e.g. hangman fracture—see 📖 p.153).

Ligature furrow

The ligature furrow is the most important visible feature on examination after hanging. It may differ from a strangulation mark caused by a ligature. The furrow is caused by the pressure of the ligature or suspension cord on the neck. It may be far more pronounced than a strangulation mark, with clear imprint patterns and an indication of the position of the highest point of the noose (with sparing of the skin where no pressure was exerted). Ligature strangulation marks are likely to result in complete encircling of the neck, with a complete encircling strangulation mark and no sparing of the skin.

Careful examination of the ligature furrow may provide an indication of the location of any knots, and the type of material which was used.

Other findings

Physical signs of attempting to escape death from hanging include, as with strangulation, visible fingernail scratches in and around the ligature mark. Laryngeal/hyoid fractures may occur. Survivors of accidental or suicidal hanging may have no obvious sequelae. Some may experience residual hypoxic brain damage ranging from profound to being only detectable by neuropsychological assessment. Others may have motor and/or sensory loss as a result of ischaemic brain damage. A small number of cases of cerebral ischaemia or neurological deficit due to delayed presentation of post-hanging carotid dissection have been described. Consideration should be given to imaging the carotid arteries in any survivor of a hanging.

Judicial hanging (see 📖 p.153)

Hanging when used for judicial execution involves a drop (often a trap-door being opened below the feet of an individual with a noose round the neck). The distance for the drop to allow a 'humane' and rapid death rather than a prolonged suspension time, but which avoids decapitation, varies according to the individual's weight. The mechanism of death is predominantly sudden distraction force on the neck, avulsing the brainstem, often in association with fracture dislocation of the neck vertebrae.

Concealed homicide

This must be considered in any hanging victim. An individual may have been killed by some other means and the body then suspended to mimic suicide. The need for rigorous assessment of the history, locus, and autopsy is essential to ensure that criminal acts are not missed.

Compression asphyxia

Background

Asphyxia can be caused by compression or external forces that prevent an individual being able to breathe. The neck and head may be spared. The key element is enough compression of chest and/or abdomen to prevent adequate respiration. This is sometimes known as *crush* or *traumatic asphyxia*. Deaths caused by large crowds where groups of individuals are pushed together so tightly that they cannot inspire and expire can result in rapid death. This is the mechanism responsible for death in many mass crowd disasters. Such events may also occur in other settings—for example, in motor vehicle repair accidents (jacks collapsing), industrial accidents (walls collapsing), farm accidents (tractors overturning), and natural disasters (earthquakes, landslips).

Findings

In such cases, typical findings (irrespective of other injuries) include intense purple congestion and swelling of the face and neck, and/or petechial haemorrhages of the skin of the face and/or conjunctivae.

Positional (or postural) asphyxia

Compression asphyxia also embraces all types of positional or postural asphyxia where the circumstances cause a victim to be placed in a position where breathing is compromised by inability to use the thorax and/or diaphragm. This may be the result of the victim's own actions or those of others. An example of the first is an intoxicated individual falling across a fence or trying to crawl through an open window and becoming stuck. An example of the latter is the use of restraint in someone arrested by police and placed prone, with handcuffs behind the back and pressure exerted (e.g. with knees) in the small of the back.

Risk factors

The risk of positional asphyxia is increased with factors such as obesity and heart disease, but there is still uncertainty as to the physiological mechanisms (over and above splinting of the respiratory muscles) that may have influence in these settings. Positional asphyxia has resulted from inadvertent positioning that compromised respiration due to intoxication, multiple sclerosis, epilepsy, Parkinson disease, Steele–Richardson–Olszewski syndrome, Lafora disease, and quadriplegia. The key element of a fatal outcome is that the victims of positional asphyxia are unable to get themselves out of the compromised situations due to impairment of cognitive responses (e.g. through alcohol and drugs) and/or other reasons of impaired coordination. The latter can include neurological diseases, loss of consciousness, physical impairment, or physical restraints. It is crucial that police or other personnel whose jobs includes restraint are aware of the risks of postural asphyxia and its potential fatal outcome.

Smothering

Smothering—whereby the nose and mouth are occluded with the intention of causing death—may leave no signs in survivors, but may show classic signs of asphyxia in the deceased. The mode of smothering and the physical capability of the victim can influence the physical findings. If the victim is physically compromised (e.g. a child, elderly person, or an individual under the influence of drugs), they may be unable to struggle. Close examination at a very early stage may be required to document any signs that are present, which include reddening or bruising around the nose and face due to hand compression. If an object such as a pillow is used, no physical signs may be apparent. However, retention of such objects alleged to have been used may have evidential value. Saliva, for example, may be identified on a pillow used in an attack and DNA matching may corroborate the account given.

Choking

Accidental (unintentional) or intentional ingestion of objects or food can cause choking. Prompt treatment is required in order to preserve life. In those suspected of choking, the Resuscitation Council guidelines (see ℘ http://www.resus.org.uk) should be followed as detailed in ▱ Chapter 7.

Autoerotic asphyxia

Definition

The term describes death when an individual has died during some form of solitary sexual activity, as a result of an accident caused by failure of associated items or objects used for sexual gratification. Many other terms have been used to describe these deaths, including sexual asphyxia, sex hanging, asphyxiophilia, Kotzwarrism, autoasphyxiophilia, and hypoxyphilia. The recurrent feature tends to be some form of device, appliance, or restraint that causes neck compression, asphyxia, or hypoxia which is used in an attempt to heighten the sexual response. Death occurs as a result of failure of the device or the failsafe mechanism used to self-limit the experience. Such deaths occur predominantly, but not exclusively, in males. There are a number of features of such deaths which may point to an appropriate diagnosis:

- Evidence of solo sexual activity.
- Private or secure location.
- Evidence of previous similar activity in the past.
- No apparent suicidal intent.
- Unusual props including ligatures, clothing, and pornography.
- Failure of a device or set-up integral to the activity causing death.

Causes of such asphyxial deaths include hanging when neck compression occludes major neck veins and arteries, blocks the airway, or stimulates the carotid sinus reflex. Techniques used include: suspension from ligatures around the neck and limbs; occlusion of the mouth and nose by rubber masks, tape, or plastic sheeting; plastic bags placed over the head; and other objects such as plastic balls held in the mouth. The variety is limited only by human imagination. As with suicidal hanging, the autopsy and surrounding events and known history are crucial to ensure that the death has not been staged to conceal homicide.

Stigma

There is a certain stigma attached to attributing death to autoerotic asphyxia. This can occasionally result in some pressure on the coroner to attribute death to another cause (see 📖 p.51).

Drowning

Background

Although most drowning deaths reflect accidents or suicides, some may result from homicide. It is most important to note that the presence of a body in water does not necessarily indicate drowning. Certain clues when a body is recovered (e.g. ligatures to hands and feet) may suggest foul play. Drowning may occur in only a few inches of water and when investigating a possible drowning death, as much knowledge as possible of the circumstances and locus is needed to make a proper and accurate determination of the cause of death. Jumping or diving into water may result in head and/or neck injuries that render a person incapable of swimming. The cause of death may not be due to water ingestion.

Initial effects of immersion

The effects of immersion vary according to the type of water. Entry into cold water initiates the 'cold-shock' response—an initial gasp of air intake, followed by hyperventilation and sensation of breathlessness. Breath-holding time is also reduced to merely a few seconds. This may increase the risk of aspiration in water where waves and spray are present. Increased heart rate and cardiac output follows, with an increased risk of cardiac arrhythmias in those with specific risk factors. The diving response (characterized by apnoea, peripheral vasoconstriction, and bradycardia) is seen if the face is immersed in cold water. Not all individuals exhibit this to a great degree. However, both cold-shock and diving responses together increase the risk of cardiac arrhythmias.

Cold water immersion

As time in cold water proceeds, so does the likelihood of hypothermia. As hypothermia develops, cognitive function becomes impaired increasing the risks of wrong decisions and aspiration of water.

Pathophysiology

Drowning is a mixture of both mechanical presence of water within the respiratory system (causing mechanical asphyxia) and fluid and electrolyte changes which vary according to the medium (sea water as opposed to fresh water) in which immersion has occurred. Hypotonic fresh water intake results generally in haemodilution with hypervolaemia, hyponatraemia, and haemolysis with hyperkalaemia. Hypertonic sea (salt) water results in water transfer into alveoli with haemoconcentration, hypovolaemia, and hypernatraemia.

Both of these pathophysiological mechanisms result in surfactant destruction and pulmonary oedema, with metabolic acidosis and associated respiratory failure. After initial immersion, where breath-holding occurs, CO_2 accumulates and respiration is stimulated, which may result in further aspiration of water with subsequent coughing, vomiting, and relatively rapid onset of loss of consciousness.

Investigation of drowning

Any investigation of a drowning incident needs to establish the following:
• Was the individual dead before entry into the water?
• What was the cause of death?
• How did the individual get into the water?
• What prevented survival?

A rigorous assessment including investigation of premortem movements, examination of locus, and autopsy should address these questions.

Factors affecting appearance

Postmortem appearance after water immersion is dependent on many factors including:
• Water type (fresh or sea water)
• Sea or water bed type
• Tidal movement
• Temperature
• Predators
• Insects.

Appearances are very variable and on extraction from water, rapid changes occur in physical appearance. Any identifying marks or objects should be retrieved and documented. It is generally not possible to determine the time of immersion from the physical appearance of the body. Certain external features may be observed after immersion including:
• Maceration (washerwoman's hands).
• Loss of epidermis.
• Loss of pigment layers.
• Postmortem abrasions (often caused by body movements over the water bed).
• Water-based animal or insect predation marks.

Autopsy findings

Postmortem findings after drowning are non-specific and may include:
• Foam around nose and mouth.
• Frothy fluid in the airways.
• Emphysema aquosum (caused by overinflation of the lungs and air trapping in the alveoli—lungs appeared ballooned, voluminous and bulky) with overlap of medial edges of two lungs at autopsy.
• Presence of foreign material, including sand and silt in lungs, airways, stomach, and small intestine.

Diatoms are a class of algae of many different types. Smaller diatoms enter the systemic circulation having been filtered via the lung alveoli and can be demonstrated in body tissue such as bone marrow. Comparison of these diatoms with those in the water from which the body is recovered is considered to be useful corroborative evidence to support death by drowning (as opposed to death and then immersion).

Forensic pathology of physical injury

Injury classification

Within a forensic context, the interpretation and classification of injuries is important in helping to gain an insight into how they were caused.

Is it an injury?

Certain natural disease processes can masquerade as injuries. On occasions, normal appearances can be mistaken for an injury. On this basis, the first important question to be answered is whether there really has been an injury. This question particularly applies in the field of child abuse, where there are two classic errors:

- A Mongolian blue spot over the lower back of some children may be mistaken for bruising.
- Thrombocytopenia, purpura, and bleeding tendencies from any cause may also be mistaken as bruising of purely traumatic origin.

Avoid inappropriate terminology

The importance of applying the correct terminology when describing injuries in a medicolegal context cannot be overstated. Many practitioners in forensic and other fields have learnt this to their cost, embarrassment, and sometimes even ridicule (as occurred when Emergency Medicine specialists wrote in the *British Medical Journal* about a 'neatly incised laceration'). Inherent in the meaning of certain terms used to describe an injury is an implication regarding the mechanism responsible for causing that injury. This particularly applies to skin wounds, where some descriptive terms imply that the injury resulted from blunt force (e.g. laceration, abrasion), whereas others imply sharp force (e.g. incised wound). The potential medicolegal implications are obvious. It is more than simply sloppy to describe an incised skin wound which resulted from a person being stabbed by a knife as a 'laceration'—it is incorrect. In a courtroom setting, if one aspect of the testimony of a witness is shown to be wrong, doubt may be cast over the remainder of his/her testimony and credibility. Sometimes it can be difficult for a non-expert (or even an expert) to judge whether a particular skin wound is an incised wound or a laceration—in this instance, it may be prudent to carefully document the findings (as outlined on 📖 p.120) and describe it simply as a 'skin wound'.

Problems with terminology

Having warned against use of inappropriate terminology to describe injuries, it is only fair to acknowledge that the meanings of some terms used to describe injuries are not generally agreed (and for this reason some are perhaps best avoided). Even the meaning of the term 'wound' is not universally agreed—some authorities apply it to any injury, whilst others restrict its use to injuries which involve a breach in the skin. As many jurisdictions have precise definitions of a 'wound', the term should be used with caution.

Terms used to describe injuries

Given that language is designed to aid communication, it may appear surprising that there is such an array of terms used to describe injury from a forensic perspective. Some might interpret this as a conspiracy to maintain medical 'elitism'—a view not contradicted by the fact that definitions of many of the terms are not generally agreed! The following principal terms used to describe injuries are discussed in more detail in subsequent pages.

Abrasions to the skin typically reflect blunt force trauma applied tangentially (also known as 'grazes' or 'scrapes'), denuding the superficial skin. The term may also be used to cover damage to the superficial layers of skin by compression—these include patterned abrasions, where the imprint of an item is stamped onto the skin.

Avulsion is the term applied when a structure is ripped forcefully away from its normal attachments. It may be applied in a variety of situations (e.g. when the kidney becomes detached from its vascular pedicle, or when a piece of bone is plucked away by a tendon).

Blast injuries reflect transmission of a narrow wave of very high pressure.

Blunt force trauma describes a general mechanism of injury.

Bruises are extravascular collections of blood which are more than a few mm in diameter.

Burns usually reflect thermal skin injury, although the term is also applied to chemical skin damage and thermal damage to other epithelial surfaces (e.g. the pharynx).

Chop wounds, such as those caused by an axe or machete, have features of both blunt force and sharp force trauma.

Contusions are bruises, although use of this term has no particular advantage.

Cuts are skin wounds, but the term means different things to different people—some consider them to be incised (particularly slash) wounds, whilst colloquially the term often covers any sort of skin wound.

Defence injuries are patterns of injury which imply that an individual was trying to defend him/herself against attack. These include an isolated ulna shaft fracture resulting from an individual raising an arm to protect him/herself from attack from a baseball bat ('nightstick injury') and incised wounds to the palm of the hand as a victim being attacked by a person wielding a knife tries to grab it.

Ecchymoses are small bruises.

Entry and **exit wounds** reflect interpretations of causation relating to penetrating trauma.

Factitious wounds are self-inflicted wounds which are caused in an attempt to create the false impression of having been sustained in an assault by someone else.

Firearm injuries include a number of highly characteristic injuries.

Fractures is a term which covers all types of breaks to bones, although the term can also be applied to other organs (e.g. the erect penis).

Haematomas are large collections of blood following haemorrhage.

Haemorrhages are areas of bleeding.

Incisions or **incised wounds** follow sharp force trauma.

Lacerations are full thickness skin wounds which follow blunt trauma where the tissues are crushed and/or torn or split apart. The term may also be applied to damage to rupture of solid internal organs.

Penetrating trauma is usually applied to the situation when objects pierce the skin.

Perforating injury describes events in which an object penetrates into a cavity or where a normally contained organ (such as the stomach) bursts open.

Petechial haemorrhages are tiny areas of bleeding (typically of <2mm diameter), and often follow indirect trauma. There is a traditional association between this term and asphyxial injury (see 📖 p.103).

Puncture wounds can affect a number of organs, but when applied to the skin, form a part of some bite injuries. The term implies relatively deep penetration with a small skin wound.

Scalds are thermal injuries to the skin caused by hot liquids/steam.

Scratches may include a variety of different injuries, but are typically applied to skin wounds caused by fingernails (*'scratch abrasions'*—narrow linear abrasions to the skin), but also cover other injuries (e.g. *'point scratches'*—superficial incised wounds caused by the tip of a sharp object such as a knife).

Sharp force trauma describes the mechanism of injury. It includes knife stab and slash wounds.

Slash wounds are incised wounds which are longer than they are deep.

Stab wounds are deeper than they are long, and are mostly caused by sharp force (typically knives).

Transfixing injury describes through and through penetration of part of the body.

Wounds usually affect the skin, but the term is often applied to injuries elsewhere. Its meaning may depend to some extent upon who uses it and in what context. Note that in English law, for example, 'wounding' is defined as an injury which penetrates or breaks all of the layers of the skin.

Describing injuries

It is important for the forensic practitioner to record injuries in an accurate fashion. It is worth trying to develop a system which ensures that all of the important elements are considered and recorded. Wherever possible, appropriate body diagrams should be used. This particularly applies to the occasions where there are complex or numerous injuries—here it is advisable to number the injuries and cross-reference written descriptions with numbers applied to a body diagram (see 📖 p.122).

All of the following elements need to be considered.

Type and nature of injury

The findings should be described exactly as they appear.

- *Bruises*—the colour needs to be recorded and most particularly, whether there is any yellow colour present (this has implications in relation to dating the injury—see 📖 p.126). A ruler needs to be used to accurately measure the dimensions, including both length and width (employing metric measurements). For example: 'the yellow/ brown bruise measured 4.5cm (horizontally) x 2.5cm (vertically)'. Any particular patterns or shapes should be described, but reference to size in terms of everyday objects should be avoided (e.g. stating that a bruise is the 'size of an egg' is unhelpful, especially considering that eggs come in different sizes. The presence/absence of any swelling and/or tenderness should be specifically searched for and documented.
- *Skin wounds*—these need to be measured accurately with a ruler, with comment on the depth and stating if deep structures are visible and if there is any contamination with dirt or other foreign material. The orientation of the wound (vertical, horizontal, oblique, etc.) also needs to be recorded. If possible, an attempt should be made to judge the nature of any wound and ascribe the appropriate term (e.g. 'laceration' or 'incised wound'). However, if the exact nature of an injury is unclear, this should be documented. For those wounds which have been treated and closed at hospital, it is appropriate to record the number and nature of the sutures used and/or any adhesive paper strips.
- *Abrasions*—the size, orientation, and depth should be described and the presence of any patterns or skin tags recorded.
- *Burns*—the colour and nature of the burn (including any blistering) should be recorded. In the conscious patient, it is important to check for sensation over the burnt skin which will assist attempts to make a judgement about depth.

Location of injury

The exact position of an injury should be recorded using standard anatomical terms and the distance of the injury from a definite point measured (e.g. 'the distal extent of the skin wound was situated along the ulnar border of the mid-forearm at a distance of 9cm from the proximal palmar crease').

Associated functional damage

Clinical evidence of underlying damage (e.g. inability to weight bear suggesting fracture, reduced air entry implying pneumothorax) needs to be carefully searched for, as it might not be otherwise immediately apparent. In the case of skin wounds which penetrate the skin, it is important to check as appropriate for nerve, tendon, or vessel injury and test for distal sensation, movements, and pulses.

Photographs

In certain instances, photographs can convey an enormous amount of useful information about the nature and extent of injuries. They have a particularly important role in the investigation and analysis of suspected bite wounds (see 🕮 p.292). Photographs taken by SOCOs usually employ a standard L-shaped ruler in order that distortion in two planes can be accounted for. Digital photographs are increasingly being used. It is worth remembering that colour reproduction is not necessarily accurate and that colours 'on screen' might be significantly different to the originals.

Body diagrams

An example of a standard recommended body diagram is shown in Fig. 5.1. Copies of standard diagrams can be obtained from the (publications section of the) Faculty of Forensic and Legal Medicine's website (𝔖 http://www.fflm.ac.uk).

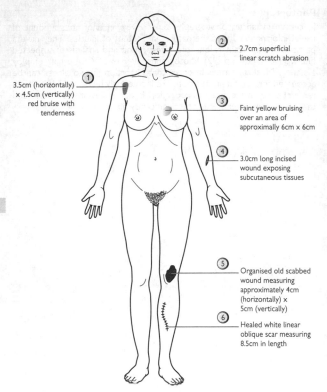

② 2.7cm superficial linear scratch abrasion

① 3.5cm (horizontally) x 4.5cm (vertically) red bruise with tenderness

③ Faint yellow bruising over an area of approximally 6cm x 6cm

④ 3.0cm long incised wound exposing subcutaneous tissues

⑤ Organised old scabbed wound measuring approximately 4cm (horizontally) x 5cm (vertically)

⑥ Healed white linear oblique scar measuring 8.5cm in length

Fig. 5.1 An example body diagram (anterior surface).

Injuries (see Fig. 5.1)

1 3.5cm (horizontally) x 4.5cm (vertically) red bruise with tenderness.
2 2.7cm superficial linear scratch abrasion.
3 Faint yellow bruising over an area of approximately 6cm x 6cm.
4 3.0cm long incised wound exposing subcutaneous tissues.
5 Organized old scabbed wound measuring approximately 4cm
   (horizontally) x 5cm (vertically).
6 Healed white linear oblique scar measuring 8.5cm in length.

Bruising

Bruising results from damage to blood vessels which have bled into adjacent tissues. It is associated principally with blunt force trauma. Although usually applied to damage to the skin and subcutaneous tissues, bruising can affect deep organs also.

Terminology

Forensic medicine has many areas of confusing terminology, perhaps no more so than in relation to the descriptions of bruises. The cynic might be forgiven for thinking that the multitude of terms in use is designed to confuse the non-specialist. The aim should be to record findings using simple descriptive terms with the expectation that these may need to be explained in a court! See 📖 p.118 for explanations of various terms in common use, including contusion, ecchymosis, haematoma, petechiae. 'Bruise' is the basic term which covers most forms of bleeding larger than a few mm in diameter.

Characteristic skin bruising

The appearance of bruising reflects a variety of factors other than simply the mechanism of injury. In particular, bruising looks different depending upon the thickness, colour, and nature of the overlying skin.

Intradermal bruises
Bruising confined to the superficial parts of the skin may cause an accurate imprint (e.g. the sole of a boot which inflicted a stamp).

Fingertip imprints
Bruising from gripping fingertips is often seen on the inner aspect of the upper arms of individuals who have been restrained.

Finger marks
The slap from an open hand may result in an identifiable pattern.

Tramline bruising
Two parallel straight lines of bruising separated by a pale central part reflect blunt trauma from a cane, rod, snooker cue, or other linear object (see Fig. 5.2).

Bruising in specific sites

Battle's sign
Bruising which appears over the mastoid process behind the ear in the absence of any direct trauma indicates base of skull fracture. The bruising is not immediately apparent, but typically takes several days to 'come out'.

Raccoon (panda) eyes
Bruising limited to within the orbital margins on both sides is another sign indicating a base of skull fracture.

Bruising after death

Movement of red blood cells in the early period after death follows a relatively predictable course, as covered on 📖 p.32. However, quite distinct from this process, much attention has previously been devoted to a different phenomenon—that of postmortem bruising. Although it has been reliably described, bruising occurring within the first few hours after death appears to be really quite unusual.

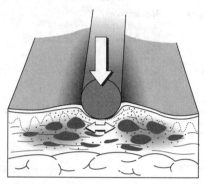

Fig. 5.2 Tramline bruising.

Progression of bruising with time

Ageing bruising

It is often very important from a medicolegal perspective to try to ascertain exactly when injuries occurred. Unfortunately, there is a dearth of reliable science to assist with this, although the testimony of certain experts over the years may not always have given this impression! Bruises do not follow the traditional account of the progression through various colours, which may be summarized as follows:

Time after injury   *Appearance*
- 0–2 days   Swollen, tender, red/blue
- 3–5 days   Blue/purple
- 5–7 days   Green
- 7–10 days   Yellow
- 10–14 days   Brown
- 14–28 days   Resolution

Added to the difficulty of assessing the age of bruises are the following:
- Different individuals will have different interpretations of the colours that they see.
- Bruising looks different in different lighting.
- Bruises often become more prominent hours or even days after the initial injury.
- Similar bruises in the same individual may go through colour change at a different rate.
- Different colours in a bruise may coexist.
- Research from one of the authors suggests that in one family, most bruises amongst three siblings disappeared within 3 days!

Consistently, evidence does indicate that with the possible exception of young infants:

A yellow colour in a bruise implies that it is >18h old.

Other factors which may help an expert make an informed guess about the age of bruising include:
- Tenderness and/or swelling tend to imply a relatively recent origin.
- A fresh patterned bruise superimposed upon an area of fading bruising implies separate injuries occurring at very different times (potentially important from a forensic perspective).
- Bruising in certain sites tends to move slowly with time under the influence of gravity—hence an injury to the mid-calf not infrequently results in bruising around the ankle a few days later. Much more useful information is available from examination of a 'live' individual, rather than inspection of photographs.

Lacerations, abrasions, and scratches

Skin lacerations (Fig. 5.3)

Lacerations to the skin are caused by blunt force trauma in which the skin is torn apart by a crushing/shearing force. Skin lacerations may exhibit the following features:

- Ragged, irregular skin edges.
- Bruising of the skin edges which have obviously been crushed.
- Contamination of the wound (sometimes by forensically important and collectable trace material).
- Varying depths and breadths of the wound in different places.
- Bridging of tissues within the wound, reflecting certain stronger elements within the wound remaining intact (e.g. nerves and blood vessels).
- Abrasion of part of the wound margin.
- Presence of intact hairs which cross the wound.

Lacerations of the skin tend to occur at sites where there are underlying bony prominences. Lacerations around the eyebrows are relatively common in individuals who fall and hit the ground under the influence of alcohol: the scalp being split apart as it is crushed between skull bone and hard ground. Once a wound has been cleaned and satisfactorily closed, it may be very difficult to determine with confidence whether it was a laceration or an incised wound. Therefore, it is important that this issue is considered prior to closure.

Skin abrasions

Abrasions are 'grazes' or 'scrapes'. Most result from blunt force trauma being applied tangentially. They are typically superficial in that they do not involve the full thickness of the skin, although occasionally fully thickness wounds occur. Contact against a wide rough surface causes wide abrasions which are sometimes referred to as '**brush abrasions**'. It may be possible to determine the direction in which the abrasion occurred by observing small epidermal skin tags at that edge of the wound which was last in contact with the abrading surface.

The terms '**impact**' and '**patterned**' **abrasions** are sometimes used to describe blunt force injuries which are at right angles to the skin.

Ageing of abrasions

Histologically, infiltration of polymorphs is obvious by 4–8h after injury—the important issue is that this implies that the injury occurred whilst the patient was alive. Similarly, macroscopically, scab formation reflects injury during life. Abrasions can occur after death, in which case there is no inflammatory response apparent histologically. Macroscopically, postmortem abrasions are yellow (rather than red) and tend to appear translucent.

Scratches

This is another slightly ambiguous term, which has been defined in different ways. However, most forensic practitioners are happy with the idea that linear abrasions may defined as scratches.

Scratch abrasions caused by fingernails are the most frequent scratches seen in clinical practice. Typically, several relatively narrow linear wounds of similar depth may run together in parallel or slightly converging fashion. Note that it may be possible to collect forensically important trace material (DNA) from under the fingernail of the person who inflicted the injury.

Point scratches are incised wounds of superficial nature which are caused by the tip of a sharp object (e.g. knife or broken glass) running across the skin.

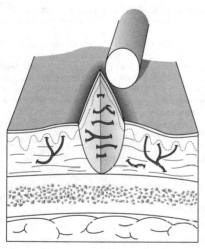

Fig. 5.3 Laceration.

Incised wounds

As already mentioned earlier in this chapter, from a forensic perspective, the key issue when interpreting an injury is often to diagnose the nature of the injury in order to determine whether a wound was caused by blunt or sharp force trauma. Incised wounds follow sharp force injury and may be caused by any object which has a sharp edge, most usually knives and the sharp edges of broken glass. Incised wounds typically exhibit the following characteristics:

- The skin wound is linear in nature.
- There is an absence of adjacent bruising of the skin edges.
- There is an absence of 'bridging' tissue extending from one side to the other within the wound (as is often seen in lacerations).
- In the case of hair covered areas, such as the scalp, there may be divided hairs lying free in or around the wound.

Note that incised wounds which penetrate obliquely (tangentially) through the skin will inevitably result in one skin edge being 'undercut' when compared with the other.

It can sometimes be very difficult to judge whether a particular wound is an incised wound or a laceration—in this instance, simply record and describe the findings, and document it as a 'wound'. It is worth bearing in mind the fact that skin wounds which overlie bone can sometimes have relatively 'clean' edges, so it is important to look carefully for other features, such as underlying structural damage, particularly linear 'scoring' of the periosteum resulting from sharp force injury.

Traditional nomenclature divides incised wounds into 'slash' wounds and 'stab' wounds as follows:

- **Stab wounds** are deeper than they are long.
- **Slash wounds** are longer than they are deep.

It may be best to avoid use of the term '*cut*' which can be confusing, is really rather non-specific, and is frequently used by members of the general population to cover any skin wound which bleeds, whether it is an incised wound, laceration, or abrasion.

Characteristic incised wounds

There are occasions when the wound resulting from an injury is so characteristic that it can provide a 'forensic' match for a particular weapon and mechanism. The pattern of injury, combined with findings on examination may suggest defence injuries (see 📖 p.139), or self-inflicted injuries (see 📖 p.136).

Surgical wounds

It is no surprise that surgeons typically choose to inflict incised skin wounds upon their patients. With minimal damage to adjacent tissues, these wounds combine the potential advantages of rapid healing, minimal scarring, with a low risk of infection.

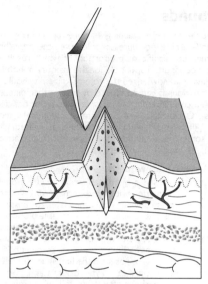

Fig. 5.4 Incised wound.

The best known incised wounds in history?

On the Ides of March (15 March) 44 BC, the Roman dictator (Gaius) Julius Caesar was assassinated in Rome. He was killed by a group of 60 conspirators who inflicted a total of 23 stab wounds on him. According to one report, a physician who examined him afterwards stated that it was a wound to his chest that was the fatal injury. Legend has it that when Caesar saw Brutus amongst the conspirators, he said to him 'You too, Brutus?', an account which was immortalized in Shakespeare's *Julius Caesar* as 'Et tu, Brute?' Other less dramatic but possibly more accurate accounts, reported that Caesar said nothing during the attack, but simply used his toga to hide his face.

In addition to the incised wounds that killed him, Caesar's name is strongly and obviously associated with medical incisions in the form of a 'Caesarean section'. The exact origin of the term, however, remains somewhat obscure.

Stab wounds

For most people, the term 'stabbing' conjures up an image of an assault involving a knife. This is not unreasonable, given the prevalence of knife injuries, a small but significant proportion of which result in fatalities. Indeed, knife wounds are responsible for the majority of homicidal deaths in the UK. Having acknowledged the role of knives, it should be remembered that stab wounds can be caused by many other different types of pointed implements (including scissors, screwdrivers, pencils, and even stiletto heels). Occasionally, stabbings are unintentional ('accidental') or self-inflicted. Although understandably classed as incised wounds, stab wounds can sometimes be inflicted by objects with a relatively blunt tip (e.g. a pencil), provided that sufficient force is used.

The trouble with stab wounds

In most instances, concerns around stab wounds reflect obvious potential for severe internal injuries, with the external (skin) wound identifying this possibility. The most obvious concern relates to massive concealed **internal haemorrhage** due to direct damage to large blood vessels. In the case of the chest, pneumothorax (particularly **tension pneumothorax**) and **cardiac tamponade** present additional threats. Neck stabbings may cause airway obstruction, air embolism, or spinal cord injury. Stab wounds to the neck and/or trunk (as opposed to the limbs) understandably arouse most concern. However, significant hypovolaemia and even death from massive **external haemorrhage** may occur following limb stabbing, particularly where the victim is not in a position to seek or receive appropriate medical attention (e.g. those heavily under the influence of alcohol and/or drugs).

Forensic examination of stab wounds

From a forensic perspective, scrutiny of the skin wound can provide crucial information about how an injury was caused. The classical picture is of a victim with an obliquely orientated incised skin wound over the front of the left chest which was inflicted by a right-handed assailant directly facing the victim and holding the knife in a traditional dagger fashion (thumb gripping furthest away from the blade). However, many simple factors, such as movement of the two parties can alter this.

- **Knife wounds** are considered in detail on 📖 pp.134–5.
- **Scissors** can produce a variety of wounds depending upon their design and whether they are open or closed at the time of injury. A closed pair of scissors typically has a relatively blunt tip and so tends to split the skin causing a Z-shaped wound. A protruding screw in the blades of the scissors may also cause a small laceration in the middle of one wound.
- **Broken bottles** can cause numerous grouped incised skin wounds of varying shapes, sizes, and depths.
- **Traditional screwdrivers** and **chisels** typically produce rectangular wounds with abraded margins.
- **Cross-head screwdrivers** cause characteristic X-shaped wounds.

Emergency treatment after stabbing

Forensic practitioners are not often directly involved in providing emergency care for victims of stabbings, but do need to appreciate the principles of standard treatment.

Prehospital care

When faced with a patient who still has the stabbing object *in situ*, it should be left in place, as the foreign object may be providing tamponade—release might result in torrential haemorrhage. Concepts underpinning management of penetrating trauma have changed considerably in recent years. The principal risk is acknowledged to be haemorrhage. In the past, treatment focused around intravenous fluid replacement and haemodynamic stabilization prior to transfer. However, research evidence has shown that patients with significant haemorrhage have a better outcome if intravenous fluid replacement is kept to a minimum and they are transported as rapidly as possible for definitive treatment (usually surgery at hospital). On this basis, having provided oxygen, decompressed any tension pneumothorax, and applied pressure to external bleeding, ambulance services now tend towards a policy of 'scoop and run' rather than 'stay and play' at the scene.

Hospital treatment

Hospital staff aim to quickly identify and treat immediately life-threatening injuries. Any pneumothorax is drained using a large intercostal tube—unfortunately, hospital staff still sometimes continue to insert these through stab wounds, thereby destroying the forensic evidence and increasing the risk of infection. Continuing the aim of the prehospital services, hospital staff look to provide those patients who require definitive surgery for haemorrhagic shock with this treatment as soon as possible.

Procedure after death is declared at hospital

Many of those who die having been stabbed are taken to hospital, either with a pulse or without, for resuscitative efforts. Cardiac arrest at hospital following penetrating trauma is an indication for emergency thoracotomy. This, combined with other attempts at resuscitation, will necessarily result in significant effects on the body as far as subsequent forensic examination is concerned. The following may help hospital staff faced with this situation:

- Attempts at resuscitation should take precedence over initial concerns about gathering forensic evidence.
- Once death is declared, police will advise about collection of evidence.
- All lines, tubes, and therapeutic devices should be left in place, together with any embedded foreign body (e.g. knife).
- Resuscitating staff need to make detailed contemporaneous notes (using diagrams), particularly of resuscitative efforts and injuries. This will help the forensic pathologist to distinguish injuries which were inflicted as part of any assault from those associated with resuscitative efforts (e.g. insertion of intercostal chest drains).
- The hospital press officer should expect considerable interest.

Knife anatomy (Fig. 5.5)

Knives come in many different shapes and designs. As a result, when used as weapons, different knives inflict very different patterns of injury. The typical 'anatomical' features of knives are shown in the figure below. The two basic components are the blade (almost universally metal) and the handle (made of a variety of materials). Knives and in particular, blades, come in numerous shapes, sizes and designs. The tip or point may be sharp or blunt, and there may be one or two sharp edges—in the case of just one sharp edge, the opposite side is a blunt back. As the blade extends towards the handle it typically widens and the sharp edge finishes. This results in an area of the blade adjacent to the handle with two blunt edges (ricasso). Where the blade meets the handle, there is tradition-ally an expansion of the handle into a guard. The main part of the handle serves as the grip.

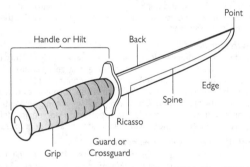

Fig. 5.5 Labelled diagram of a knife. Reproduced from DiMaio VJ and DiMaio D, *Forensic Pathology*, 2nd edn, Copyright 2011. Taylor & Francis Group LLC – Books. Reproduced with permission of Taylor & Francis Group LLC.

Identifying the weapon

It is clearly easiest to identify the knife responsible for an injury when it is left embedded in the body! Not infrequently, part of the blade breaks off and is left behind as the remainder of the weapon is removed—this then opens the potential for a match. In most other instances, however, it is impossible to make a certain match solely based upon the nature of the wound. The most that can usually be said is that a particular knife would have been capable of ('consistent with') causing a particular wound. However, certain wound characteristics imply certain knife features, as considered in the following section. Forensic examination of a knife may reveal vital clues, in terms of DNA and fingerprints.

Range of injuries from knives

In addition to stab wounds, knives can inflict slash wounds and superficial point scratch abrasions (see 📖 p.129), as well as blunt trauma from the handle. Features of stab wounds reflect a variety of factors, as follows:

- *Orientation* of skin wounds affects appearance in that wounds tend to gape more when they cross Langer's lines, but remain narrow slits when parallel to them.
- *Double sharp-edged blades* can cause linear wounds with two 'pointed' or V-shaped ends.
- *Single sharp-edged blades* can result in one pointed end and one 'fish-tail' or 'squared off' wound, the latter reflecting localized blunt trauma from the blunt edge, with localized tearing and bruising of the skin. Note, however, that some single-edged knives have a sharp edge on the back at the very tip, so that the initial penetration is from a double edged weapon, and if the knife is then moved down towards the large sharp edge, the blunt edge makes no contact, so the wound has two pointed ends.
- *Serrated blades* may cause characteristic serrations of the stab wound or adjacent skin.
- *Movement* (of the knife or victim) alters the shape of wounds. An L-shaped wound may reflect the knife being twisted in the body, or movement of the body as the knife is withdrawn. Within the limits of 1mm or 2mm skin elasticity, the skin wound is at least as long as the blade is wide at any particular point, but clearly it can be much longer—measure the wound with the edges apposed.
- *Compression* of the subcutaneous tissues by a knife thrust with some force may allow a blade to penetrate a depth which is longer than the blade, when measured under normal (non-compressed) conditions. This applies more to the abdomen and buttocks than to the chest.
- *Penetration to the ricasso* may result in double fish-tails at wound ends.
- *Imprints and/or bruising* from the guard may also result from complete penetration—the area of maximal prominence bruising may indicate whether the knife was inserted with up- or downwards force. In the latter case, there will be more bruising above the wound.

How much force was required?

This is a frequently asked question in a court-room setting as the answer may have implications relating to the mechanism of injury and *mens rea*. However, it is possible to answer this question in general terms only, rather than with scientifically quantifiable certainty. It has traditionally been stated that having penetrated the skin, most underlying tissues (except bone and cartilage) offer relatively little resistance. Similarly, it is easy to imagine how a sharp knife might easily penetrate the skin, but a less sharp knife which also penetrates thick clothing will obviously require a considerably greater amount of force.

Survival time after fatal stabbing

The issues of how long the victims of a fatal stabbing lived for after injury, and how much physical activity they were capable of during this time, are difficult, but often important medicolegally.

Slash wounds

Incised wounds which are longer than they are deep are termed 'slash wounds'. Sometimes a cutting force follows an initial stabbing injury to produce a long 'stab–slash' injury. Slash wounds may result from a variety of different forms of sharp force, but knives or broken glass are usually responsible. Despite a lack of depth, slash wounds in certain sites (e.g. the neck) can pose a real threat to life. Some characteristic slash injuries are considered here.

Facial slash wounds

Slash wounds to the face commonly follow assault and are generally disfiguring rather than life threatening. Depending upon the exact location, there may be associated damage to important structures such as the parotid gland and duct and the branches of the facial nerve (supplying muscles of facial expression). Standard treatment of uncomplicated facial slash wounds comprises careful cleaning and closure of the skin with fine interrupted nylon sutures, with the latter removed at an early stage (e.g. 3 days) to be replaced with adhesive paper strips.

Neck slash wounds

Slash wounds affecting the anterior triangle of the neck may threaten life by one or more of the following mechanisms:
• Exsanguination from damage to large vessels.
• Air embolism resulting from air being sucked into damaged large veins by negative intrathoracic pressure.
• Damage to the larynx and upper airway.

Immediate treatment involves the direct application of pressure (to prevent haemorrhage) and urgent transfer to the care of a surgical team to explore under anaesthetic in theatre. Generations of junior doctors have learnt to avoid 'gentle exploration' of neck wounds in the Emergency Department—torrential bleeding may (re)commence and be rather tricky to stem. Slash wounds to the neck can follow assaults or be self-inflicted. The latter classically have 'hesitation marks' (or 'tentative' wounds) adjacent to a tentative wound.

Wrist slash wounds

Are also typically (but not exclusively) self-inflicted, in which case they tend to run parallel on the flexor aspect of the non-dominant wrist, possibly with evidence of healing or healed old scars around the same region. Unintentional ('accidental') slash wounds of the wrist and forearm not infrequently follow an individual (perhaps under influence of alcohol) putting his/her arm through a pane of glass. Injury from broken glass is notorious for causing significant damage to important deep structures (nerves and tendons) and for resulting in retained foreign bodies.

Hand slash wounds

These include the classical defence injuries incurred when a victim grasps the knife being wielded by an assailant or raises the hand in defence (see 🔲 p.139).

Chop wounds

This term is usually applied to those wounds caused by sharp-edged heavy weapons such as axes and meat cleavers. Axes are very powerful weapons and it is no surprise that they hold a significant place in the history of warfare. Resulting injuries combine a sharp force injury to the skin with dramatic injury to underlying structures, including bone.

Skin wound healing

From a pathophysiological point of view, the healing process of skin wounds is divided into three stages which chronologically overlap:

- **Early vascular phase:** the coagulation process involves production of fibrin (interestingly, this may occur after death). An inflammatory response continues with release of cytokines and associated substances. This coincides with vascular changes of reduced tissue perfusion and enhanced vascular permeability.
- **Cellular reaction:** neutrophils are attracted to the wound, followed later by macrophages, which are responsible for degradation of red blood cells. Monocytes join other white blood cells in releasing factors which promote activity of fibroblasts.
- **Proliferative changes:** fibroblasts become very active—collagen is laid down and new blood vessels appear (the combination forming 'granulation tissue'). The epidermis is replaced by keratinocytes.

Factors affecting wound healing

The wound healing process can be adversely affected by a number of factors which may coexist: poor generalized nutrition, reduced local blood flow and oxygenation, contamination with foreign material, and infection (the risk of infection is highly dependent upon the presence of the other factors). In general, wounds tend to heal more rapidly in younger individuals, who are more prone to exaggerated healing responses, resulting in **keloid** and **hypertrophic scars**.

Skin wounds and scarring

Skin wounds heal with characteristic scarring. In the early stages, an organized scab is replaced by a pink scar, which typically fades over weeks and months to leave a white scar. Note that wounds which are inadequately treated and which contain coloured foreign material may result in (often unsightly) discoloration ('**tattooing**'). The final appearance of a scar depends upon the exact location and nature of the wound, as well as how it was treated. The best chance of a good long-term cosmetic result requires the wound to heal with its skin edges neatly apposed. Surgical skin wounds which are closed using staples or interrupted sutures ('stitches') often exhibit evidence of this in the form of two lines of small 'dot scars' adjacent and parallel on either side of the principal scar. The full thickness skin wounds which tend to heal with the best long-term appearance are linear incised wounds which penetrate at right angles to the skin surface (rather than one wound edge being undercut) and which are aligned along natural skin creases ('**Langer's lines**'). The orientation of these natural skin creases is particularly appreciated by surgeons, who generally attempt to follow them when making surgical incisions.

Defence injuries

Certain types and patterns of injury suggest that they were inflicted on an individual who was attempting to protect him/herself (Fig. 5.6). Interpretation of such injuries carries obvious medicolegal implications. Although certain injuries and patterns of injury are characteristic of having been sustained in self-defence, always be aware of other possible explanations.

Blunt force defence injuries

Ulna shaft fractures

Individuals who are being attacked with weapons such as baseball bats or truncheons typically raise their hands up in front of their faces in an attempt to protect themselves. This exposes the ulnar aspects of the forearms—direct blows may cause isolated fractures of the ulna shaft (the so called 'nightstick injury').

Other injuries

When under attack from fists and/or boots, a common response is to protect the face and if lying on the ground, to curl up into a ball. As a result, bruises and abrasions occur over the extensor aspect of the hands and forearms and also over the exposed lateral aspects of the upper arms.

Sharp force defence injuries

Palmar knife wounds

An individual who is being attacked by an assailant who is wielding a knife may attempt to grasp the blade of the knife (Fig. 5.6a). This typically results in palmar incised wounds. However, injuries to the extensor aspect of the hand and forearm may also result from defensive actions during an attack (Fig. 5.6 b & c).

(a)　　　　　　　　　　(b)

(c)

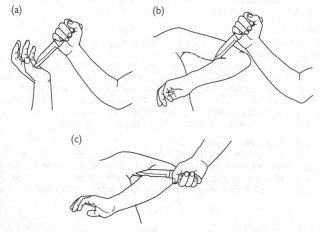

Fig. 5.6 Defence injuries.

Intimate partner violence and abuse

Background and definitions

The term 'intimate partner violence and abuse' is in the process of replacing older terms such as 'wife battering', 'spouse abuse', and 'domestic violence'. This new terminology takes into account the following facts:

- There is more to abuse than physical violence.
- Violence and abuse does not just occur between married couples, but in other relationships also.
- Men can be victims as well as women (and may be particularly embarrassed and reluctant to admit to being abused).

In the past, a combination of legal and cultural factors conspired to almost legitimize the abuse of women by their husbands. Changes in attitude have been accompanied by changes in legislation. These include the introduction of equal rights for women and the acceptance of the concept of rape within marriage.

Scope

Intimate partner violence and abuse is much more than physical injury inflicted by one partner on the other. It often involves control by one partner of the other and can involve one or more of the following elements:

- Physical injury
- Threat of physical injury (to partner and/or children/dependants)
- Sexual abuse
- Verbal abuse and isolation
- Emotional abuse
- Economic abuse.

It is acknowledged that children who are brought up with a background of intimate partner violence and abuse suffer as a result.

Prosecution—the victim and the police

Traditionally, in the UK, the police have not successfully prosecuted as many cases of intimate partner violence and abuse as they might have done. Once reunited back in the home, the injured party (traditionally the woman), retracted her statement, possibly in fear and in the belief that this was the best course of action for her own safety and that of her children and the police did not follow through a prosecution. Attitudes have now changed in that the police will consider prosecution even if the injured party no longer wishes this to occur.

Medical presentations

Many victims fail to seek medical attention for their injuries. When they do, the reported history of injury may hide what actually happened. Deaths as part of abuse do occur, but appear to be relatively rare. Occasionally, perpetrators are killed in self-defence or in retribution for past attacks.

Elder abuse and neglect

An increasing proportion of the general population is elderly and with advances in medical care, this demographic change seems set to continue. Amongst this group, there are an increasing number of individuals with dementia and other chronic health problems. At the same time, abuse of the elderly has emerged as a recognizable entity. Elder abuse includes domestic elder abuse (abuse by a family member or caregiver), institutional abuse (abuse in a residential facility, usually by carer), or self-abuse (self-neglect which involves refusal to accept the basic needs of food, drink, medicine, warmth, and shelter).

There are six main forms of elder abuse:
- Physical abuse
- Sexual abuse
- Psychological or emotional abuse
- Neglect
- Abandonment
- Financial exploitation.

Being aware of the possibility of elder abuse is the key to recognition, otherwise appropriate action cannot be taken.

Torture

Definition
There are many different definitions of torture. In forensic practice, the most useful definition is the deliberate infliction of severe physical and/or psychological harm on an individual by a perpetrator who acts on behalf of a state. Paradoxically, the torture is usually administered by the very individual tasked with guarding and taking care of the detained person.

History
In medieval times, it was considered perfectly acceptable for the state to use torture in order to extract information or confessions. During the 20th century, there developed an international agreement about the unacceptability of the use of torture. Despite this, torture continues into the 21st century. Forensic practitioners may be involved in the examination and treatment of those who have been tortured and in the investigation of torture and war crimes.

Purpose of torture
Torture may be inflicted for a number of reasons, including one or more of the following:
- To obtain information
- To extract a confession
- To punish
- To spread psychological terror in a community
- To force collaboration and strengthen a regime
- Ethnic cleansing
- Personal gain and/or gratification.

Commonly employed torture methods
Torture may be classified into physical and psychological forms, although such distinctions are somewhat artificial. Commonly employed forms are:
- *Beating* which takes many forms. It includes telefono, where the ears are simultaneously struck, leading to tympanic membrane rupture. Falanga is beating of the soles of the foot, which can result in permanent difficulty walking.
- *Suspension* can cause dislocations and nerve damage.
- *Asphyxiation* includes wet submarino, which involves submersion of the head until unconsciousness ensues. Dry submarino uses a plastic bag over the head to achieve the same thing.
- *Electrical torture* typically targets the most sensitive body areas.
- *Sexual torture and rape* is common and takes many forms.
- *Administration of drugs* may weaken resistance and be used to assist with interrogation.
- *Psychological torture* may involve sleep deprivation, dehydration, food and water deprivation, forced nakedness, humiliation, social isolation, mock execution, prolonged interrogations, continuous noise, and/or bright lights.

Medical examination of victims

Acute findings

When examined soon after injury, it is particularly important to carefully and accurately document injuries, as long-term evidence may diminish or disappear.

Chronic findings

Many of the forms of torture which are used are specifically chosen to leave little or no long-term evidence. It is usually advisable for assessment, examination, and treatment of both physical injuries and psychological effects to be undertaken by respective experts in examination of torture victims. Specialist investigations, such as MRI and nerve conduction studies may be useful in the detection of soft tissue injuries and nerve damage respectively.

Forensic investigation of war crimes

Forensic pathologists and forensic physicians may play a key role in the investigation of alleged war crimes and torture on behalf of the United Nations and/or international community. Exhumation and forensic examination of bodies has been used in a number of different parts of the world, including Rwanda and the former Yugoslavia.

Scalp injury and skull fracture

Background

The head comprises the brain, surrounded by a strong supportive and protective 'box' (the skull), with the relatively delicate and complex bones and soft tissues of the face attached at the front. Injury to the brain is the key determinant of outcome, both in terms of survival/death and function. Fracture of the skull is, however, strongly linked with significant damage to the brain.

Scalp injury

Incised wounds follow sharp force trauma, typically in the form of knives or broken bottles. Blunt force causes lacerations, haematomas (including those under the galea aponeurosis—*subgaleal haematomas*), and occasionally even degloving injuries. These last injuries may occur, for instance, when long hair is caught up in machinery.

Most scalp injuries do not in themselves threaten life, but it is worth noting that in infants significant haemorrhage can result from scalp injury. At autopsy, scalp injuries are not always easy to identify, unless it is reflected back in dissection and/or the hair is shaved (see 📖 p.78).

Skull fracture

As with fractures elsewhere, fractures of the skull may be 'closed' or 'open' (compound) to the air. They may be compound via scalp wounds or occasionally, by communicating elsewhere (e.g. by extending into the frontal sinus or middle ear). Sometimes, only the outer table of the skull vault is breached and the inner table remains intact. Underlying a skull fracture, there may be contusions and/or lacerations to the cerebral (brain) tissue. The presence of a skull fracture significantly increases the chance of other associated intracranial injury being present or developing, most classically acute extradural haematoma occurring as a result of damage to the anterior branch of the middle meningeal artery (Fig. 5.7; see also 📖 p.149):

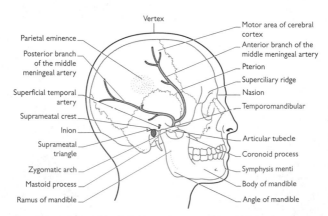

Fig. 5.7 Lateral view of the skull showing the course of the middle meningeal artery.

Skull fractures take many shapes and forms, as outlined here:

Linear fractures

Running in a line, these fractures are the most common, typically affecting the vault after the application of blunt force. Fractures which damage an underlying meningeal artery cause extradural haemorrhage (see 🕮 p.149). Secondary fracture lines may radiate away in a *stellate* ('star shaped') fashion. Repeated blows to an already fractured skull may result in *comminution* (multiple bony fragments).

Base of skull fractures

These include the devastating *hinge fracture*, in which a transverse fracture through the petrous temporal bone allows the two parts of the skull to open up like a hinge. Unsurprisingly, this injury is often seen at autopsy. Other skull base fractures were often not seen on X-ray (although now may be seen on CT), but may be apparent clinically in a variety of ways, including: bilateral 'raccoon' eyes, haemotympanum, otorrhoea, rhinorrhoea, Battle's sign (bruising over the mastoid appearing late after injury).

Ring fractures

Fractures around the foramen magnum in a ring usually reflect significant trauma, often in the form of a fall from a height or high-speed motorcycle crash (with impact to the top of the head).

Depressed fractures

Inward displacement of the inner table of the skull may reflect force applied to a relatively small area of the skull (e.g. hammer blow), or the application of extreme amounts of force to a larger area (e.g. assault by an axe). In those who survive any form of depressed fracture, epilepsy is common. Other more dramatic penetrating injuries follow gunshot injuries and explosions—fragments of skull bone may be forced into the brain. *Bullets* typically punch out sharp-edged defects in the outer skull table, with larger defects in the inner table.

Contrecoup fractures

Injury to the back of the skull (occiput), typically when an individual falls backwards, may cause a fracture of the thin orbital plates at the front of the base of the skull due to the 'rebound' of the brain.

Diastasis

Separation of normal suture lines before they have fused may occur in children as a result of brain swelling (not a fracture), but this can also occur as a fracture in older individuals.

Puppe's rule—fractures from two or more injuries

This rule was devised to assist forensic interpretation when there is more than one fracture from more than one blunt force injury. Puppe's rule is that fracture lines resulting from the second injury will not cross those from the first, thereby helping identification of which fracture occurred first. The rule has been recently applied to analysis of radial fracture lines caused by multiple bullet wounds to the head.

Primary brain injury

The brain may be injured by the *primary insult* (contusions, diffuse axonal injury, lacerations, and penetrating wounds) or the subsequent development of *secondary effects* (cerebral oedema, haematoma, infection, fits).

Cerebral contusions

Bruising to the brain occurs both at the site of injury ('coup contusion') and at the opposite pole ('contrecoup'), with the latter reflecting injury to the brain as it decelerates against the internal skull surface. Contusions typically affect the cortical surface, when there is associated haemorrhage into the adjacent subarachnoid space. Contusions may also occur deep in the brain tissue or as a result of massive brain swelling and movement (*herniation contusions*). In those who survive, cerebral contusions heal to leave cavitated scars.

Lacerations and massive crush injuries

Massive crush distortion of the brain, avulsions, and lacerations are usually unsurvivable. Although avulsions affecting the brainstem (e.g. at the pontomedullary junction) and lacerations elsewhere (e.g. corpus callosum) may follow closed head injury, most lacerations result from the effects of fracture fragments or penetrative foreign material.

Diffuse axonal injury

Diffuse axonal damage throughout the brain may follow hypoxic insult as well as serious head injury. For this reason, within the context of head injury, it is properly referred to as '*traumatic diffuse axonal injury*'. Shearing of axons (and adjacent small blood vessels) occurs during acceleration/deceleration and there is often some associated subdural haemorrhage. Many individuals do not survive, but in those who do, it can be a difficult diagnosis to make. Autopsy findings are characteristic, both macroscopically and microscopically. Macroscopically, there may be haemorrhages in the corpus callosum and basal ganglia. Microscopically, it may be difficult to identify changes if the individual has died within the first few hours after injury. Following this, injured axons swell and then when completely disrupted, form 'retraction bulbs', visible using standard haematoxylin and eosin staining. Histologically, staining with antibodies to detect the presence of beta-amyloid precursor protein within axons has been used to identify injury to them within 24h.

Traumatic intracranial haemorrhage

The brain is surrounded by a number of layers, collectively called the meninges, comprising (from inside out) the pia mater, arachnoid mater, and dura mater. Bleeding following trauma may occur between these various layers as outlined next.

Subarachnoid haemorrhage

The subarachnoid space contains cerebrospinal fluid which helps to 'cushion' and protect the brain. A small amount of bleeding into this space accompanies most cortical contusions. Larger amounts of haemorrhage can occur, particularly in association with serious (often unsurvivable) injuries to the base of the skull. Traumatic subarachnoid haemorrhage needs to be distinguished from non-traumatic ('spontaneous') bleeding from other causes (e.g. from rupture of berry aneurysms in the circle of Willis or haemorrhage from arteriovenous malformations).

Subdural haemorrhage

Bleeding under the dura mater results from damage to bridging veins that drain into the venous sinuses. There may or may not be associated skull fractures and/or cerebral contusions. Bleeding may be acute or chronic.

Acute subdural haematomas

These may follow very minor trauma in the elderly, alcoholics, and/or those with a bleeding disorder. Individuals who are taking anticoagulants (e.g. warfarin) are at particular risk. Bleeding tends to track around the brain and when significant, can cause shift of the midline and transtentorial or uncal herniation (see later in this section).

Chronic subdural haematomas

Typically develop over days or weeks as a gradual accumulation of blood and are seen in the elderly and very young. The accumulation may result from further haemorrhage and/or possibly the osmotic effect of a slowly liquefying haematoma. There may be no history of injury available, rendering it a clinically difficult diagnosis. Attempting to establish the time of injury can be of considerable medicolegal importance at autopsy, but it is extremely difficult to do this with any degree of certainty. Haematomas which are more than a week old tend to turn brown in colour and develop a surface membrane, and start to liquefy after about 3 weeks. Sometimes the diagnosis is only made at autopsy, but when the diagnosis is made during life, it can be difficult for neurosurgeons to decide if and when to time surgical intervention.

Extradural haemorrhage

This injury, also known as epidural haemorrhage, usually results from a skull fracture which damages a meningeal artery (e.g. the anterior branch of the middle meningeal artery) as it courses along the inner aspect of the skull. The resulting bleeding strips the dura mater away from the skull to rapidly produce a unilateral lens-shaped collection of blood which may cause midline shift and fatal compression of the brainstem. The classic presentation is of an initial injury (with or without loss of consciousness), followed by a lucid interval of several hours, before unconsciousness (and if not surgically evacuated) death ensues. Extradural haemorrhage may occur in the absence of a skull fracture, as in the case of actress Natasha Richardson (see box).

Extradural haemorrhage in a historical context

The famous actress Natasha Richardson died on 18 March 2009, aged 45 years, from an extradural haemorrhage, sustained in what appeared initially to be a relatively minor fall on a beginners' ski slope at Mont Tremblant in Quebec. For the first hour after the injury she was reported to be 'fine', but then deteriorated. Commentators reported this lucid interval as 'talk and die syndrome' and called for helmets to be used more widely during skiing.

Another well-known individual to succumb to extradural haemorrhage was Dr Robert Atkins, famous for the 'Atkins diet', which focuses upon the control of carbohydrate intake. He slipped and fell on his way to work, aged 72 years.

One death which some have postulated to be due to extradural haemorrhage was that of the biblical giant Goliath at the hands of David. It is generally agreed that Goliath was almost certainly suffering from visual field defects resulting from a pituitary adenoma. Speculation continues, but many now believe that original sources indicate that his temples were protected by a metal helmet and that he sustained a frontal blow which resulted in pituitary haemorrhage.

Further complications of brain injury

Cerebral swelling
Massive swelling of part or all of the brain (and/or haemorrhage) can follow serious injury and cause a dramatic increase in intracranial pressure. This can lead to unconsciousness and death, with the final pathway often involving herniation of part of the brain down and out of its normal position, resulting in compression and pressure on vital brain centres. For example, as a result of pressure from above on one side, the midbrain may be pushed against the free edge of the tentorium, causing a characteristic (Kernohan's) notch in the cerebral peduncle. Dramatic and symmetrical pressure from above may cause the cerebellar tonsils to be forced into the foramen magnum (so called 'coning').

At autopsy, cerebral oedema is apparent macroscopically as there is a greatly increased weight and filling out of the normal sulci ('valleys'), with smoothing of the gyri ('ridges').

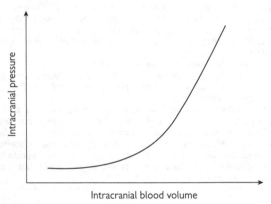

Fig. 5.8 Monro doctrine: intracranial pressure according to intracranial blood volume.

Meningitis and brain abscesses
Bacterial meningitis can result from any compound skull fracture. Brain abscess is particularly associated with compound skull fractures involving penetration of the brain by foreign material or bony fragments.

Post-traumatic fits
Seizures may occur after head injury, either in the early period or later as a long-term problem. Penetrating brain injury, lacerations, haematomas, and contusions are risk factors.

Chronic brain injury—boxing

Boxers can take a very large number of blows to the head during a career. The 'punch drunk' clinical presentation is of Parkinsonism, dysarthria, ataxia, and dementia ('dementia pugilistica'). There are characteristic chronic changes within the brain: degeneration of the substantia nigra, fenestration of the septum pellucidum, scarring of the cerebellum and other parts of the brain.

Boxing death after world title fight

The potential for boxing to cause acute head injury was clearly demonstrated when US boxer Leavander Johnson died in Las Vegas in September 2005. Having failed to successfully defend his world title, he was able to leave the ring unassisted, although he visibly struggled to reach the dressing room. He collapsed shortly afterwards and died despite undergoing prompt surgery for an acute subdural haematoma. Inevitable calls to 'ban boxing' followed and the sport has continued to court controversy to the present time.

Facial injury

The bony skeleton of the face is an intricate construction of relatively delicate bones. A variety of fractures can result from injury and there are frequently medicolegal implications. Very often, injuries reflect assaults, typically taking the form of punches, kicks, or blunt injury from weapons (bottles, baseball bats). Many blunt force injuries to the face do not cause a fracture, but result in bruising to the soft tissues, with the classic example being a periorbital haematoma ('black eye'). The soft tissues of the face are often targeted in assaults involving sharp force trauma, with scars having very significant cosmetic effects.

Le Fort facial fractures

Very serious facial fractures can follow blunt force trauma, such as high-speed car crashes (particularly when no seat belt is worn and the front seat occupant smashes into the inside of the windscreen). All result in some instability of the middle third of the face. Le Fort fractures are classified into three types:

- **Le Fort I fracture** is also known as a Guérin fracture. It involves the premaxilla above the apices of the teeth, rendering the upper front teeth a mobile unit.
- **Le Fort II (pyramidal) fracture** refers to a fracture line which extends through the maxilla (cheek bone) on both sides, meeting in the middle at the nose.
- **Le Fort III fracture** is a high transverse injury which reflects the face being essentially 'sheared off' from the face (craniofacial separation). Bleeding and/or airway compromise may be dramatic and even be the principal cause of death.

René Le Fort (1869–1951)

This French surgeon conducted a series of somewhat bizarre experiments on the skulls of cadavers. Having applied a variety of forms of blunt trauma, he carefully observed the resulting fracture patterns, from which he devised his classification of three types of midfacial fractures.

Other facial fractures

Isolated fractures to the nose, maxilla, and mandible are all relatively common injuries. They each often follow interpersonal violence (see 📖 p.286).

Spinal injury

Cervical spine injury

Fractures and dislocations can result in complete transactions of the medulla oblongata or cervical spinal cord. Damage to the upper cord is fatal without medical intervention (the phrenic nerve supplying the diaphragm is derived from C3,4,5 spinal roots). **Complete cord damage** to the cord below this typically results in paralysis, loss of sensation, neurogenic shock (bradycardia and hypotension from loss of sympathetic tone to the heart), spinal shock (flaccidity and loss of tendon reflexes), priapism. There are many clinical patterns of **partial spinal cord damage**, perhaps the most intriguing being spinal cord injury without radiographic abnormality (SCIWORA).

Common patterns of cervical bony injury are summarized as follows:
- **Jefferson fracture** is a compression fracture of the ring of C1 (the atlas), often without neurological damage.
- **Odontoid peg fractures** are the commonest fractures to affect C2 (the axis), perhaps reflecting the slightly unusual anatomy.
- **Hangman fracture** affects the posterior part of C2 (both pedicles or pars interarticularis), usually from an extension mechanism, with or without distraction.

Judicial hanging

Until the mid 19th century in the UK, judicial hanging involved a short fall (a few feet), with death occurring painfully by asphyxiation. The drop distance was increased to 4–6 feet with the aim of causing a (hangman) fracture and severance of the spinal cord, resulting in rapid unconsciousness and death. The concept of a 'measured drop' was introduced in 1872, whereby the height of the drop was tailored to the individual. An excessive drop, however, can result in decapitation, as occurred during the execution of the Iraqi al-Tikriti in January 2007.

Fracture—dislocations of the cervical spine
Unifacet or bilateral facet joint subluxations/dislocations are usually associated with significant neurological damage.

Thoracic and lumbar spine injuries

The most vulnerable part is the thoracolumbar junction, with injuries to the vertebral body of L1 often occurring during falls from a height. The spinal cord terminates around the level of L1, but damage below this can injure the cauda equina (collection of nerve roots). **Cauda equina syndrome** is characterized by bladder and bowel dysfunction.

The vertebral bodies of the lumbar spine are particularly prone to osteoporosis-related collapse. A specific severe injury to the lumbar spine is a **Chance fracture**—a transverse fracture through the vertebral body/disc, reflecting significant trauma, usually distraction in flexion, and often associated with intra-abdominal injury and neurological damage.

Chest injury

Serious chest injury may follow penetrating or blunt injury.

Penetrating chest injuries include knife stab and bullet injuries, which often result in pneumothorax. Death may follow damage to the heart or great vessels, resulting in massive haemothorax and/or cardiac tamponade. Significant defects in the chest wall may cause sucking chest wounds.

Blunt chest injuries include falls and motor vehicle collisions. Rib fractures are common and the sharp broken rib ends can cause pneumothorax and sometimes also damage to great vessels and/or the heart. Multiple rib fractures can result in a flail segment. Massive shear forces can result in rapidly fatal aortic rupture.

Sternal fracture

Isolated fractures often occur as a result of seat belt restraint in car crashes. There is sometimes associated myocardial injury.

Rib fracture

Isolated rib fracture is a common (clinical) diagnosis (see 📖 p.299), often resulting from a low fall. Ribs typically break at the posterolateral junction and heal well within a few weeks, albeit with deformity.

Flail segment

Fractures of three or more ribs in two places can result in a mobile (flail) segment of chest wall. A massive flail segment including the sternum can occur when large numbers of anterior ribs are broken bilaterally. A flail segment moves in opposite direction to the rest of the chest (i.e. moving in on breathing in), adding considerably to the work of breathing.

Pneumothorax

Once a lung is punctured (e.g. by a broken rib or knife), a connection is established between the (inter)pleural space and the lung air spaces, causing the lung to collapse. Occasionally, the connection acts as a one-way valve, causing pressure to build, the lung to collapse completely, and the mediastinum to start to shift (away) from the *tension pneumothorax*. Mediastinal shift in a tension pneumothorax results in kinking of the great veins, thereby obstructing venous return and reducing cardiac output.

Sucking chest wound

A significant defect (hole) in the chest wall may result from impalements and gunshots. The defect, connecting with underlying pneumothorax, may offer much less resistance to air flow than the usual air passages and thereby prevent the normal inflation/deflation of the lungs.

Aortic injury

Rapid deceleration which occurs in a very high fall or high-speed motor vehicle collision can result in transection of the thoracic aorta at the point where the mobile arch meets the fixed descending part (at the level of the ligamentum arteriosum). The traditional explanation for the injury relates to differential movement ('shearing') of the mobile and fixed parts, but there are alternative pathophysiological theories. One is that the clavicle and first rib move down to pinch the aorta ('osseous pinch theory'). Whatever the exact mechanism, the result of a complete transection is usually rapidly fatal torrential haemorrhage. Occasionally, there may be contained haemorrhage, allowing survival to hospital.

Other great vessel damage

Bleeding from great blood vessels and their branches may follow direct penetration (e.g. from knife, bullet, or broken rib) or tearing. There may be a resultant massive haemothorax (collection of blood in the pleural cavity). The chance of survival depends upon the exact nature of the injury.

> ### The death of Princess Diana
> In the early hours of 31 August 1997, Princess Diana was the rear seat passenger in a car which was involved in a high-speed collision in a Paris underpass. The exact sequence of events that led to the crash remains the subject of much speculation, although the combination of excessive speed and alcohol in the bloodstream of the driver, Henri Martin, has been blamed. Autopsy confirmed that the cause of Diana's death to be haemorrhage from a torn pulmonary vein. There is considerable controversy about the treatment that she received at the scene, with many observers commentating that her injuries were potentially survivable. Fingers have been pointed at the system which resulted in a delay of about 2h from the time of the crash to her reaching hospital (🖑 http://www.wethepeople.la/diana4.htm). Others have focused upon the fact that she was not wearing a seat belt at the time of the crash.

Myocardial injury

Direct penetration into a cardiac chamber or blunt cardiac rupture can cause significant bleeding or *cardiac tamponade*. The latter reflects a collection of blood in the pericardial cavity, which prevents filling of the heart, thereby preventing cardiac output.

Blunt injury to the chest can cause fatal ventricular arrhythmia (*commotio cordis*), even when the heart is healthy. This may occur when a hard ball or kick is applied to the front of the chest in a sporting context.

Abdominal injury

The upper abdominal contents are partly protected by the lower ribs, but the lower abdomen is relatively unprotected.

Liver and splenic injury

Although protected by overlying ribs, fractures to lower ribs are associated with liver and splenic injury. The principal risk of trauma to the liver and spleen is haemorrhage, which may be torrential and rapidly life-threatening. Occasionally, there is an initially contained haematoma which ruptures and causes problems days later.

The spleen, malaria, and murder
Disease can render the spleen much more likely to bleed after injury. This fact has been used historically by assassins in the Far East, who have targeted the enlarged malarial spleen by attacking their victims with a blunt metal object called a larang. Applied with force into the left upper abdomen, the victim bleeds to death from splenic rupture, with little in the way of external marks being left on the body.

Diaphragmatic rupture

Massive force applied to the lower chest/upper abdomen may result in rupture of the diaphragm, thereby forcing intra-abdominal contents into the chest, causing amongst other things, serious respiratory compromise. On the left side, it is the stomach and spleen which are often forced upwards; on the right side, the liver.

Intestinal injury

The intestine may rupture as a result of either penetrating or blunt trauma. Perforation of any part of the intestine carries a risk of infection, particularly when diagnosis is delayed.

Pancreatic injury

Severe blunt injury to the upper abdomen can cause transection of the pancreas or acute pancreatitis.

Injury to the renal tract

Blunt force trauma can result in renal damage, including avulsion of the renal pedicle. The bladder and urethra are at risk of injury in association with pelvic fracture.

Fractures of the pelvis and extremities

Pelvic fracture

Apart from the relatively minor fractures involving the pubic rami, fractures to the pelvis carry significant risks, particularly of haemorrhage. Fractures follow a variety of different patterns, including 'vertical shear' (especially after high falls), 'open book' (typically anterior–posterior crush injury), acetabular fractures (also known as central hip dislocations, often seen in high-speed road traffic collisions). Despite the best modern treatment, including external fixation and embolization, it may prove impossible to stop haemorrhage (typically from internal iliac veins).

Extremity fractures

Most limb fractures reflect force applied to normal bones, but some (pathological) fractures occur after minimal force is applied to diseased bone (e.g. metastatic cancer, Paget's disease). Five fractures are associated with osteoporosis in the elderly: Colles' distal radius, hip, surgical neck of humerus, pubic rami, and lumbar spine compression fractures.

Fractures caused during life inevitably result in haemorrhage. In some cases, the extent of this bleeding can be life threatening. For example, it is estimated that a femoral shaft fracture is associated with approximately 1–2L of blood loss.

Terminology

Most bone fractures result in two bony fragments ('simple'), but occasionally, there is more than one fracture line, resulting in three or more bony fragments, when the fracture may be described as 'comminuted'.

Fractures with an overlying skin wound are described as 'compound' (or 'open') and are at risk of becoming infected. Fractures with no overlying wound are termed 'closed'. Fractures may be described as transverse, longitudinal, oblique, spiral, crush, or avulsion ('tension'). The type of fracture may provide an indication as to how they were caused (e.g. spiral fractures reflect the application of a twisting force).

Fracture healing

Healing occurs faster in children than adults, so, for example, a fractured distal radius in an adult is typically treated in a cast for 6 weeks, but only 3 weeks in a 10-year-old. Interestingly, fractures in young adults do not heal faster than those in the elderly. Pathophysiologically, there is an initial haematoma around the fracture, with subsequent inflammation, then osteoblasts produce new bone to form callus. Callus is visible radiologically within a few weeks of injury (2 weeks in children). It is difficult to exactly age healing fractures either radiologically or at autopsy, but it is frequently possible to conclude that there are fractures of different ages (i.e. occurring at different times)—this can be of considerable medicolegal significance, especially in suspected child abuse.

Fractures after death

Bones may be broken after death, in which case there will be a lack of vital reaction, inflammation, or evidence of healing. Note that bodies that are burned after death may sustain 'heat fractures' (see 📖 p.159).

Burns

Although the body can be burned by chemical or even microwave burns, most burns result from physical heat. In some instances, there is a short-lived ignition causing 'flash burns', whilst in others, exposure to the burning agent is more prolonged. Burns from hot liquids or steam are 'scalds'.

Depth of burns

The extent of damage to the skin from a burn depends principally upon the temperature of the burning agent and the length of exposure.

Burns are traditionally classified according to the following system:

• *First-degree burns* are superficial and comprise erythema.
• *Second-degree burns* are 'partial thickness' burns, often characterized by erythema and preserved sensation. They heal without scarring.
• *Third-degree burns* are 'full thickness' burns in which all layers of the skin are burnt, sensation is absent, and healing occurs with scarring. The burnt skin ('eschar') often appears leathery.
• *Fourth-degree burns* are very severe burns which extend deeper than the skin to involve underlying tissues (e.g. fat, muscle, bone).

Deaths from burns

A previously quoted rule of thumb was that a person was likely to survive a burn if the sum of their age and the % area burnt was <100. Improvements in treatment may have changed this, but it underlines the fact that younger individuals can tolerate larger burns. Deaths from burns are associated with airway burns and extensive burns.

Airway burns

The upper air passages, including the pharynx and larynx, are particularly susceptible to becoming rapidly and dramatically swollen when damaged by hot gases. This swelling may result in complete airway obstruction, which without prompt medical intervention has fatal results.

Breathing compromise

Circumferential full thickness burns of the chest can prevent normal chest movement and require surgical incision ('escharotomy') to allow the chest wall to move properly with respiration.

Circulatory collapse

Burns cause fluid loss which can be dramatic in larger burns, requiring many litres of intravenous fluid (± blood) to restore circulating volume. Specialists calculate the amount of fluid required in the initial 24h using the % area burnt and patient's weight (Muir and Barclay formula).

Multiorgan failure

Individuals who survive the initial insult of a large burn are at risk of later complications, including renal failure, pneumonia, generalized sepsis, disseminated intravascular coagulation, and multiorgan failure.

Smoke inhalation

Most domestic fire deaths result from smoke inhalation, particularly carbon monoxide, rather than the direct effects of burns.

Extent of burns

In clinical practice, the extent of the body surface burnt is traditionally estimated by the 'rule of 9's' and use of Lund and Browder charts. The patient's palm is said to be approximately 1% body surface area.

Rule of 9's: the following estimates are used in adults: head 9%; each arm 9%; each leg 18%; front of trunk 18%; back of trunk 18%; perineum 1%.

Note that in children, the percentages of body surface area are in different proportions to adults (e.g. the head covers a relatively larger area—in infants, it accounts for 20% of body surface area).

Autopsy findings

Severe burns result in hair being completely burnt away and full thickness skin burns. Contractures of muscles after death result in a 'pugilistic' (boxer's) posture. Given that fire has been used by murderers in an attempt to destroy evidence, it is important to try to search for injuries which may have occurred before the effects of a fire. However, several effects may be erroneously attributed to injury other than heat injury:

- Splits in the skin (contractures) may appear to be knife wounds.
- The skull and other bones may fracture due to the heat.
- An 'epidural heat haematoma' may form after death, but be mistaken for an antemortem injury.

Timing of death

It can be important to try to establish if death occurred before or after a fire started. The presence of carbon (soot) particles in the upper airways and high levels of carboxyhaemoglobin in the blood imply that a person was alive (at least for a short time) during the fire.

Identification

In many deaths involving fire, identification of a body can be very challenging. Once facial features and fingerprints have been destroyed, reliance is placed upon comparison between X-rays and dental records.

> **Plane crash at Faro**
> On 21 February 1992, a Dutch DC-10 aircraft crashed at the Portuguese airport of Faro. A British passenger, Nicola Gunner, was initially believed to have died, but was identified 9 days later by dental records to be alive in a hospital in Rotterdam. She had sustained 65% burns and unfortunately died the following year.

Spontaneous combustion

The myth of 'spontaneous combustion' has a degree of popular appeal, but has little scientific basis. It is true, however, that on occasions, a body can burn away almost completely, with relatively little fire damage to surrounding structures.

Explosive injuries

Explosions may occur in industrial (e.g. factory) or domestic (e.g. gas) settings, or reflect war or terrorist activity (e.g. bombs, grenades). Incidents almost inevitably have significant forensic/legal implications and result in understandable media interest.

Primary injuries

An intense, short-lived pressure wave lasting only a few milliseconds, expands outwards from the explosive focus. It reflects compression of air at the interface of rapidly expanding hot gases. Blast waves can be reflected from buildings. Injuries may result from the following:

- Disruption at air/tissue interfaces, especially lungs and ears, resulting in blast lung and tympanic membrane rupture respectively. Initial haemorrhage characteristic of 'blast lung' may be followed in those who survive initially by adult respiratory distress syndrome (ARDS).
- Shearing at tissue/tissue interfaces, causing subserous and submucosal haemorrhage.
- Implosion of gas-filled organs (resulting in gastrointestinal perforations and air embolism).

Blast winds

Rapidly moving columns of air following the initial blast wave can inflict tremendous damage, including amputation and even dismemberment.

Secondary ('fragmentation') injuries

Objects from within a bomb (e.g. nails, nuts, bolts) may cause abrasions, bruises, puncture lacerations, and other wounds. They can also carry debris (e.g. glass, masonry) which act as secondary missiles causing injuries.

Tertiary injuries

Individuals may be injured when thrown by the blast or strike large objects thrown by the blast and sustain ('translational') injuries. Structural collapse of buildings may also cause serious injuries.

Quaternary injuries

Heat and/or fumes from the explosion may cause burns. These are typically superficial, affecting exposed skin in individuals are located close to the explosion. Severe burns usually reflect secondary fires resulting from the initial explosion. Smoke inhalation may also occur.

Quinary injuries

These include the health effects caused by materials added to bombs, including bacteria, chemicals, and radiation. Fragments of human remains (e.g. bones from a suicide bomber) may be included in this category.

Psychological effects

It is hard to overestimate the psychological effects of being involved in a serious explosion. These effects are magnified when there are multiple casualties and/or deaths.

The attacks of 11 September 2001

On the morning of 11 September 2001, four passenger aeroplanes were taken over by hijackers with the intention of undertaking coordinated suicide attacks on buildings with international significance. The hijackers used knives to kill cabin crew and then fly towards their targets. All of the planes crashed, killing everyone on board and several thousand on the ground:

- The 110th floor North Tower of the World Trade Center in New York was struck first (at 0846 hours), caught fire, and collapsed within 2h.
- The South Tower was struck at 0903 hours, collapsing within an hour.
- The third target was the Pentagon, into which a passenger jet crashed at 0937 hours.
- The fourth hijacked plane crashed into a field in Pennsylvania at 1003 hours after passengers attempted to wrestle control of the aircraft back from the hijackers.

The attacks on the twin towers took the heaviest death toll. Most of the individuals died when the towers collapsed, although many died at the time of the initial impact and some later due to the effects of fire, with a number falling or even jumping to their deaths in an effort to escape the fire and smoke.

The short and long-term effects of the '9/11' attacks were considerable—the impacts were felt worldwide, in economic, social, and political form.

For forensic experts, the challenge of trying to identify those who died in the collapse of the twin towers was enormous. After a vast investigation, an impressive 57% of the victims were positively identified using a combination of DNA, dental records, and jewellery. However, this did leave >1000 victims who remain to be identified.

Investigations after an explosion

Forensic investigations after a suspected terrorist or other explosion will initially take second place to treating victims.

Number of fatalities

When deaths occur in any explosion, the first job is to try to establish how many people have died and exactly who they are. On those occasions when there are numerous victims with very serious injuries, it can be a considerable challenge to ascertain the number of individuals who have been killed. The process may involve a painstaking search and close examination of the retrieved body parts.

Identification

The easiest means of identification is visual confirmation of a person's identity by a relative, although corroboration by a second individual is a sensible precaution. For some casualties, visual identification may be impossible due to the extreme nature of the injuries sustained, so reliance may need to be placed upon other means, including a combination of the following:
• Fingerprints
• Tattoos
• Dental records
• Scars
• DNA (e.g. a blood sample).

Cause of death

The presence of serious injuries in the context of an explosion might lead to the simple conclusion that the explosion caused death. However, it is very important to consider the possibility that death may have occurred in another way prior to the explosion. Analysis of the injuries on each individual will help to provide an idea of the relative positions at the time of the explosion. It can be helpful to X-ray bodies prior to autopsy in order to establish where foreign material (shrapnel etc.) is embedded.

Suicide bombers

The use of suicide as a way of killing the enemy is not new, as underlined by Japanese ('kamikaze') pilots targeting allied warships in World War II. In more recent times, suicide bombers have been used against both civilian and military targets. The methods employed have varied, ranging from individuals detonating devices which are strapped to their bodies when standing close to their targets, to the use of vehicles or (as in the attacks of 11 September 2001, see p.161) aeroplanes. In most instances, the suicide bomber sustains overwhelming injuries, which may be so severe that little of the body is recovered. Occasionally, as in the case of the Exeter bomber in 2008, injuries may be relatively minor.

The 7 July 2005 London bombings

Four suicide bombers targeted London in the most deadly bomb attack on the city since World War II, in what subsequently became known as the '7/7' bombings. Three explosions occurred on the London Underground (two on the Circle line, one on the Piccadilly) and one on the top deck of a double-decker bus in Tavistock Square. In addition to the four bombers, 52 people died in the attacks. The bombers were British Muslims who appear to have been motivated to attack other members of the British public due to Britain's involvement in the war in Iraq.

The bombs

Home-made organic peroxide devices carried in rucksacks were used in the attacks. The explosive mixture comprised chapatti flour and liquid hydrogen peroxide.

Firearms

Types of weapons

Shotguns

Also known as 'smoothbore weapons', shotguns fire a bundle of lead pellets (shot) which travel down a smooth metal tube (barrel) to emerge via the muzzle. Some weapons have a double barrel, with one barrel employing a distinct taper (choke), which affects the spread of pellets. The barrels may be shortened in order to render them less conspicuous in armed crime ('sawn-off shotgun').

Rifles

The long barrel of a standard rifle contains spiral grooves ('rifles') which impart a rotation on the bullet with the intention of providing some stability as it travels through the air, thereby increasing accuracy and range. The inner aspects of the barrel between the grooves are known as the 'lands'. Minor imperfections in the rifling causes characteristic imprints on the bullet as it passes by, resulting in marks on the bullet which can be as specific as fingerprints and allow a 'match' to be made between a bullet and the weapon that fired it. The calibre of a weapon is usually defined as the inner diameter of the barrel. Military weapons are 'self-loading' (gun continues to fire each time the trigger is pulled) or 'automatic' (the weapon continues to fire once the trigger is held). Bullets which travel at >300m/s are regarded as 'high-velocity' missiles.

Handguns

Modern handguns also have rifling of the barrel. They include revolvers and automatic pistols. Revolvers have a cylinder which rotates (revolves) each time the trigger is pulled, bringing the next shell into line. Automatic pistols have spring-loaded magazines, which achieve the same.

Ammunition

This typically comprises the bullet, attached to the cartridge case, with gunpowder and primer between. When the gun's firing pin strikes the base of the cartridge, the primer is detonated and thence the gunpowder. Detonation of the gunpowder forces the bullet down the barrel at speed. At the same time, some of the gunpowder (and burnt gunpowder in the form of soot) emerges from the muzzle, causing characteristic tattooing of the skin at close range (see 📖 p.168).

- *Bullets* come in various materials, shapes, and sizes.
- *Shotgun cartridges* (shells) contain numerous lead pellets.

Anatomy of guns (Fig. 5.9)

(a)

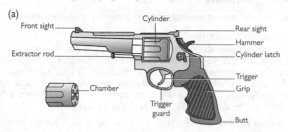

(b)

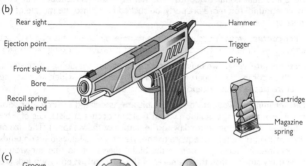

(c)

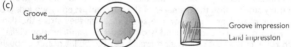

Fig. 5.9 Anatomy of guns: a) parts of a revolver; b) parts of a semi-automatic revolver; c) left, cross-sectional view of a rifled barrel, right, bullet fired from a weapon having a right-handed twist to its rifling.

Rifled gunshot injuries

Careful analysis of gunshot wounds can yield important forensic information.

Entry wounds from rifles

Close contact between the muzzle of the weapon and the skin results in characteristic contact wounds, which depend upon the type of weapon, the part of the body injured, and the angle of contact. Firm contact forces the bullet and associated hot gases under the skin and leaves a muzzle imprint on the skin. Depending upon the part of the body affected, in some instances, the skin may split open at this entry point.

Loose contact wounds typically result in a dark ring of soot. Note that in close and near contact wounds, material from the target (hair, skin, etc.) may 'rebound' (or, more properly, be sucked back) into the muzzle of the weapon.

Near contact wounds occur when the muzzle is close, but is not in direct contact with the skin. There is no significant powder tattooing of the skin.

Intermediate range wounds result in gunpowder tattooing of the skin, which becomes less apparent and spread out over a wider area as the distance between the weapon and skin increases.

Distant gunshot wounds do not exhibit any associated tattooing or soot staining of the skin, a situation which typically occurs at distances of >1m (although it does vary according to the nature of the weapon). The size of the (entry) hole does not equate to the size of the bullet, as the skin tends to become stretched just before the bullet pierces it, so that the wound is typically smaller than the diameter of the bullet. Most entry wounds are circular or oval, depending upon the angle at which they strike the skin. The skin around the entry wound is discoloured as an 'abrasion collar', which reflects the heat and friction created as the bullet passes through the skin.

Exit wounds

It is important to try to distinguish entry from exit wounds. This task is not usually very difficult. Exit wounds tend to be larger and more irregular than entry wounds, as the bullet is likely to be deformed and travelling in less predictable fashion as it exits the body. There is usually no abrasion collar, although this can occur when the skin at the point of exit is pressed against a hard surface—the resulting wound is referred to as a 'shored wound'.

Autopsy procedures

It is standard practice to X-ray the body of anyone who is found dead after gunshot injury, in order to identify the number and position of bullets prior to autopsy. Probes may be helpful in demonstrating the paths taken by bullets.

Behaviour of bullets inside the body

Gunshot wounds are regarded as medium- and high-energy injuries. As the bullet travels through the body tissues, it crushes tissues, stretches adjacent tissue, and creates a large temporary cavity, which can cause widespread damage. This damage is much greater with high-energy weapons, where the vacuum effect of the temporary cavity can suck clothing and other foreign material into the wound. Bullets behave differently according to the tissues through which they pass:

- Bone may shatter as it is struck by a bullet, resulting in numerous fragments which cause damage as secondary missiles.
- Head injuries from gunshot can be devastating, particularly when high-energy weapons are used, when the skull can 'explode'. As a bullet passes through the skull bone, the internal defect is usually larger than the external one, giving a 'cratered' (or 'funnelled') appearance at autopsy. Bullets may ricochet inside the skull.
- Chest injuries are often fatal, due to overwhelming damage to the heart and large vessels. Bullets which pass through the lungs produce an inevitable pneumothorax (see 📖 p.154), but due to the less dense nature of the lungs, less energy tends to be transferred to the tissues.
- Abdominal injury from gunshot injury can also be devastating, depending upon the structures damaged. Damage to the bowel adds considerably to the potential for infection.

Bullet emboli

Occasionally, bullets enter the vascular system (either venous or arterial system) and a distance around the body. This can result in an initial impression of a 'missing bullet'.

The shooting of John F. Kennedy

Perhaps the best-known gunshot wounds in history were those inflicted on the US President, John F. Kennedy. The 46-year-old suffered fatal gunshot wounds whilst travelling in a motorcade in Texas on 22 November 1963. An autopsy performed at Bethesda Naval Hospital concluded that he sustained two gunshot wounds: one (the 'fatal' injury) to the back of his head and the other to his upper back. A man named Lee Harvey Oswald was arrested a little more than an hour later on suspicion of having been responsible for the assassination, but he was himself shot and killed before he could stand trial. An official report at the time concluded that Oswald was responsible, but this did not stop a myriad of conspiracy theories. Many of these theories persist to this day, perhaps being partly fuelled by apparent discrepancies in previous accounts and doubt being cast upon the validity of the autopsy findings.

Shotgun injuries

Shotguns fire multiple lead pellets ('shot') via a smoothbored barrel. The pellets initially emerge from the muzzle grouped closely together, but gradually spread out and disperse as they travel away from the weapon. The extent to which the pellets spread out varies from weapon to weapon and depends upon the taper ('choke') of the barrel, as well as the type of ammunition which was used. In addition to the pellets emerging from the muzzle, so do wads (typically made of cardboard or felt), powder, and soot, which cause characteristic marks when the shotgun is discharged at close range.

Shotgun entry wounds (Fig. 5.10)

Contact wounds produce a skin wound of approximately the size of the internal diameter of the barrel, although in certain circumstances, larger wounds can occur (especially over the skull, when overlying skin can be torn away). As with rifled injuries, there may be a muzzle imprint. Sometimes, carbon monoxide in the hot discharge gases may bind to myoglobin and haemoglobin in the wound, causing pink/cherry red discoloration.

Near contact (close range) shotgun wounds of <15cm are circular defects, with soot staining and powder tattooing of adjacent skin, which may be burnt (and have burnt hairs)—see Fig. 5.10(f). The wad is usually to be found buried in the wound.

Intermediate range wounds comprise less perfect circular skin defects, perhaps with some pellets making individual (satellite) holes outside this (reflecting minor dispersal of the pellets). Usually with the wad is buried in the wound. The skin edges tend only to be blackened if the range is within 30cm and similarly, skin tattooing occurs only for distances less than 1m.

Longer range shotgun wounds exhibit a wider spread of pellets (Fig 5.10(a)), although a central defect may still be seen at ranges <10m (Fig. 5.10(b)). Determination of the exact range may require test firing of the weapon using identical ammunition.

Direction of shotgun injury

When a shotgun is discharged at right angles to the skin, the resulting central defect will be circular, but will become an ellipse when the weapon is applied tangentially. In the case of the latter, one edge of the wound will be undercut. It can be difficult to trace the exact paths of shotgun pellets, especially when there is deflection/ricochet off other structure, notably bone.

Shotgun exit wounds

Because of the relatively small size and velocity of the pellets, they rarely completely penetrate the adult trunk, but can penetrate the limbs and neck. When fired in suicidal fashion through the open mouth, a shotgun is capable of a devastating destructive lesion in which much of the brain is expelled from a large defect in the skull.

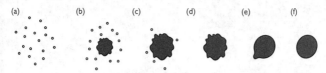

Fig. 5.10 Shotgun entry wounds, ranging from near contact wounds (f) through to longer range wounds (a).

The police custody unit

The custody unit

Depriving individuals of their liberty is a serious matter and the grounds for arresting and detaining individuals are carefully prescribed in law. You can be arrested and taken into police custody with or without a warrant. A warrant for someone's arrest can be issued if, for example, he/she is suspected of a serious offence such as murder, but the police can also take him/her into custody without a warrant to take fingerprints or if they have 'reasonable grounds' to suspect that he/she committed an offence.

In England and Wales, the rules governing powers of arrest and detention are set out in the Police and Criminal Evidence Act 1984 (PACE)—see 🕮 p.176.

Designated police stations

Every police force has a list of 'designated police stations', which are deemed to be fit for purpose by the force's chief police officer. Cells in designated stations are intended for single occupancy and cell sharing should only occur on an exceptional basis. Cells should provide basic amenities, such as a mattress, clean bedding, and access to a toilet and washing facilities. They should be designed to a nationally approved standard that ensures there are no ligature points for self-suspension.

Increasingly, closed-circuit television (CCTV) is being used to monitor activity in police stations. CCTV-equipped cells may be used to monitor vulnerable individuals whilst in custody.

The custody officer

There has to be at least one custody officer appointed to every designated police station. Custody officers are in charge of ensuring the welfare of those in police custody. They are police officers of the rank of sergeant or above who cannot be involved in the investigation of the offence for which a person has been arrested. They are responsible for:
- Authorizing a person's detention.
- Ensuring that he/she is given rights and entitlements.
- Opening a custody record for each detainee.
- Making sure the investigation into the offence for which the person has been arrested is carried out diligently.
- Deciding, in conjunction with the Crown Prosecution Service (CPS), whether there is sufficient evidence to charge a person and if so, whether that person should be released on bail or kept in custody to appear before the next available court.

In Scotland, where PACE does not apply, the Scottish Police Service still has a statutory duty to care for persons in custody under the Criminal Procedure (Scotland) Act 1995. Under this legislation, suitably skilled and trained Police Custody and Security Officers (PCSOs) are able to exercise powers and undertake duties that include ensuring the well-being of detainees. The role of the PCSO in this respect is essentially the same as the custody officer in England and Wales.

Detention officers

The custody officer is assisted by detention officers, who may be police officers or specially trained civilians. Detention officers play a key role in attending to the welfare needs of detainees, including providing them with food and drink, allowing them washing facilities, conducting regular cell visits, and arranging for the attendance of a healthcare professional as necessary. Detention officers may also assist investigating officers by undertaking tasks such as fingerprinting and photographing detainees and obtaining saliva samples for drug testing.

Designated detention officers

Designated Detention Officers were introduced in England, Wales and Northern Ireland under the Police Reform Act 2002. One of their functions is to conduct drug testing on detainees arrested for trigger offences, but they also assist custody officers in many aspects of their work.

Independent custody visitors (ICVs)

The ICV scheme, which operates in England, Wales, and Northern Ireland, represents an important safeguard for detainees, as it involves unannounced visits and private consultations by impartial members of the public. ICVs are volunteers whose role is to attend police stations to check on the treatment of detainees and the conditions in which they are held, and to establish that their rights are bring observed. Responsibility for organizing and overseeing the delivery of independent custody visiting lies with police authorities, in consultation with chief constables.

ICVs can visit a police station at any time and must be given immediate access to all custody areas unless doing so would place them in danger. A report is completed after very visit and copies are provided for the police, police authorities, ICV groups, and the Home Office. Independent custody visiting was introduced into Scotland on a non-statutory basis in 2000.

Drug arrest referral schemes

Drug arrest referral schemes should operate in most custody suites to encourage drug misusers in contact with the police service to voluntarily participate in confidential programmes of advice, information, and treatment. The schemes are facilitated by drug arrest referral workers who work in custody units and seek to help detainees who misuse drugs to address their problem and find a solution for their drug misuse.

Purpose of detention

As soon as is practicable after arrival at the custody unit, the custody officer must determine whether there is sufficient evidence to charge an individual with the offence for which he/she has been arrested. The custody officer may detain a person for as long as is necessary to make such a determination—this may include waiting for others arrested at the same time to be interviewed.

As soon as the custody officer determines that there is sufficient evidence to charge a person, he/she should either be charged or released without charge, the latter may be on bail or without bail. If released without charge, the custody officer is obliged to inform the detainee if the decision about whether he/she is to be prosecuted for the offence has not yet been taken.

Detention without charge

If the custody officer decides that there is insufficient evidence to charge a detainee, then he/she must be released either on bail or without bail. The only exception to this is when the custody officer has reasonable grounds for believing that detention without charge is necessary:

• To secure or preserve evidence relating to the offence for which a person has been arrested, for example by seizing clothing or taking forensic samples.
• To obtain such evidence by questioning.

In these circumstances, the custody officer may order further detention, but must make a record in writing of the grounds for detention and tell the detainee what these grounds are.

Detention without charge cannot be authorized in a person's own interest (e.g. to receive medical treatment that has been recommended by a healthcare professional), or to prevent the repetition or continuation of an offence.

Review of detention

Periodic reviews of detention must be carried out for all persons in police custody, pending the investigation of an offence. If a detainee has been charged, the review is carried out by the custody officer. If a detainee has not been charged, it is carried out by an officer of at least the rank of inspector, who has not at any stage been directly involved with the investigation. The general rule is that the first review should be conducted not later than 6h after an individual's detention was first authorized, and subsequent reviews must take place at intervals of not more than 9h.

Before deciding whether to authorize detention of an individual, the review officer must give him/her (unless asleep) and his/her legal representative an opportunity to make oral or written representations. An inspector may, in certain circumstances, carry out reviews by telephone or using video-conferencing facilities.

The detention clock

The length of time for which a person may remain in police detention is limited by legislation. Such limitations are based of the passage of time from a particular point—that point being referred to as the 'relevant time'. As a general rule, the detention clock starts running from the time a person arrives at the first police station to which he/she is taken after arrest, rather than from the time of arrest. If arrest takes place at the police station, the time starts when that arrest occurs.

The detention clock stops when a person in police detention is taken to hospital for medical treatment and only restarts when the person arrives back at the police station. However, the detention clock is not suspended when a person receives medical treatment at a police station or when a forensic practitioner recommends a period of 'sobering up' before a person is fit to be interviewed.

Detention limits

The basic rule is that a person may not be held in police detention for >24h without being charged. This period can be extended for a maximum of 12h by an officer of the rank of superintendent or above in circumstances where:
- The officer has reasonable grounds for believing that the offence is an indictable offence.
- The investigation is being conducted diligently and expeditiously.
- Detention without charge is necessary to secure or preserve evidence of an offence for which a person is under arrest or to obtain evidence by questioning.

The authorization cannot last beyond 36h from when the detention clock first started running. Further extensions of detention can only be made if application is made to a Magistrates' Court sitting in private. The court may authorize further detention of up to 36h from the time that the application is granted and a further extension of up to 36h may be granted if a similar procedure is adopted. The total maximum period of detention is 96h from the original 'relevant time'—except under the Terrorism Act 2006, where the maximum is currently 28 days.

Detention after charge

The custody officer must order a detainee's release once a person has been charged, unless one of the following conditions apply:
- A detainee's name and address is unknown or doubted.
- Detention is necessary to prevent him/her committing an offence or causing physical injury to any other person.
- Detention is necessary to prevent his/her failing to appear in court on bail or his/her interfering with the administration of justice or the investigation of the offence.
- Detention is necessary to take a sample of urine or saliva to determine whether he/she has specified Class A drugs in his/her body (see 📖 p.458).
- Detention is necessary for his/her own protection.

A person who is detained after being charged must be taken to court as soon as practicable and not later than the first sitting after charge.

Police and Criminal Evidence Act 1984

At the time it was enacted, the Police and Criminal Evidence Act 1984 (PACE) represented a long overdue reform and modernization of the law governing the investigation of crime in England and Wales and it still provides the primary legal framework in relation to:
- The powers and duties of the police.
- The handling of persons in detention.
- Confession evidence.
- Police discipline and complaints against the police.
- Other associated matters.

Codes of Practice

The Codes of Practice are issued by the Home Secretary under provisions set out in PACE and provide a clear statement of the rights of the individual and the powers of the police. They deal with contacts between the police and public in the exercise of police powers to stop and search, to search premises, and with the treatment, questioning, and identification of suspects and the tape recording of interviews. The Codes regulate police powers and procedures in the investigation of crime and set down safeguards and protective measures for members of the public.

There are currently eight Codes, 'A'–'H', of which Codes 'C' and 'H' are the most relevant to healthcare professionals. Code 'C' sets out the requirements for the detention, treatment, and questioning of persons detained by the police for offences other than terrorism. Code 'H' sets out the same group of requirements as they apply to suspects arrested for terrorism.

A person's rights when in custody

Under the Codes of Practice, the custody officer must tell any person detained in police custody that they have the following basic rights:
- The right to have someone informed of his/her arrest.
- The right to consult privately with a solicitor and the fact that independent legal advice is available free of charge.
- The right to consult the Codes of Practice setting out the powers, responsibilities, and procedures of the police.

At the time of being booked into custody, the custody officer is required to ask detainees whether they would like legal advice and whether they want someone to be informed of their detention. Detainees are asked to sign the custody record to confirm their responses to these questions.

The custody officer is also obliged to provide detainees with a written notice setting out the previously listed three rights; to explain the procedure for obtaining legal advice; and to inform them that they have the right to have a copy of their custody record when they leave detention. An additional written notice setting out their entitlements while in custody should also be provided and detainees are asked to sign the custody record to acknowledge receipt of these written notices.

The custody record

Requirements of the custody record

The Codes of Practice set out in the Police and Criminal Evidence Act 1984 require the custody officer to open a custody record as soon as practicable for any person brought to a police station under arrest (or who is arrested at the police station having attended voluntarily). The custody record logs the circumstances and reasons for the arrest, the outcome of the risk assessment conducted by the custody officer, and all interactions with the detainee during his/her period of detention (Fig. 6.1).

The custody officer is responsible for the custody record's accuracy and completeness. All entries have to be timed and attributable to the person making the entry (i.e. handwritten entries need to be signed and computerized records need to contain the identification of the operator). In cases of detention under the Prevention of Terrorism Act, warrant or other identification numbers should be used, instead of names.

The custody officer is also responsible for ensuring that the record or a copy of the record accompanies a detained person if he/she is transferred to another police station. The record needs to demonstrate the time and reason for any such transfer.

Computerized records

Traditionally, custody records were all handwritten. However, police forces in the UK are now moving over to fully computerized custody records. The National Strategy for Police Information Systems (NSPIS) acknowledges that there are opportunities for increasing police effectiveness by integration of IT systems both within and between police forces. Accordingly, the Home Secretary has advised that all police forces adopt NSPIS Custody, a bespoke software system that incorporates the custody record and also detained persons' medical and medication forms. However, there have been delays in implementation of NSPIS Custody because of concerns about its fitness for purpose.

Audio or video recording

It should be noted that any audio or video recording made in the custody area is not part of the custody record but may be used in court.

Custody Record—Continuation Sheet

Custody No: ST/4778/10
Name: A Detainee

Date	Time	Include full details of any action/occurrence involving the detained person. Other than in terrorist cases show full particulars of all officers. Individual entries need not be restricted to one line. Except in terrorist cases, all entries to be signed by the writer (include rank and number)
4/7/08	06.00	DP was brought into custody in handcuffs having assaulted two officers at scene of arrest. DP states that he is a heroin addict and currently appears to be under the influence of drugs. He denies any injuries or other medical problems. Handcuffs removed and placed in male cell 6, a CCTV monitored cell. For ½ hourly rousing. DP's property listed. DP's clothing removed as part of the investigation—provided with boiler suit. Doctor called to examine DP at 06.05 hours. PS 222 Smith
	06.18	Provided with drink. DO 123 Jones
	06.30	Checked and roused in cell—all in order. DO 123 Jones
	06.40	Taken from cell to medical room to be seen by doctor. DO 123 Jones
	06.58	Returned to cell. DO 123 Jones
	07.10	Doctor advised that DP is currently intoxicated with opiates. Fit to detain but will need to be checked and roused every ½ hour until medical review in 4 hours. Not currently fit for interview. PS 222 Smith
	07.30	Checked and roused in cell. DO 123 Jones
	07.38	Spoke to solicitor on phone. DO 123 Jones

Fig. 6.1 Example of a custody record.

Conditions of detention

The conditions of detention a person is entitled to whilst in police custody are set out in the Codes of Practice. As a general principle, detainees should be provided with:

- Reasonable standards of physical comfort.
- Adequate food and drink.
- Access to toilets and washing facilities.
- Suitable clothing.
- Medical attention if required.
- Exercise when practicable.

The police cell

The Home Office issues guidance on cell design, stipulating the minimum size and making recommendations to eliminate the existence of ligature points from which suicidal detainees can hang themselves. So far as is practicable, the cells should be single occupancy only. They must be adequately heated, cleaned, and ventilated. Adequate lighting should be provided which is capable of being dimmed in order to allow people detained overnight to sleep. Bedding and mattresses supplied must be of a reasonable standard and in a clean and sanitary condition.

Access to toilets and washing facilities must be provided and detainees should be able to call custody staff by means of a bell or alarm in their cell.

Increasingly, CCTV is being used to monitor a number of cells in each custody unit so that vulnerable individuals (such as those at risk of self-harm) can be more closely monitored. Positioning of CCTV cameras should be such that the detainee is out of sight when using the cell toilet.

Food and exercise

At least two light meals and one main meal should be provided in any 24-h period and these should, as far as practicable, be offered at recognized meal times or at other times that take account of when the detainee last had a meal. Meals provided should offer a varied diet and meet any specific dietary needs or religious beliefs the detainee may have. Drinks should be provided at meal times and upon reasonable request between meals. As the appropriate healthcare professional, forensic practitioners may be asked to advise custody staff on medical and dietary matters.

Brief outdoor exercise should be offered daily where practicable.

Clothing

On occasions, it may be necessary for the police to remove a detainee's clothing for forensic analysis as part of the investigation into the alleged crime. Clothing may also have to be removed for cleaning or for hygiene and health reasons. In all such circumstances, the police are obliged to provide replacement clothing of a reasonable standard of comfort and cleanliness. The PACE Codes of Practice specifically state that a detainee must not be interviewed unless adequate clothing has been offered.

Medical attention

The Codes of Practice used to require the police to call a 'police surgeon' if a detainee needed clinical attention (the Codes still refer to police surgeons although the preferred term is now 'forensic physician' or 'forensic medical examiner'). However, following a revision of the Codes in 2003, the police may now call upon the services of a police surgeon or an appropriate healthcare professional. A 'healthcare professional' is defined as a clinically qualified person working within the scope of practice as determined by their relevant professional body, and is intended to include nurses and paramedics. Whether a healthcare professional is 'appropriate' depends on the circumstances of the duties they carry out at the time.

Risk assessment

In order to determine whether a detainee requires medical attention, the custody officer is obliged to perform a risk assessment as soon as practicable. Risk assessments follow a structured process that seeks to establish whether detainees:

- Are suffering from any illness, injury, or other medical or mental condition.
- Are receiving any treatment or medication for a medical or mental condition.
- Have ever tried to harm themselves.
- Need the assistance of an appropriate adult (see 📖 p.186).

The results of the risk assessment have to be included in the custody record.

The forensic physician

Forensic physicians (FPs) are registered medical practitioners who are appointed to provide independent and impartial clinical forensic medical services to the police. Many FPs are GPs, providing clinical forensic medical services as part of a portfolio career; some have primary careers in other specialties such as paediatrics, gynaecology, and emergency medicine; whereas a few doctors, primarily in the busier metropolitan areas, work exclusively as FPs.

Types of medical attention required in police stations

Fitness for detention (see 📖 p.204)
- Assessment of injuries/illness/drug and alcohol problems.
- Advice to custody staff on general care whilst in custody.
- Provision of necessary medication.
- Referral to hospital.
- Assessment under mental health legislation.
- Provision of a report of any illness or injury requiring attention to be passed to other healthcare professionals upon detainee transfer.

Fitness for interview (see 📖 p.428)
- Assessment of risk to physical or mental state posed by conducting an interview.
- Assessment of competence to understand and answer questions.
- Advising on the need for an appropriate adult.
- Advising on any special provisions required during interview or need for reassessment after interview.

Forensic examination
- Assessment and recording of injuries.
- Interpretation of injuries.
- Collecting forensic samples.
- Comprehensive examinations to assess whether a person is unfit to drive through drink or drugs.

Transfer and care
Assessment of a detainee's fitness and need for special care on transfer:
- From one custody suite to another.
- From police stations to court.
- From police stations to prison.

Special functions of forensic physicians

In addition to the basic custody functions previously listed, FPs with sufficient training and experience may be requested to:
- Examine adult complainants and suspects in alleged sexual assault.
- Examine alleged child victims of neglect, or physical or sexual abuse.
- Become Section 12 approved practitioners (Mental Health Act 1983) and perform formal mental health assessments under the Act.
- Provide expert opinion in court for both prosecution and defence.

Multidisciplinary team working

Increasingly, FPs work in multidisciplinary teams alongside nurses and other healthcare professionals. Most of the clinical duties defined under the PACE Codes of Practice are now permitted to be performed by either a doctor or an appropriate healthcare professional, although the Codes do stipulate that only a doctor can supervise the administration of certain controlled drugs (see 📖 p.213). Intimate searches can be performed by a doctor or a nurse, but not by a paramedic (see 📖 p.194).

Terminology

It is intriguing that there are so many different names for doctors who undertake clinical forensic work—this probably reflects the rapidly changing nature of the specialty of clinical forensic medicine. For the purposes of this text, the term 'forensic practitioner' is used to include forensic physicians (doctors), nurses, and paramedics who undertake clinical forensic work in custody (it also includes those healthcare professionals who perform forensic work in other settings).

Advice required from the healthcare professional

Whenever a forensic practitioner is called to give medical advice in accordance with the provisions of the Codes of Practice, the custody officer should ask his/her opinion about:
- Any risks or problems that the police need to take into account when making decisions about the detainee's continued detention.
- When to carry out an interview if applicable.
- The need for any safeguards.

Further reading

Association of Forensic Physicians and British Medical Association (2009). *Healthcare of detainees in police stations*, 3rd edn. London: BMA.

Faculty of Forensic and Legal Medicine. *The Role of the Independent Forensic Physician*. Available at 🔊 https://fflm.ac.uk/upload/documents/1184164719.pdf

Vulnerable persons in custody

Enshrined within the PACE Codes of Practice are special statutory provisions and safeguards for certain groups of people who may be particularly vulnerable during police detention.

Juveniles

For the purposes of PACE, a juvenile is anyone under the age of 17 years (or anyone who appears to be under the age of 17 in the absence of clear evidence that they are older). By virtue of their age, juveniles are at greater risk of providing false confessions to the police and are more likely to be vulnerable to the distress and pressures caused by the experience of arrest and police detention. Safeguards within the Codes of Practice that apply to juveniles include:

- They should not be arrested or interviewed at their place of education except in exceptional circumstances.
- On arrival in custody, the custody officer must try to ascertain the identity of the person responsible for the juvenile's welfare and inform them about the arrest and where the individual is detained.
- Arranging for an appropriate adult to attend the police station (see 📖 p.186).
- A requirement that juveniles should only be placed in a police cell if:
  - No other secure accommodation is available and the custody officer considers it is not practicable to supervise them if they are not placed in a cell, or
  - A cell provides more comfortable accommodation than other secure accommodation in the station.
- They may not be placed in a cell with a detained adult.
- They should be visited more frequently than ordinary detainees.

The mentally ill and mentally vulnerable

Individuals with mental illness may come into contact with the police for a variety of reasons. As a group, they have a number of vulnerabilities while in police custody. Comorbidity is a particular problem, especially coexistent drug and alcohol misuse. The risk of suicide and self-harm in custody is much higher amongst those with a history of mental illness, and these individuals are also at risk of providing false confessions during police interview. As with juveniles, arrangements should be made for an appropriate adult to attend the police station as soon as practicable after a mentally ill or mentally vulnerable individual has been booked into custody.

For the purposes of the PACE Codes of Practice, if an officer has any suspicion, or is told in good faith, that a person may be mentally disordered or otherwise mentally vulnerable, then they should be treated as such unless there is clear evidence to dispel that suspicion. Mental vulnerability is defined as applying to any individual who, because of their mental state or capacity, may not understand the significance of what is said, of questions, or of their replies.

Court diversion schemes

Over the last decade, a number of schemes have been developed which aim to divert mentally disordered offenders away from the criminal justice system as early as possible. The objectives of such schemes are:

- To divert mentally disordered offenders from prosecution by assessing them in police custody, on remand in prison, or bail.
- To provide information to the CPS on the nature and severity of the mental disorder to enable the CPS to exercise its right not to prosecute or to discontinue proceedings on the grounds of public interest.
- To reduce the number of mentally disordered offenders remanded to prison for psychiatric reports.
- To reduce the number of mentally disordered offenders serving a custodial sentence.
- To re-establish links between mentally disordered offenders and community psychiatric services when contact has been lost.
- On release from prison, to seek to prevent further offending by liaising with appropriate services for provision of a suitable package of care.

As a forensic practitioner, it is important to be aware of any court diversion schemes operating in the local area. Forensic practitioners can play an active role in supporting the objectives outlined earlier, whilst remembering that the ultimate decision regarding the diversion of a mentally disordered offender from police custody rests with the custody officer, whose decision must take into account wider public safety issues.

Other special groups

Those with communication difficulties

If a detainee appears deaf or there is doubt about their hearing or speaking ability or ability to understand English, and the custody officer cannot establish effective communication, then the custody officer must, as soon as practicable, call an interpreter for assistance. In many parts of the country access to interpreters is extremely limited, so this statutory requirement is met by using telephone-based interpreting services.

The visually impaired

If a detainee is blind, seriously visually impaired, or unable to read, the custody officer must make sure that his/her solicitor, relative, appropriate adult (if otherwise necessary), or some other person likely to take an interest in them (and not involved in the investigation) is available to help check any documentation. The detainee may, if they prefer, ask this person to sign documents and consent forms on their behalf.

Appropriate adults

'Appropriate adults' offer support to individuals who may be vulnerable whilst in police custody by virtue of their young age, mental illness (including learning disability), or mental vulnerability. They are required to be present during the cautioning, interviewing, and searching of vulnerable individuals, when their role is to:

- Look after the detained person's welfare.
- Explain police procedures.
- Provide information about their rights and ensure that these are protected.
- Facilitate communication with the police.

As soon as practicable after the vulnerable person has arrived at the police station under arrest, the custody officer must inform the appropriate adult of the grounds for the person's detention, their whereabouts, and ask the adult to come to the police station to see the detainee.

If a juvenile or a person who is mentally disordered or otherwise mentally vulnerable is cautioned in the absence of the appropriate adult, the caution must be repeated in the adult's presence.

Only in exceptional circumstances (when delay might seriously compromise the investigation or lead to harm to others) can a juvenile or person who is mentally disordered or otherwise mentally vulnerable be interviewed regarding their involvement or suspected involvement in a criminal offence or offences, or be asked to provide or sign a written statement under caution or record of interview, in the absence of the appropriate adult.

When acting for a juvenile or person who is mentally disordered or otherwise mentally vulnerable, the appropriate adult should consider whether legal advice from a solicitor is required. If the vulnerable person indicates that they do not want legal advice, the appropriate adult has the right to ask for a solicitor to attend if this would be in the best interests of the person. However, the detained person cannot be forced to see the solicitor if he/she is adamant that he/she does not wish to do so.

An appropriate adult is not subject to legal privilege and may be required to disclose the content of discussions with the detainee in court. Therefore, a detainee should always be given an opportunity, when an appropriate adult is called to the police station, to consult privately with a solicitor in the appropriate adult's absence if they want.

When an appropriate adult is present at an interview, the police are obliged to inform the adult that:

- They are not expected to act simply as an observer; and
- The purpose of their presence is to:
  - Advise the person being interviewed.
  - Observe whether the interview is being conducted properly and fairly.
  - Facilitate communication with the person being interviewed.

Who can be an appropriate adult?

They are responsible adults who are independent of the police. The PACE Codes of Practice list who can act as an appropriate adult for different vulnerable groups and specifically state that a solicitor or independent custody visitor present at the police station in that capacity may not be the appropriate adult.

Juveniles

In the case of a juvenile, the appropriate adult means:

- The parent, guardian, or, if the juvenile is in local authority or voluntary organization care, or is otherwise being looked after under the Children Act 1989, a person representing that authority or organization.
- A social worker of a local authority social services department.
- Failing these, some other responsible adult aged 18 or over who is not a police officer or employed by the police.

The police are required to exercise discretion when selecting the 'appropriate adult'; case law has held that the 'appropriate adult' should not have been a person with whom the juvenile had no empathy. If a juvenile's parent is estranged from the juvenile, they should not be asked to act as the appropriate adult if the juvenile expressly and specifically objects to their presence.

Mentally ill and mentally vulnerable detainees

In the case of a mentally disordered or mentally vulnerable detainee, the appropriate adult means:

- A relative, guardian, or other person responsible for their care or custody.
- Someone experienced in dealing with mentally disordered or mentally vulnerable people, but who is not a police officer or employed by the police.
- Failing these, some other responsible adult aged 18 years or over who is not a police officer or employed by the police.

Appropriate adults and the forensic practitioner

The responsibility for calling an appropriate adult rests with the custody officer, but if a forensic practitioner becomes aware of the need for an appropriate adult, he/she should pass this information to the custody officer and record it in the custody record. As the courts have the power to rule confession evidence inadmissible if a mentally disordered or mentally vulnerable detainee is interviewed in the absence of an appropriate adult, it is important to consider the likely effect of any mental illness or mental vulnerability on the reliability of the detainee's confession (see 📖 p.429). Whenever there is any doubt about an individual's vulnerability, it is best to err on the side of caution and recommend the presence of an appropriate adult.

Solicitors and legal representatives

A person arrested and held in police custody has the right to consult a solicitor privately at any time (although the police have powers to delay access to a legal advice if there are grounds to believe that immediate access may seriously compromise the investigation or expose persons to the risk of physical harm). Legal advice can be provided by solicitors, trainee solicitors, or legal representatives (non-lawyers who are accredited to represent solicitors on behalf of detainees).

The purpose of legal advice

The purpose and significance of legal advice and assistance is:

- To maintain a balance between the powers of the police and the protection of the rights of the detainee.
- To relieve the detainee of pressures which can induce false confessions and cause a miscarriage of justice.
- To ensure that detainees are aware of their rights and are treated fairly and in accordance with the PACE Codes of Practice. At times, this may include advising detainees to exercise their right to silence or assisting them to give an account of the activities for which they are under suspicion.
- To allow the legal advisor to keep accurate and full contemporaneous records that, together with the custody record, can result in the exclusion of prosecution evidence at trial.

The role of the solicitor

The solicitor's role may include:

- Explaining the powers and duties of the police as they affect the detainee.
- Ensuring that the detainee understands what facts are being alleged, what criminal offences are under investigation, and the legal elements necessary to prove them.
- Assisting the detainee to decide whether to give no comment during police interview or to respond to the allegations by means of denial, explanation, or admission.
- Attending any interview to ensure it is conducted fairly.
- Explaining police powers in relation to statutory powers to obtain or preserve evidence (e.g. obtaining intimate samples or attending identification parades),
- Making representations to the police at reviews of detention.
- If charges are preferred, advising on the formalities where appropriate (e.g. fingerprinting and DNA samples) and making representations on the issue of bail.
- Discussing with the detainee whether legal representation at court is advisable.
- Requesting medical attention for the detainee if this is appropriate.
- Protecting throughout the well-being of the detainee.
- Making appropriate records.

Consulting with a solicitor present

It is for the detainee to decide whether he/she wants his/her solicitor to be present during a medical examination—the forensic practitioner should respect any such wish as long as it does not introduce an unreasonable delay in undertaking the examination. There may be occasions when the forensic practitioner considers it prudent to provide the detainee with an opportunity to ask the solicitor to leave the medical room, such as when performing intimate examinations.

Further reading

Edwards A (2003). *Advising a Suspect in the Police Station*, 5th revised edn. London: Sweet & Maxwell.

Fingerprints and drug testing

The police have a number of statutory powers to take samples from suspects of crime for identification purposes and to detect those who may misuse drugs.

Fingerprints

Fingerprints have been used as an identification aid by the police since 1902 and may now be taken to:
• Compare with fingerprints found at the scene of a crime.
• Check and prove convictions.
• Help to ascertain a person's identity.

Fingerprints (and palm prints) may not be taken without the suspect's consent, unless an officer of at least the rank of inspector authorizes it and there are reasonable grounds to believe that the suspect has been involved in a criminal offence and the fingerprints will tend to confirm or disprove that involvement, or assist in establishing their identity. Fingerprints may also be taken without consent if the suspect is charged with a recordable offence, or informed that they will be reported for such an offence.

Fingerprint technology

Under Home Office guidance there used to be a minimum requirement for 16 ridge characteristics to be in agreement between mark and impression in order for a 'match, to be declared. However, since 2001, matches can be declared on a case-by-case basis with no predetermined or set numerical 'standard'.

 The way fingerprints are taken has moved away from the old inkpad and paper process to embrace modern computer technology. In most police forces, fingerprint impressions are now taken by computer scanners (the 'Livescan' system) and then transmitted electronically to the national fingerprint database where immediate identity checks are performed. Responses return to the terminal in <5min.

Drug testing on arrest

Under new powers contained in the Drugs Act 2005, the police can now test offenders for heroin, crack, and cocaine, on arrest for certain acquisitive crime offences, such as robbery or burglary. Those who test positive will then be required to attend a compulsory drug assessment by specialist drugs workers to determine the extent of their drug problem and help them into treatment and other support, even if they are not charged.

 Testing is performed using oral fluid obtained with a collection pad. Suspects must consent to testing, with those who fail to provide a sample or comply with a required assessment facing a fine of up to £2500 and/or up to 3 months in prison.

DNA and the national database

Historical aspects

The application of DNA profiling to criminal law enforcement has been the biggest development in the field of human identification since the discovery of fingerprinting at the start of the 20th century. The sensitivity and discriminatory powers of DNA profiling; the wide range of biological material that can be subjected to DNA analysis; and the fact that minute amounts of material can be successfully analysed, has meant that since its introduction in the early 1990s, DNA analysis has virtually replaced all other methods of trace analysis.

In 1995 the government set up the UK national DNA database. Before 2001, the police could take DNA samples from suspects during investigations, but had to destroy the samples and records derived from them if the people concerned were acquitted or charges were not proceeded with. The law was changed in 2001 to remove this requirement, and changed again in 2004 so that DNA samples can now be taken from anyone arrested for a recordable offence and detained in a police station.

DNA sampling

DNA samples may also be obtained from volunteers in order to eliminate them from a police enquiry. In addition to agreeing to the immediate use of the DNA in a particular crime, those who volunteer samples for elimination purposes may also be asked to sign a consent form for their profile to be added to the database. This consent cannot subsequently be revoked and any stored profile may subsequently be used for speculative searches against samples left at scenes of crime (including both serious and more minor offences).

Samples are taken by means of a mouth swab and can be taken without consent in accordance with the law governing other non-intimate samples. The samples are taken by police officers.

The national DNA database

The UK's national DNA database is the largest of any country: 5.2% of the UK population is on the database, compared with 0.5% in the USA. The database stores DNA samples obtained at crime scenes and from people detained at police stations and allows comparisons to be made. In 2005–2006, 45 000 crimes were solved as a result of matches against records held on the DNA database, including 422 homicides and 645 rapes.

Non-intimate and intimate samples

Forensic physicians may be called upon to take a number of different forensic samples from both those suspected of criminal offences and their victims. The statutory powers that govern the taking of samples distinguish between non-intimate and intimate samples.

Non-intimate samples

These comprise:
- Hair other than pubic hair, which includes hair plucked with the root.
- A sample taken from a nail or from under a nail.
- A swab taken from any part of a person's body including the mouth, but not any other body orifice.
- Saliva.
- A skin impression, other than a fingerprint, including foot impressions.

Non-intimate samples can only be taken from suspects with their written consent, unless an officer of the rank of inspector or above authorizes it and there are grounds to believe that the sample will tend to confirm or disprove the suspect's involvement in a recordable offence.

Normally, non-intimate samples are taken by police officers, but forensic practitioners may be asked to take such samples, usually as part of an examination that they have otherwise been asked to undertake.

Intimate samples

Whereas non-intimate samples can be taken without the consent of the detainee, intimate samples can only be taken with written consent from the suspect and following authorization by an officer of at least the rank of inspector. The authorizing police officer must consider that the taking of the samples will tend to confirm or disprove the detainee's involvement in a recordable offence.

The rules with regard to obtaining intimate samples from a detained person require 'appropriate consent' in order for the intimate sample evidence to be admissible. The identity of the person able to give 'appropriate consent' varies depending on the age of the detainee:
- In relation to a person who has attained the age of 17 years, the consent of that person.
- In relation to a person who has not attained that age, but has attained the age of 14 years, the consent of that person and his/her parent or guardian.
- In relation to a person who has not attained the age of 14 years, the consent of his/her parent or guardian.

Where the consent of a parent or guardian is required it is not necessary for the parent or guardian to be at the police station to give that consent. Where the detainee is mentally disordered or mentally handicapped, the consent is only valid if given in the presence of the appropriate adult.

Refusing to give consent

If the taking of an intimate sample is refused without good cause, the court may draw inferences from the fact of the refusal and the refusal may 'be treated as, or as capable of amounting to, corroboration of any evidence against the person in relation to which the refusal is material'.

PACE classifies the following as 'intimate samples':
- Swabs from any body orifice other than the mouth
- Pubic hair
- Blood
- Urine
- Semen
- Any other tissue fluid
- Dental impression.

The majority of intimate samples can only be obtained by a 'registered medical practitioner or a registered healthcare professional'. The exceptions are urine, which can be taken by a police officer, and dental impressions, which can only be obtained by a 'registered dentist'.

Labelling samples

It is the responsibility of the person who obtains the intimate or non-intimate sample to ensure it is appropriately labelled.

Swabs, sheaths, and bottles should be labelled with the following information:
- Name of person from whom the sample is taken.
- Description of the sample (e.g. penile shaft swab).
- Unique identification number.
- Date on which the sample was taken.
- Urine and blood only—time at which the sample was taken.

Where two swabs have been taken from the same site, it is imperative that there is a clear indication on the label regarding the order in which the swabs were obtained. This is most easily done by describing the first of the two samples as sample A and the second as sample B.

Tamper evident bags should be labelled with the same information as the swabs, sheaths, and bottles they contain. In addition, they should be signed by the person who first handled the exhibit and thereafter signed by all other persons who handle the exhibit.

Intimate searches

An intimate search consists of the physical examination of a person's body orifices other than the mouth and must be authorized by an officer of inspector rank or above, who has reasonable grounds to believe that the person may have concealed on him- or herself:

• Anything which he or she could and might use to cause physical injury to the person or others (a 'safety search').
• A Class A drug which he or she intends to supply to another or to export (a 'drug offence search').

Safety searches may be performed by a registered medical practitioner, a registered nurse, or a police constable of the same sex (if authorized to do so by an officer of the rank of inspector or above), whereas drug offence searches may only be performed by a registered medical practitioner or a registered nurse. Drug offence searches must be undertaken in a hospital, surgery, or other medical premises (with resuscitation facilities), but one for weapons can also be undertaken in a police station.

Consent

A fundamental ethical principle guiding medical practice is that no examination, diagnosis, or treatment of a competent adult should be undertaken without the person's consent. The ethical obligation to seek consent applies even where this is not a legal requirement. Consent is not legally required for an authorized safety search and forcible restraint may be used if necessary. Although any doctor or nurse carrying out an authorized safety search without consent would not be acting unlawfully, they would be acting contrary to the ethical principles of their professional bodies. Therefore, forensic practitioners should not conduct a safety search without the consent of the detainee (not least because conducting such a search in an uncooperative patient could expose both the patient and the forensic practitioner to risk). Whenever carrying out an intimate search for weapons or other objects that could be used to cause physical injury, the forensic practitioner should assess and take steps to protect his/her own safety during the search.

Under the Drugs Act 2005, written consent is required to carry out an intimate body search for Class A drugs (Class A drugs include heroin, cocaine, ecstasy, methadone, and injectable amphetamines, but not cannabis—see 📖 p.458). If consent is refused without good cause, a court can draw such inferences as appear proper. In the case of refused consent, the forensic practitioner should discuss the possible risks to the detainee's health should the suspected drugs be absorbed (including the risk of overdose if a package splits). Alternative methods of identification or retrieval of concealed material should also be discussed.

X-rays and ultrasound scans

The Drugs Act 2005 has amended PACE to allow persons suspected of having concealed on themselves a Class A drug which they intend to supply to another or to export to have an X-ray taken or an ultrasound scan performed (or both). An X-ray or ultrasound may be performed only by a registered medical practitioner or a registered nurse and only at a hospital, surgery, or other medical premises. Failure to consent without 'good cause' may harm the detainee's case if it comes to trial. The forensic practitioner may be asked to explain what is involved in the procedures and to discuss/allay any concerns the detainee may have about the effect an X-ray or carrying out an ultrasound scan might have on them. The PACE Codes of Practice state that if appropriate consent is not given, evidence of the explanation that the forensic practitioner has given may, if the case comes to trial, be relevant to determining whether the detainee had a good cause for refusing.

Further reading

Faculty of Forensic and Legal Medicine and British Medical Association (2007). *Guidelines for doctors asked to perform intimate body searches*. London: BMA.

Approach to custody work

General considerations

The relationship between a forensic practitioner and detainee is a unique one—the forensic practitioner needs to explain the important differences from the normal doctor–patient relationship. For example, he/she should advise that the usual rules of confidentiality are not as robust in custody and clarify that the purpose of the examination may not be purely therapeutic. It is important that forensic practitioners recognize that they have a special responsibility toward detainees, who are vulnerable by virtue of having their liberty infringed. Thus, if they believe that the basic human rights of a detainee are being ignored or abused, they have a duty to report the concern to the appropriate person in authority (e.g. duty inspector or the head of criminal justice unit).

Forensic practitioners should be sensitive to the fact that the detainee has no choice over the identity of the doctor called to attend. At all times, the forensic practitioner should introduce him/herself, identify his/her role and remain courteous. He/she should appreciate that detainees have the same rights and expectations of medical care as any patient, and these include the right to privacy and confidentiality. He/she should respect the right of the detainee to withhold consent and should personally check the validity of any consent given.

Consent

It is assumed that all adults are competent and have capacity to consent. Valid consent is that which is freely given, without fear, duress, or fraud and which is appropriately informed. To give valid consent, detainees need to understand in broad terms the nature and the purpose of the proposed intervention so the forensic practitioner should inform them of any 'material' or 'significant' risks in the proposed intervention, any alternatives to it, and the risks incurred in doing nothing.

As a police station is one area where consent may appear to be tainted by fear or pressure, the forensic practitioner must satisfy him/herself that consent has been given freely before commencing the intervention in question.

Form of consent

Although implied and verbal consent are just as valid as written consent, many forensic physicians prefer to obtain written consent to interventions in police custody. This is particularly important when the intervention has a forensic as opposed to purely therapeutic element. In cases where the forensic practitioner perceives that subsequent questions may be raised about the validity of the consent, it may be appropriate to have the patient's consent witnessed by a third party.

Consent from children and young people

Under the Family Law Reform Act 1969, children attain adult status at age 16 years and are entitled to consent to their own medical treatment. Although not decided in law, it is reasonable to assume that young people aged 16 or 17 years have the capacity to consent to a forensic examination just as they do to a therapeutic examination. However, forensic practitioners need to be aware that there are additional procedural considerations with regard to forensic examinations of young people.

In the eyes of the PACE, juveniles become adults at age 17 and thus 17-year-olds can give consent. When dealing with detainees under this age, the police are required to follow certain rules to ensure that evidence obtained from juveniles in custody is legally admissible in court. The rules with regard to obtaining intimate samples from a detained person require 'appropriate consent' in order for the intimate sample evidence to be admissible. 'Appropriate consent' is defined in section 65 of PACE as meaning:

- In relation to a person who has attained the age of 17 years, the consent of that person.
- In relation to a person who has not attained that age but has attained the age of 14 years, the consent of that person and his/her parent or guardian.
- In relation to a person who has not attained the age of 14 years, the consent of his/her parent or guardian.

Where the consent of a parent or guardian is required, it is not necessary for the parent or guardian to be at the police station to give that consent. Where the consent of the juvenile is required it must be obtained in the presence of an appropriate adult, who may be the parent or guardian or some other suitable person over the age of 18 years.

Confidentiality

Respecting a patient's confidentiality poses particular problems in clinical forensic medicine and when obtaining consent to an examination from both detainees and victims the forensic practitioner should ensure that they are aware of what use will be made of the information obtained.

When conducting therapeutic examinations of detainees, forensic practitioners should record in the custody record only that information which is relevant to the safe care of the detained person. This will include directions to the custody staff for the medical care of the detainee, the giving of any medication, and an assessment of fitness for detention, interview, charge, transfer, or release. Clinical information that is not relevant to the safe care of the detainee should be retained in the forensic practitioner's private notes and not divulged to the custody staff. By contrast, as the purpose of forensic examinations is to glean information for use as evidence, details of examination findings need to be revealed to investigating officers. When seeking consent from a suspect or victim to a forensic examination, the forensic practitioner must explain the purpose of the examination and the fact that findings will be subsequently disclosed. The individual then has the opportunity to either agree or refuse to be examined.

Personal safety

Research evidence suggests that verbal and physical violence are common in the custodial setting. Forensic practitioners should be aware of how to assess and minimize the risk of such violence.

Assessing the risk of violence

The only safe way in which to approach an unknown detainee is to assume that he/she may become violent without warning. Clinical practice should therefore be based on a safety-first principle, in terms of ensuring personal protection.

The risk of violence may be categorized as:
- High risk—an obvious threat.
- Unknown risk—an undiscovered threat.

There should be no such thing as 'no risk'.

Risk factors

Certain individuals are more likely to initiate violence than the average person. Risk factors include:
- Mental illness, particularly paranoid psychosis.
- Drug and alcohol intoxication.
- Past history of violence (past behaviour is a good predictor of the future).
- Altered mental state due to physical illness (e.g. head injury) or metabolic disturbance (e.g. hypoglycaemia).

Warning signs of imminent aggression

Non-verbal cues that suggest that a detainee might be about to initiate violence include:
- Lips tightening to produce a tight-lipped mouth.
- Head position shifting from tilted back to a down position to protect the neck.
- Eye contact changing from a direct stare as a means of intimidation to breaking eye contact before looking at the target of the attack.
- Assuming a 'fighting stance' in which the hands become fists and the shoulders square onto the target.

Reducing the risk of violence

Before the examination

The forensic practitioner needs to consider the risk of violence and collect as much information as possible about the detainee's current and past behaviour from custody staff, arresting officers, PNC warnings, and, where appropriate, family, friends, and healthcare providers.

Planning the examination

When considering where to conduct the examination, it is always worth taking advice from the custody staff. Although most examinations take place in the medical room, it may be more appropriate to examine a detainee in his/her cell if the risk of violence is considered high. Having decided to conduct the examination in the medical room, the forensic practitioner needs to check it to minimize the risk of violence by:

- Ensuring that the detainee is sat furthest from the door so he/she cannot block the route of escape.
- Locating the panic button.
- Ensuring that there are no objects that could be used as weapons within the reach of the detainee (including a medical bag and its contents).

Presence of police officers during the examination

When examining any detainee, the forensic practitioner needs to balance that detainee's right to confidentiality with his/her personal safety. Where the risk of violence is not considered to be high, it is usually good practice to be accompanied by an escort, either a police officer or civilian jailer, who should remain outside the medical room within calling distance, but out of earshot.

When the risk of violence is considered high, the forensic practitioner should be accompanied throughout the examination by a police officer/civilian jailer of the same sex as the detainee. The officer's role is to supervise the detainee and ensure the safety of the forensic practitioner.

If the detainee refuses to be examined in the presence of a police officer, the forensic practitioner should consider the risk to him/herself before deciding whether to proceed with the examination.

It is important to remember that the presence of a police officer may, on occasion, provoke the detainee and increase the likelihood of physical or verbal assault.

During the examination

It is possible to reduce the risk of assault by adopting certain strategies during the examination:

- Explaining the forensic practitioner role fully, emphasizing independence from the police.
- Remaining calm and avoiding becoming annoyed or confrontational. The forensic practitioner's attitude affects his/her behaviour which in turn affects the examinee's attitude and subsequent behaviour.
- Sitting at an angle to the examinee rather than directly opposite, as this is perceived to be less confrontational.
- Listening and responding in a non-critical way, expressing sympathy and understanding where appropriate.
- Suspending the examination whenever the risk of violence appears to be escalating beyond control.

The medical room

It is essential that there are adequate facilities and equipment within police stations for healthcare professionals to perform their tasks effectively. To this end, there should always be a designated medical room or suite in police stations that regularly hold detainees and this room or suite should be used exclusively for that purpose. While there are certain core requirements, the precise nature and amount of equipment and medication kept in the medical room will depend to some extent on local needs and preferences.

Operational guidelines for medical rooms

- The room should be locked when not in use.
- The room should only be used for medical purposes.
- The room should have all surfaces cleaned (including the floor) on a daily basis.
- The room should have a lockable drug cupboard and a pharmaceutical waste bin should be provided for the safe disposal of unused prescribed drugs.
- The room should not be used for the storage of other items.
- A named person should have responsibility for checking and restocking the room on a regular basis (at least once a week).
- There should be a wall-mounted clinical waste bin with foot lever to open. This must be emptied at least once a week, regardless of how full it is and appropriate arrangements made for the safe disposal of this waste.
- The sharps disposal bin should be replaced when three-quarters full.

Equipment for medical rooms

In addition to stock items, each medical room should have:
- Desk with laminated surface and drawers for stationery.
- Three wipeable chairs.
- Examination couch.
- Lockable floor units with laminated worktops, labelled to identify what they contain.
- Lockable wall units, labelled to identify what they contain.
- Washbasin with elbow operated taps.
- Wall mounted examination light.
- Telephone.
- Panic button(s) that is accessible if sat or stood.
- Waste bin.
- Clinical waste bin (wall mounted).
- Good heating, lighting, and ventilation.
- Sharps disposal bin.
- Pharmaceutical waste bin.
- Paper towels and liquid soap dispenser.
- Access to a small fridge (not used for food).

Medication

All forensic physicians should have available to them a personal doctor's bag containing those drugs normally carried when on call in general practice. The bag should be checked regularly and its contents kept in date. In addition, provided a suitable locked medicine cabinet is available in the medical room, a small number of frequently used drugs may be kept as stock items at the police station. Such stock items may include:

- Analgesics:
  - Paracetamol
  - NSAI (e.g. ibuprofen)
  - Co-dydramol (or similar)
  - Dihydrocodeine.

- Anxiolytics:
  - Diazepam
  - Chlordiazepoxide.

- Hypnotics:
  - Nitrazepam
  - Zopiclone
  - Glucagon for injection.

- Acute behavioural disturbance:
  - Lorazepam.

- Antipsychotics:
  - Olanzapine.

- Antibiotics:
  - Co-amoxiclav
  - Erythromycin.

- Antiepileptics:
  - Carbamezepine
  - Sodium valproate.

- Gastrointestinal system:
  - Antacids
  - Ranitidine
  - Omeprazole
  - Domperidone
  - Loperamide.

- Cardiovascular system:
  - Glyceryl trinitrate spray
  - Aspirin.

- Injectables:
  - Naloxone
  - Adrenaline (e.g. Epipen®)

- Seizures:
  - Diazepam rectal solution.

- Vitamins:
  - Thiamine.

- Respiratory system:
  - Salbutamol inhaler.

- Other:
  - Loratadine
  - Levonelle®-1500
  - Histoacryl® tissue adhesive
  - Hypostop® gel.

All prescriptions issued for detainees (unless they are the doctor's own NHS patients) must be issued on a private prescription and obtained at police expense.

Further reading

Faculty of Forensic and Legal Medicine. *Operational procedures and equipment for medical rooms in police stations and victim examination suites.* Available at ✆ http://www.fflm.ac.uk

Documentation

It is vital that all healthcare professionals working in the forensic field keep a permanent record of their clinical findings. By the very nature of their work, they can expect their clinical notes to be the subject of rigorous scrutiny at times and it is well to remember this even in the dead of night. Notes should be made at the time of the examination or immediately afterwards. They should be complete with both relevant positive and negative findings and they should be legible.

The form of the clinical note

Although computerized clinical records are relied on increasingly in general practice and hospital medicine, the written record remains the preferred option in clinical forensic medicine. Some forensic physicians record their examination findings in hard-backed books. These are easier to store than loose leaf paper and can demonstrate the contemporaneity of the entry by virtue of the note's position in the book. However, it is not easy or tidy to store additional material or documents, such as consent forms or body charts, in hard-backed books and increasingly, the preferred manner of recording notes is in loose leaf pro formas. These have the advantage of acting as an aide-memoire and can be easily stored in conjunction with other relevant documents. Pro formas usually include a consent form—obtaining the detainee's written consent is a simple way of demonstrating that the note was made contemporaneously. A selection of excellent pro formas is available from the Faculty of Forensic and Legal Medicine (℞ http://www.fflm.ac.uk/library)

The content of the clinical note

For each encounter with a detainee or victim the following should be recorded:
- Details of the person examined.
- The time, date, duration, and place of examination.
- Details of who requested the examination, who provided briefing at the police station, what information they gave, and what was asked of the forensic practitioner.
- The consent for the examination.
- The history and examination.
- A list of any samples that may have been taken.
- The management and treatment plans made by the forensic practitioner, including any advice about the need for review of the patient.
- Details of any information given to the patient or custody staff.

Recording injuries (📖 p.120)

The documentation, management, and interpretation of injuries are core activities of the forensic practitioner. It is vital that accurate records of any injuries noted are kept. Body charts are an invaluable additional resource for recording injuries. When recording an injury the following should be noted (see 📖 p.120): site, size, shape, colour, orientation, specific features (e.g. direction of skin tags in abrasions; bruised and abraded edges of a laceration), subjective features (e.g. tenderness).

Storing clinical notes

Health records, such as clinical notes, are classed as sensitive data under the Data Protection Act 1998—stringent rules apply to the processing of this data. Security of the data should be commensurate with the nature of information covered. As clinical notes are likely to include sensitive information, such as personal data and sensitive information relating to previous medical history, a high level of security must surround the data in terms of its collection and storage. Thus, medical records must be stored securely and in a manner that allows easy retrieval for later reference when writing statements or appearing in court.

Access to records

Patients in the UK have a statutory right of access to information about themselves (enshrined in the Data Protection Act 1998) and this extends to the information held in forensic clinical records. Competent patients, including young people, may apply for access to, and copies of, their own records. They may also authorize third parties, such as their solicitor, to access their records on their behalf.

The custody record

Forensic practitioners should be aware that the Codes of Practice of PACE require that a written record must be made in the custody record of any clinical directions and advice given by a doctor or healthcare professional about the care and treatment of a detainee. Good practice dictates that forensic practitioners should make such written records themselves, as this will prevent errors in interpretation that may occur if police officers record verbal instructions that have been given. The instructions about care and treatment should be recorded in the computerized custody record (NSPIS). If directions are given that a detainee requires constant observation or supervision, there should be an accompanying explanation to precisely describe what action needs to be taken to implement such directions.

Forensic practitioners will keep their own contemporaneous notes of consultations with detainees and are obliged to record in the custody record that they have retained these records.

Under PACE, 'the detainee, appropriate adult or legal representative shall be permitted to inspect the original custody record after the detainee has left police detention provided they give reasonable notice of their request'.

Assessing fitness to detain

The request by a custody officer to see if a detainee is fit to be detained in police custody is probably the commonest problem a forensic physician encounters. The request is usually made in response to the custody officer's duty under PACE Codes of Practice C9.5:

> **C9.5**—The custody officer must make sure a detainee receives appropriate medical attention as soon as reasonably practicable if the person:
>
> (a) appears to be suffering from physical illness; or
> (b) is injured; or
> (c) appears to be suffering from a mental disorder; or
> (d) appears to need clinical attention.
>
> This applies even if the detainee makes no request for clinical attention and whether or not they have already received clinical attention elsewhere. If the need for attention appears urgent, e.g. when indicated as in *Annex H*, the nearest available healthcare professional or an ambulance must be called immediately.

Although the requirement to seek clinical attention for a detainee does not apply to minor ailments or injuries that do not require such attention, the Codes of Practice emphasize that any doubt must be resolved in favour of calling an appropriate healthcare professional.

Advice of the forensic practitioner may also be sought if a detainee:
- Appears to be suffering from an infectious disease or condition (C9.7).
- Requests a clinical examination (C9.8).
- Is required to take or apply any medication that was prescribed before their detention (C9.9).
- Has in their possession, or claims to need, medication relating to a heart condition, diabetes, epilepsy, or a condition of comparable seriousness (C9.12).

Responsibilities when assessing fitness to detain

In all cases, the forensic practitioner is duty bound:
- To practise good medicine and treat all persons with courtesy and respect.
- To consider the health, safety, and well-being of the detainee to be of paramount importance (overriding forensic considerations).
- To obtain appropriate consent and explain to the detainee the implications of the examination.
- To respect confidentiality within the constraints of personal safety and public duty.
- To provide proper instructions to the police to enable them to care for the detainee.

The purpose of the examination

- To assess illness, injuries, and drug and alcohol problems.
- To advise the custody staff about general care for the detainee whilst in custody.

- To provide necessary medication.
- To identify those detainees who are not fit to be detained and assist with arrangements regarding their appropriate diversion from custody.
- To liaise with other key health workers.
- To make mental health assessments.
- To advise on the risk of self-harm.
- To advise on the need for clinical review of the detainee.

Making an assessment

Liaison with custody staff

This is essential before examining the detainee. The following information should be obtained and recorded:

- Why the person has been arrested.
- Any relevant details about the arrest (e.g. whether restraint was used, whether the person sustained injury at time of arrest or exhibited abnormal behaviour).
- Any significant items in the detainee's property when booked into custody (e.g. medication, drug injecting paraphernalia).
- What the custody officer is concerned about and what questions need to be answered (e.g. fit to be detained, fit for interview, fit for transfer).
- What are the time constraints.
- Are any specialized forensic assessments required (e.g. taking of samples, interpretation of injuries).
- Any significant warnings on the PNC.
- Any relevant information from others (e.g. prisoner escort record [PER] form, family, friends, hospital).

History and examination

Having obtained information from the custody staff, the forensic practitioner needs to decide, in conjunction with the police, where to examine the detainee. After introducing him/herself and obtaining appropriate consent, the forensic practitioner should proceed to take a standard medical history, including a careful drug history. It is worth bearing in mind that detainees may have a different agenda from that classically encountered in patients in the community.

Outcome of the assessment

Common sense should prevail when deciding whether a detainee's particular medical condition renders him/her unfit to be detained in police custody. A useful question to consider is, if the consultation had occurred in general practice, would it still be reasonable to keep the patient at home under the care of his/her family? If not, he/she is unlikely to be fit to be detained in custody, because custody staff cannot be expected to carry out sophisticated observations over and above those expected of other members of the public.

Instructions to custody staff

PACE Codes of Practice require custody officers to seek advice on the management and care of detainees who have been examined by healthcare professionals:

> **C9.13**—Whenever the appropriate healthcare professional is called in accordance with this section to examine or treat a detainee, the custody officer shall ask for their opinion about:
> - Any risks or problems which police need to take into account when making decisions about the detainee's continued detention;
> - When to carry out an interview if applicable; and
> - The need for safeguards.

Following assessment of a detainee, it is essential that the forensic practitioner provides custody staff with clear and detailed instructions about any medical supervision required, including the frequency of visits needed. The information should be written down in the custody record to ensure it is available to staff after changes in shift. It is worth bearing in mind that police officers are not medically qualified, so it is best to avoid complicated medical terminology and acronyms. Due account should be taken about confidentiality—information about a detainee's health should only be provided when it is necessary to protect their health or that of others who come into contact with them. The PACE Codes of Practice 'do not require any information about the cause of any injury, ailment or condition to be recorded on the custody record if it appears capable of providing evidence of an offence' (Code C.9G).

Frequency of visits by custody staff

When advising custody staff about the frequency of visits you need to be aware of their obligations in this respect under PACE Codes of Practice.

> **C9.3**—Detainees should be visited at least every hour. If no foreseeable risk was identified in a risk assessment … there is no need to wake a sleeping detainee. Those suspected of being intoxicated through drink or drugs or whose level of consciousness causes concern must, subject to any clinical directions given by the appropriate healthcare professional, *see paragraph 9.13*:
> - Be visited and roused at least every half hour.
> - Have their condition assessed as in *Annex H*.
> - And clinical treatment arranged if appropriate.

Whenever possible, juveniles and mentally vulnerable detainees should be visited more frequently than every hour (C.9B).

If the forensic practitioner considers that a detainee should be checked more often than half hourly, serious consideration must be given to whether it is safe for the detainee to remain in custody. Forensic practitioners should not recommend a frequency of checks that is impractical in a busy custody suite.

Rousing detainees

Code C Annex H sets out how custody staff should assess the level of rousability based on the '4Rs'.

Annex H—Detained Person: Observation List

1 If a detainee fails to meet any of the criteria listed below, an appropriate healthcare professional or an ambulance must be called.

2 When considering the level of rousability, consider:

Rousability—can they be woken? Go into the cell, call their name, shake gently.

Response to questions—can they give appropriate answers to questions such as—What's your name? Where do you live? Where do you think you are?

Response to commands—can they respond appropriately to commands such as—Open your eyes! Lift one arm and then the other.

3 Remember to take into account the possibility or presence of other illnesses, injury or mental condition, a person who is drowsy and smells of alcohol may also have the following: diabetes, epilepsy, head injury, drug intoxication or overdose, stroke.

Custody staff need to be advised that 'the purpose of recording a person's responses when attempting to rouse them using the procedure in Annex H is to enable any change in the individuals consciousness level to be noted and clinical treatment arranged if needed' (C.9H).

Levels of observation by custody staff

These are set out in the national *Guidance on the Safer Detention & Handling of Persons in Police Custody (2006)* for police officers, which suggests four different levels of observation for detainees. It is helpful if you use similar terms when making recommendations on the level of observation detainees require:

Level 1

General observation

This is the **minimum** acceptable level for all detainees. It requires the following:

- Detainees are checked **at least every hour**.
- Checks are carried out sensitively in order to cause as little intrusion as possible.
- If no reasonable foreseeable risk is identified, staff need not wake a sleeping detainee.
- If the detainee is awake, the officer should engage with the detainee.
- Visits and observations, including the detainee's behaviour/condition, are recorded in the custody record.
- Any changes in behaviour/condition must be reported to the custody officer immediately.

The use of technology does not negate the need for physical checks and visits.

Level 2

Intermittent observation

This is, subject to clinical direction, the **minimum** acceptable level for those suspected of being intoxicated through drink or drugs or having swallowed drugs, or whose level of consciousness causes concern. It requires the following:

- The detainee is visited and roused **at least every 30min**.
- Physical visits and checks must be carried out. CCTV and other technologies can be used in addition.
- In response to clinical direction, a person detained in relation to drugs swallowing need not be roused.
- The detainee is positively engaged at frequent and irregular intervals.
- Visits to the detainee are conducted in accordance with Codes of Practice, Code C, Annex H.
- Visits and observations, including the detainee's behaviour/condition, are recorded in the custody record.
- Any changes in behaviour/condition must be reported to the custody officer immediately.

Level 3

Constant observation

If the detainee's risk assessment indicates the likelihood of self-harm they should be observed at this level. It requires the following:

- The detainee is under constant observation and accessible **at all times**.
- Physical checks and visits must be carried out.
- Constantly monitored CCTV and other technologies can be used.
- Issues of privacy, dignity, and gender are taken into consideration.
- Any possible ligatures are removed.
- The detainee is positively engaged at frequent and irregular intervals.
- Visits and observations, including the detainee's behaviour/condition, are recorded in the custody record.
- Any changes in behaviour/condition must be reported to the custody officer immediately.
- Review by the healthcare professional.

Level 4

Close proximity

Detainees at the highest risk of self harm should be observed at this level. It requires the following:

- The detainee is physically supervised in close proximity.
- CCTV and other technologies do not meet the criteria of close proximity but may complement this level of observation.
- Issues of privacy, dignity, and gender are taken into consideration.
- Any possible ligatures are removed.
- The detainee is positively engaged at frequent and irregular intervals.
- Observations, including the detainee's behaviour/condition, are recorded in the custody record.
- Any changes in behaviour/condition must be reported to the custody officer immediately.
- Review by the healthcare professional.

Detainees requiring continuing healthcare

The average length of detention of those held in police custody is ~6h. Therefore, for the majority of detainees, there is no requirement for the provision of continuing care or referral for specialist treatment. However, the following are instances where some form of continuing care is necessary:

- Persons arrested towards the beginning of a weekend or bank holiday period who are to be held until the 'next available court'.
- Home Office prisoners held in police custody.
- Prisoners held under the prevention of terrorism legislation.
- People whose immigration status has been challenged or are awaiting deportation or transfer to immigration centres.

Obtaining reliable information about the past medical history of such detainees is often extremely difficult, although the introduction of the PER form has eased this problem in respect of prisoners transferred to the police from a court or prison. The PER should record the outcome of any risk assessment, together with information about the prisoner's ongoing need for medical care, observation, examination, or medication.

Home Office prisoners

On occasions, Home Office prisoners have to be detained in police cells because of inadequate provision of prison accommodation. The management of Home Office prisoners in police cells presents particular challenges for the police and the healthcare professionals responsible for their care. The conditions of their detention and medical care require special consideration and raised levels of vigilance and staffing.

Medical records

The prison authorities should arrange for the clinical records of any Home Office prisoner to travel with them when they are transferred to police custody. The records must be stored securely at the police station and the forensic practitioner should ensure that they are kept up to date either by entering his/her assessment and actions in the records or by requesting that copies of the police medical reports are sent with the prisoner when he/she is next transferred. In the absence of the previous clinical records being available, the forensic practitioner should contact the healthcare department of the prison from which the person has come in order to obtain an understanding of that individual's health needs.

Care of Home Office prisoners

Although PACE does not apply to convicted or remanded prisoners held in police cells, the provisions in the PACE Codes of Practice on conditions of detention and treatment of detainees should be considered as the minimum standard of treatment for such individuals. It is expected that Home Office prisoners in police custody will:

- Have a full healthcare assessment on arrival at the police station when an appropriate management plan (including frequency of observation, medication needs, and review frequency) will be established.

- Be entitled to medical attention at his or her request.
- Have acceptable conditions of detention in cells that are not overcrowded, are kept clean and have adequate ventilation and lighting.
- Have daily access to fresh air and exercise for a reasonable period of time.

Terrorist prisoners

The power to detain persons suspected of terrorism offences is under Section 41 of the Terrorism Act 2000 and not PACE. The power applies to any part of the UK and currently the maximum period of detention is 28 days (as amended by the Terrorism Act 2006).

Medical implications and care

All persons detained under prevention of terrorism legislation should:
- Have an automatic medical examination on detention to assess fitness to detain and interview, together with a complete body surface examination to note any injuries. In view of the potential for hunger strikes, the detained person's weight should be measured.
- Have a medical examination before release and also before and after being removed from the premises, again including a complete body surface examination to note any injuries.
- Be offered a daily medical assessment by a forensic physician, who should consider and advise on the detainee's dietary and exercise requirements.

Further reading

Faculty of Forensic and Legal Medicine (2006). *Home Office prisoners, Recommendations for forensic physicians*, and Faculty of Forensic and Legal Medicine (2007). *Medical care of persons detained under the Terrorism Act 2000*. Both available at ℘ http://www.fflm.ac.uk/library.

Prescribing medication

Principles of prescribing to detainees

Those detained in police custody are entitled to the same standard of care as those in the community. Medication prescribed in the community should be continued in custody unless it considered unsafe to do so. When prescribing to detainees, forensic practitioners should aim for a safe regimen and be wary of administering medication to those who are intoxicated by alcohol or drugs. Sufficient medication should be prescribed for the duration of the detainee's stay in custody, unless medical review is intended. As the custody staff who are likely to be administering the medication are non-clinical, it is essential that written instructions are clear to ensure that the correct medication is given, at the right dose, to the intended detainee, at the appropriate time.

How medication may be supplied

Medication may be obtained from:
- Stock items held in a locked cupboard in the medical room.
- The forensic practitioner's medical bag.
- A community pharmacy by means of a private prescription or, in the case of a controlled drug, an FP10PCD prescription.
- The detainee's property.
- Or may be brought in by a friend/relative or by the police from the detainee's home address (in these cases, the medication needs to be checked before it is administered).

Henley tablet bags (white, plastic, self-closing small bags with printed labels), preprinted envelopes, or bottles with labels to store medication can be used. Separate bags, envelopes, or bottles are used for each different medication to be supplied. Each should be labelled to show:
- Name of the detainee to whom the medication has been supplied.
- The name of the prescriber.
- Medication's name, strength, and quantity (number of tablets/capsules).
- The instructions for use.
- The date of dispensing.

Patient Group Directions (PGDs)

PGDs are legal documents that provide written instructions for the supply or administration of medicines to groups of patients who may not be individually identified before presentation for treatment. Primarily intended to authorize the supply of prescription-only medicines, they may also be used to authorize supply of general sales list and pharmacy medicines. PGDs are increasingly being used in police custody to allow nurses to prescribe in certain specific situations—offering advantages to patient care, without compromising safety. PGDs must be used within defined clinical governance frameworks. They are inflexible. Detainees must meet the specific inclusion criteria—if not, the practitioner must contact a doctor for authority to supply or administer the medication (i.e. a patient *specific* direction).

Medication forms

Details of any medication to be administered should be entered in the relevant parts of the computerized 'Detained Person's Medical Form'. These contain sections for 'Once Only Medication' and 'Regular Medication'. The date, time, and dose of each drug to be administered needs to be indicated, together with whether the medication should be given to the detainee or an escort service on his/her release/transfer from custody.

Controlled drugs

Prescribing controlled drugs

A special form (FP10PCD) has been introduced for any private prescription of schedule 2 & 3 controlled drugs which will be dispensed in the community. Forensic physicians will need to use a FP10PCD whenever prescribing schedule 2 & 3 controlled drugs to detainees in police custody. If a forensic physician has not yet been issued with a private prescriber identification number and supply of FP10PCDs, he/she should contact the local Primary Care Trust. Note that current NHS prescribers receive a separate private prescriber number in addition to their NHS prescriber number—it is important to use the correct number when prescribing NHS and private prescriptions to ensure that prescribing costs are attributed to the appropriate budget.

Administering controlled drugs in custody

Special restrictions on the administration of controlled drugs are laid down in PACE Codes of Practice C9.10:

> **C9.10**—No police officer may administer or supervise the self-administration of controlled drugs of the types and forms listed in the Misuse of Drugs Regulations 2001, Schedule 1, 2 or 3. A detainee may only self-administer such drugs under the personal supervision of the registered medical practitioner authorizing their use. Drugs listed in Schedule 4 or 5 may be distributed by the custody officer for self-administration if they have consulted the registered medical practitioner authorizing their use, this may be done by telephone, and both parties are satisfied self-administration will not expose the detainee, police officers, or anyone else to the risk of harm or injury.

In practical terms, this means that a forensic physician (but not a custody nurse or paramedic) has to be in attendance whenever detainees self-administer methadone, buprenorphine, and temazepam (but not other benzodiazepines) in custody.

Deaths in custody

Deaths in police custody, whilst small in number, have a huge impact on the public's confidence in the police. As a minimum, each death is likely to lead to an expensive inquiry, grief for the relatives of the deceased, and anxiety and stress for those involved in the care of the individual.

Definition of deaths during or following police contact

On 1 April 2002, the Home Office introduced revised categories of deaths of members of the public during or following police contact:

Category 1—Fatal road traffic incidents involving the police
This definition covers all deaths of members of the public resulting from road traffic incidents involving the police, both where the person who dies is in a vehicle and where they are on foot.

Category 2—Fatal shooting incidents involving the police
This definition covers circumstances where police fire the fatal shots.

Category 3—Deaths in or following custody
This definition covers the deaths of persons who have been arrested or otherwise detained by the police (including deaths occurring whilst a person is being arrested or taken into detention). The death may have taken place on police, private, or medical premises, in a public place, or in a police or other vehicle (including where the person dies in or on the way to hospital during transfer from police detention and where the person dies after leaving police detention and there is a link between that detention and the death).

Category 4—Deaths during or after other types of contact with police
This definition covers circumstances where a person dies during or after some form of contact with the police which did not amount to detention and there is a link between that contact and the death (e.g. where a person is actively attempting to evade arrest when the death occurs).

Deaths during or following police contact—statistics

The numbers of deaths that have occurred in England and Wales since the introduction of the revised definitions above are shown in Table 6.1.

Table 6.1 Deaths in custody—statistics for England and Wales

Year	All categories	Category 3 deaths
2002/03	104	40
2003/04	100	38
2004/05	106	36
2005/06	118	28
2006/07	82	27
2007/08	75	22

Investigating deaths in police custody

Under the Police Reform Act 2002, police forces in England and Wales have a statutory duty to refer to the Independent Police Complaints Commission (IPCC) any incident involving a death which has arisen from or during police contact. This allows the IPCC to make a decision about whether or not to investigate a case.

The IPCC is run by a Chair and ten Operational Commissioners (including two Deputy Chairs). They guarantee its independence and by law can never have served as police officers. When investigating deaths in custody, the IPCC works closely with the CPS, which is responsible for prosecuting criminal offences in relation to deaths in custody (unlawful act manslaughter, gross negligence manslaughter, and misconduct in public office).

Reducing deaths in police custody

There has been a steady reduction in the number of deaths in police custody (category 3 deaths) from a high of 56 in 1997/98. This is due to a number of factors, including:

- Designing out suicide risks from cells (e.g. absence of ligature points).
- Better monitoring (e.g. CCTV).
- Improved training of custody staff.
- Improved levels of observation of vulnerable detainees.
- Introduction of risk assessment by police.
- Improved awareness amongst FPs and nurses.
- Awareness that a significant factor in a number of deaths is a misperception by police and/or doctors that detainees are 'feigning illness'—feigning illness should be a diagnosis of exclusion.
- Increased diversion of those who are drunk and incapable away from police stations.

Life-threatening emergencies in custody

Approach to life-threatening custody emergencies

The forensic physician or nurse practitioner who works in custody for any length of time can reasonably expect to be faced with severe (life-threatening) emergency clinical problems on at least an occasional basis. The combination of relative isolation, lack of advanced facilities, and no immediately available expert assistance result in a potentially stressful situation for all concerned. Knowledge of the extent of the scrutiny of each professional's actions if things go really wrong does not help this either! It is important for forensic practitioners to ensure that they have the relevant knowledge and skills to manage life-threatening emergencies. Appropriate knowledge and expertise need to be combined with a plan of action for the more common emergencies.

Knowledge

No one can know (or be expected to know) everything, but for the purposes of treating custody emergencies, forensic practitioners should aim to 'know' anything (treatments, guidelines, protocols) which their patients need them to know and which there is not time to look up. This includes the following:

- Immediate recall of basic (and limited advanced) life support treatment algorithms, including choking.
- Knowledge of local referral (and management) protocols, including knowledge of where the nearest local hospitals are and what facilities are available there.
- Knowledge of what equipment is available within the custody centre, where exactly it is situated, and how it works.

As far as those things which forensic practitioners do not know but have time to look up, it is important that they know exactly where relevant resources are located. It is sensible to have accessible a small library of relevant texts, most particularly including the *British National Formulary*.

Skills

In addition to basic clinical skills, it is essential that forensic practitioners possess the ability to perform the following:
- Recognition of the acutely unwell (or injured) patient.
- Basic life support.
- Manoeuvres to treat choking.
- Basic airway management (assessment and basic opening procedures).
- Limited advanced airway management (use of pocket mask, bag/valve/ mask, suction, oxygen—as appropriate).
- Coordinated procedure to roll a patient into the recovery position.
- Emergency needle decompression of tension pneumothorax.
- Tamponade to stop external haemorrhage.

Local and national courses are available to gain necessary skills (see ℘ http://www.resus.org.uk, http://www.alsg.org, http://www.fflm.ac.uk)

Emergency plan of action

On the basis that they can expect to face life-threatening emergencies in custody on at least an occasional basis, it is sensible for forensic practitioners to have a plan of action of what to do. Consider the following:

- Someone should dial 999 (or 911) and request emergency assistance from the ambulance service. It may be relevant to quickly consider whether there may be other individuals who may be immediately available and of some help.
- Someone needs to obtain the relevant equipment (and where relevant, drugs) if not instantly available.
- An **A, B, C (Airway, Breathing, Circulation)** approach to initial assessment and treatment should be followed.
- Appropriate interventions need to be provided according to the situation and expertise of the practitioner.
- The forensic practitioner should wait with the patient until the ambulance arrives, then the patient handed over verbally and if possible, in writing also.
- Once the patient has left custody for hospital, notes need to be completed, then staff debriefed as appropriate.
- If the patient was in cardiac arrest in custody and/or death seems to be a likely outcome, it is important to discuss with the senior custody officer who will commence relevant procedures (see 📖 p.214).

The A, B, C approach

The A, B, C approach is widely adopted in prehospital and emergency medicine to provide a structured approach which combines assessment and treatment according to priorities and problems as they are discovered. It is often extended to A, B, C, D, E as follows:

- Airway—assessment and interventions to open the airway.
- Breathing—assessment combined with assistance if needed.
- Circulation—assessment combined with interventions.
- Disability—assessing conscious level/pupils (with interventions).
- Exposure—to identify any hidden problems.

Custody equipment

There is some variation between different regions regarding the amount of medical equipment (and drugs) which are available. This particularly applies to the provision of oxygen, suction, airway adjuncts, and automated external defibrillators, although a good case for each can be made. The forensic practitioner needs to be aware of what resources are available within each unit.

Airway obstruction 1

The importance of airway obstruction as a potential life-threatening emergency is reflected in the fact that 'A' for 'airway' is the first priority in the standard ABC assessment of any unwell patient.

Common causes of airway obstruction in custody

- Reduced conscious level due to alcohol, drugs, and/or injury or indeed, any other cause—in many instances airway obstruction is the result of the tongue falling back and obstructing the upper airway.
- Vomit and/or other secretions in the upper airway, possibly combined with reduced conscious level (with reduced airway reflexes).
- Choking from inhaled foreign body whilst eating—with the diagnosis usually obvious because of this (see 📖 Choking, p.224).

Signs of airway obstruction

These depend to a certain extent upon the cause, but include cyanosis, gurgling, snoring, and stridor. There may be some external vomit. In some patients who are struggling with complete upper airway obstruction paradoxical movements of the chest and abdomen may occur, but without audible breath sounds.

Management

Various options are available, depending upon the clinical condition of the patient and the skills and expertise available. After any intervention, reassess to establish whether there has been any clinical improvement in the patient's condition.

- In many instances, the clinical condition of the detainee will necessitate transfer to hospital, so consider the need to call 999 for an ambulance and paramedic assistance.
- The mouth needs to be opened and checked for foreign material and vomit—suction (if available) may help to remove liquid substances, but if the patient is actively vomiting, it is usually best to roll him/her onto his/her side.
- Airway opening manoeuvres. In the absence of trauma, the first manoeuvre to attempt is a *head tilt* combined with a *chin lift* by placing one hand on the patient's forehead and tilting the head back, whilst placing the index and middle fingers of the other hand under the point of the chin and lifting upwards.
- An alternative method of attempting to open the airway (useful after trauma) is to use the *jaw thrust*. This involves placing the middle and other fingers of both hands behind both angles of the mandibles and applying firm pressure upwards on both sides.
- If these measures are unsuccessful, it may be necessary to consider inserting an *oropharyngeal* (Fig. 7.1) or *nasopharyngeal airway* (Fig. 7.2).
- High-flow O_2 should be provided by mask (if available).
- Any underlying causes need to be addressed and transfer to hospital arranged as appropriate.

Oropharyngeal (Guedel) airway insertion

The oropharyngeal airway may be useful for patients with an obstructed upper airway with an absent gag reflex. It helps to stop the tongue from falling back.

- Select the correct size of airway by holding one against the patient's face: an appropriate sized airway reaches from the corner of the mouth to the external auditory canal. Typical sizes are 2 or 3 for women, 3 for most men, 4 for larger men.
- Open the mouth and insert the airway 'upside down' for ~4cm (halfway in), then rotate it 180° as it is inserted until the flange reaches the teeth. (Note that in children the oropharyngeal airway is inserted the 'right way up').
- Reassess the airway.

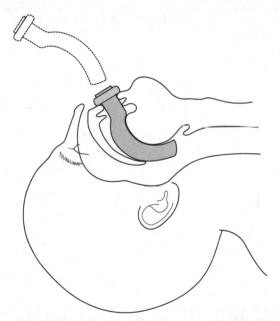

Fig. 7.1 Oral airway insertion. Reproduced from Illingworth KA *et al.* (2006). *Anaesthesia and Analgesia in Emergency Medicine*, with permission of Oxford University Press.

Airway obstruction 2

Nasopharyngeal airway insertion
The nasopharyngeal airway may be useful for patients with an obstructed upper airway whose teeth are clenched (e.g. epileptic fit). It is contraindicated in anyone with facial or head injury (risk of intracranial insertion!) and can cause nasal bleeding, particularly if excessive force is employed. A safety pin through the end prevents inadvertent displacement into the nose.

- Select the correct size of airway. Traditionally, it is said that the correct size will be the same diameter as the patient's little finger—usually 6mm diameter for women and 7mm for men.
- Lubricate the airway with water-soluble lubricant.
- Insert the tip of the airway into the right nostril and slide it in gently, aiming posteriorly until the flange meets the nostril. If there is any resistance, do not force it, but stop and try the left nostril.

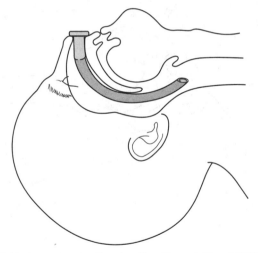

Fig. 7.2 Nasal airway insertion. Reproduced from Illingworth KA *et al.* (2006). *Anaesthesia and Analgesia in Emergency Medicine*, with permission of Oxford University Press.

Choking

Within the custody setting, choking is most likely to result from food, although other objects may be responsible, possibly in an attempt to self-harm. The Resuscitation Council 2010 guidelines for choking/foreign body upper airway obstruction in adults (see ℘ http://www.resus.org.uk) require an initial quick assessment and categorization of the severity of the problem (Fig. 7.3).

Ask the patient: *'Are you choking?'*

Mild obstruction

A patient with mild obstruction will be able to answer the question, speak, cough, and breathe. Encourage him/her to continue to attempt to clear the obstruction him/herself by further coughing.

Severe obstruction

Intervene by giving a back blow (using the heel of the hand) between the shoulder blades with the patient leaning forwards. If this fails to clear the obstruction, repeat up to a maximum of five back blows. If these all fail, try an abdominal thrust by leaning the patient forwards, standing behind them with arms encircling then thrusting sharply upwards with a fist between the umbilicus and xiphisternum. Check for a response, but if the obstruction remains, repeat up to a total of five thrusts. If the obstruction remains unrelieved, continue alternating five back blows with five abdominal thrusts.

Unconscious patient

If the patient becomes unconscious despite treatment, the standard approach is to support them carefully to the ground and commence cardiopulmonary resuscitation (starting with chest compressions). Within the custody environment, it is worth opening and checking the airway for visible and easily removable foreign body placed there in an attempt at self-harm. Ensure that someone dials 999 for an emergency ambulance.

Role of the 'finger sweep'

Use of a 'blind' finger sweep (i.e. sweep in the mouth with the fingers in the absence of visible airway obstruction) may cause further harm to the patient and/or (biting) injury to the rescuer. For these reasons, the use of a blind finger sweep is best avoided—manually remove material from the airway only if it can be seen.

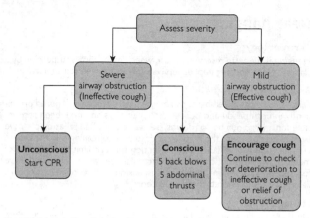

Fig. 7.3 Adult choking algorithm. Reproduced with permission of the Resuscitation Council UK (🖰 http://www.resus.org.uk).

Near hanging

Terminology

Hanging is the term reserved for use when death follows suspension by a ligature. *Near hanging* implies survival, at least for a period afterwards.

Background

Serious attempts at self-harm by hanging have historically featured prominently in both prison and police custody settings and have been responsible for a large number of deaths (see 📖 p.214). Radical attempts have been made to reduce the number of deaths by combining risk assessment with increased surveillance and prevention through limiting availability of materials which might be used. In particular, design of police cells have focused upon removing potential suspension fixture points (windows, light fittings, and 'wickets'/hatches in doors).

Management

On finding a detainee who has attempted to hang himself/herself, adopt the following approach:
- Shout for help and paramedic assistance as appropriate.
- Free the patient and gently place them supine on the floor, freeing the obstruction.
- Open and check the airway, removing any obvious visible foreign material. Theoretical concerns about possible associated cervical spine injury are remote in cases of non-judicial hanging in which the body has not fallen. Therefore, if jaw thrust (see 📖 p.220) alone fails to satisfactorily open the airway, consider using head tilt and chin lift (see 📖 p.220).
- Assess breathing and circulation: if there is no pulse and no breathing, treat as for cardiac arrest (see 📖 p.230). If the patient has a pulse but is not breathing, provide rescue breaths until breathing returns. Use upper airway adjuncts with self-inflating bag and mask (or pocket mask) with oxygen and suction as available and appropriate (see 📖 p.228), reassessing the pulse regularly. If there is a pulse and spontaneous breathing (or this returns), use airway opening techniques and monitor regularly until paramedics arrive.
- If the patient has (or regains) spontaneous respiration and circulation, but remains unconscious place him/her into the recovery position (see 📖 p.229) and continue to monitor until arrival of paramedics.
- Anticipate any successful or significant suicide attempt to be followed by a thorough investigation. Ensure that notes are written as soon after the incident as possible and that they are full and complete.

Tension pneumothorax

This serious emergency is rarely encountered in clinical forensic practice, but it is important for the forensic practitioner to be able to identify and rapidly treat it. Tension pneumothorax reflects progressive accumulation of gas in the pleural cavity and eventually causes mediastinal shift, kinking the great vessels, thereby compromising venous return and cardiac output. It occurs most frequently in victims of trauma who are being artificially ventilated, but may also occur in patients with chest trauma who are spontaneously breathing, or as a complication of asthma.

Presentation

Tension pneumothorax results in breathlessness, absent breath sounds and (hyper-)resonance on the affected side, combined with evidence of mediastinal shift (tracheal deviation away from the affected side, engorged neck veins, and tachycardia and hypotension). Diagnosis is purely clinical (even in hospital).

Treatment

- Call for emergency paramedic assistance.
- Provide O_2 by face mask (if available).
- Obtain a large bore (e.g. 14G or 16G) cannula and use it to decompress the tension pneumothorax by inserting it above the third rib (second intercostal space) in the mid-clavicular line on the affected side (see Fig. 7.4). Remove the needle and listen for a (reassuring) hiss of gas. Note that this procedure is likely to simply convert a tension pneumothorax back into a simple pneumothorax (which itself will still require to be definitively treated later).
- Tape the cannula in place and check for clinical improvement.
- If the patient deteriorates again whilst awaiting the arrival of the paramedics, reassess the patient and consider the need to insert a second cannula adjacent to the first.

Mid-clavicular line

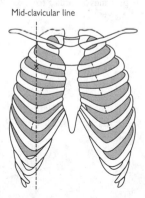

Fig. 7.4 Site for needle decompression. Reproduced from Wyatt JP et al. (2006). *Oxford Handbook of Emergency Medicine*, 3rd edn, with permission of Oxford University Press.

Respiratory arrest

There are a number of conditions in clinical forensic practice which may cause respiratory arrest and which untreated, may ultimately go on to result in cardiac arrest. Significantly reduced or absent ventilation may be caused by the following:

• Airway obstruction resulting from one or more of: external pressure; reduced conscious level with tongue falling back; foreign material including aspirated vomit.

• Reduced respiratory drive due to drugs. In particular, opioid drugs are frequently implicated, although other drugs such as benzodiazepines (especially combined with alcohol) may have similar effects on respiration.

• Respiratory inadequacy due to asthma, COPD, pulmonary embolism, tension pneumothorax.

Presentation and management

The clinical picture of a hypoxic patient with respiratory insufficiency but with a good pulse is the precursor to full cardiac arrest. Rapid assessment and intervention is required:

• Summon urgent assistance as appropriate.

• Quickly assess airway patency and use airway opening procedures (±suction—see 📖 p.220) to attempt to relieve any obstruction.

• Provide rescue breaths using a pocket mask or self-inflating bag and mask and provide oxygen (if available).

• Consider whether *opioid overdose* may be a possible underlying cause (features include pinpoint pupils and intravenous drug injection marks). If this seems a possibility, give an intramuscular injection of naloxone (suggested dose of 800micrograms, which may be repeated according to response).

• If breathing returns and circulation remains satisfactory, place the patient in the recovery position (Fig. 7.5).

• Continue to address priorities according to A, B, C (see 📖 p.218) until paramedic assistance arrives.

The recovery position

The recovery position can be helpful for patients who are breathing and have a pulse, but have reduced conscious level and no concern about cervical spine injury. It is particularly useful for patients who are at risk of vomiting and aspiration. One person can manage to move a supine patient into the recovery position as shown in Fig. 7.5—the principle is to move the patient in a controlled fashion towards the practitioner. However, within the custody setting, there are usually several people available to help with this. Having placed the patient in the recovery position, check and adjust/open the airway as necessary.

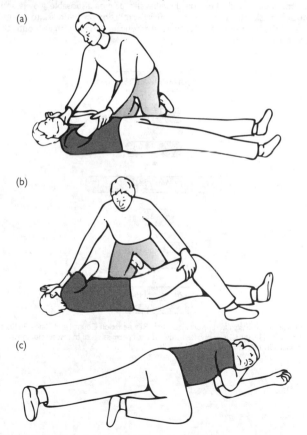

Fig. 7.5 One method of moving the supine patient into the recovery position.
Reprinted with permission from Greaves I and Porter K (1997). *Pre-hospital Medicine—The Principles and Practice of Immediate Care*, Edward Arnold (Publishers) Ltd.

Cardiac arrest in custody

Although relatively uncommon, cardiac arrest in custody does occur and on some occasions forensic practitioners are close at hand and available to commence resuscitation. Causes of cardiac arrest in custody are considered more fully on 🕮 p.214. They include some of the 'standard' medical causes (e.g. ischaemic heart disease), but a significant proportion reflect alcohol/drugs, self-harm, or other more custody-specific causes. In addition to cardiac arrest, forensic practitioners may be faced with patients who still have a pulse but have stopped breathing (respiratory arrest), particularly in the context of drug overdose. It is suggested that forensic practitioners carry with them (in their bags) a pair of disposable gloves and pocket mask—the provision of artificial ventilation pocket mask to mouth is likely to be more effective (and aesthetically pleasing) than mouth to mouth ventilation.

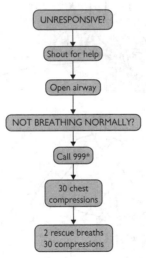

Fig. 7.6 Adult basic life support algorithm (Resuscitation Council guidelines, 2010). *For out of hospital use only. Reproduced with permission of the Resuscitation Council UK (🕾 http://www.resus.org.uk).

Basic life support in custody

The Resuscitation Council algorithm shown in Fig. 7.6 is appropriate for use out of hospital. The algorithm may be adapted for use in police custody and other forensic environments, depending upon the available facilities and expertise.

Airway opening Use a head tilt and chin lift to open the airway (as described on 📖 p.220), unless there is evidence of head/neck trauma, when a jaw thrust is more appropriate (see 📖 p.220). Remove any visible obstructions from the mouth, but leave well-fitting dentures in position.

Assessment of breathing and circulation Look, listen, and feel for breathing and check for a carotid pulse for up to 10s—it is possible for trained health professionals to perform both tasks simultaneously.

Having diagnosed cardiac arrest Once cardiac arrest has been diagnosed, the best chance of survival lies with prompt initiation of basic life support and early advanced treatment. This usually involves simultaneously commencing basic life support with calling for paramedic assistance (by dialling 999 or 911). Note that chest compressions are given before ventilations.

Chest compressions (Fig. 7.7) Depress the sternum by 5–6cm aiming for a rate of 100–120/min, allowing equal time for compression and release phases. Use a compression to ventilation ratio of 30:2.

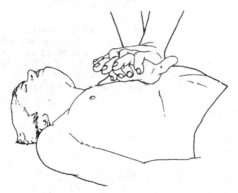

Fig. 7.7 Chest compressions. Reproduced with permission from Colquhoun MC et al. (1999). *ABC of Resuscitation* 4th edn. BMJ books, Wiley-Blackwell.

Ventilations A pocket mask or (better) bag/valve/mask attached to oxygen allows better resuscitation (given appropriate training). Each breath should last ~1s and make the chest visibly rise.

Modified advanced life support

Standard (advanced life support) management of cardiac arrest as typically practised in hospital and/or by fully equipped paramedics requires advanced training and equipment. Within the custody setting, this approach needs to be modified according to available equipment, skills, and expertise. Given that the forensic practitioner is likely to be the most trained individual present, he/she should aim to stay with the patient and commence resuscitation whilst other individuals call for help and obtain relevant equipment. Two key elements of a successful outcome following cardiac arrest are early effective **basic life support** and in the case of ventricular fibrillation or pulseless ventricular tachycardia, early **defibrillation**.

Oropharyngeal/nasopharyngeal airways

An oropharyngeal or nasopharyngeal airway may prove to be useful in helping to maintain patency of the airway. Sizing and insertion is considered on 🕮 p.221.

Suction

Wide-bore rigid suction (e.g. Yankauer suction device) can assist in the removal of blood, saliva, or other liquids from the upper airway. Given the typical lack of any wall suction, held suction devices are often employed.

Pocket mask (Fig. 7.8)

A typical custody unit is awash with pocket masks. Mouth-to-mask ventilation is more aesthetically acceptable than mouth-to-mouth ventilation and most masks offer the advantage of having a port to accept supplemental oxygen (if available, use a flow rate of 10L/min). Secure the mask in place with both thumbs and 'lift' the jaw into the mask using the remaining fingers to perform a jaw thrust. Regular practice on manikins is recommended.

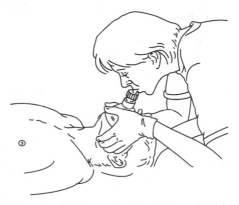

Fig. 7.8 Pocket mask use. This figure was published in Greaves I et al. (2005). *Emergency Care: A Textbook for Paramedics*, Copyright Saunders Ltd 2005.

Self-inflating bag with face mask (Fig. 7.9)

The self-inflating bag allows more controlled ventilation with air (rather than exhaled air) or high levels of O_2 if available and if combined with a reservoir bag. Use of the self-inflating bag with face mask does require some training and practice. It is generally easier (particularly for non-experts) to use a two-person technique in which one person uses two hands to apply the mask in place with the airway held open and another squeezes the bag.

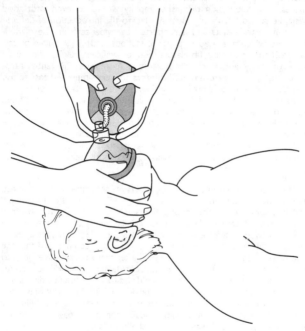

Fig. 7.9 Two-person technique for using a self inflating bag-valve-mask. Reproduced from *Advanced Life Support* (5th edition) 2006 with permission of the Resuscitation Council UK (ℜ http://www.resus.org.uk).

Other airways

The laryngeal mask airway and tracheal tube are alternative airways which are used extensively in other prehospital and hospital practice. The **laryngeal mask airway** is relatively easy to use, but there is little experience of their use in a custody setting. A correctly placed **tracheal tube** is the gold standard secure airway, but requires additional equipment, training, and practice. Given this, and the potential for harm by misplacement, it is only recommended for experts.

If cardiac arrest occurs when there is an automated external defibrillator available, follow the Resuscitation Council algorithm shown in Fig. 7.10.

Defibrillation

Patients in cardiac arrest who have the best long-term prognosis are those with heart rhythms of ventricular fibrillation or pulseless ventricular tachycardia (rather than asystole or pulseless electrical activity). Ventricular fibrillation and pulseless ventricular tachycardia may be treated with unsynchronized electrical shock from a defibrillator, but the chance of successful cardioversion diminishes rapidly with time, even with good basic life support. This argument has led to the introduction of defibrillators in custody units and is supported by evidence from use of defibrillators which are sited in airports, stations, and other public places. Old-fashioned manual defibrillators require significant training and if used inappropriately are potentially hazardous to rescuers. Recently introduced **automated external defibrillators** are very simple and easy to use and carry fewer risks. They use visual and voice prompts to guide lay rescuers and health professionals through safe defibrillation. They have been installed in many custody units, with custody police officers and detention officers being trained in their use. Forensic practitioners who work in custody units which are equipped with defibrillators need to ensure that they are familiar with their use. It is important that oxygen masks are removed and placed at least 1m away during defibrillation.

Drugs

There is little evidence that any drug affects the outcome in cardiac arrest. Treatment priorities instead focus upon good quality basic life support and appropriate defibrillation for patients with shockable cardiac rhythms. The standard treatment algorithm for cardiac arrest does advise on the use of intravenous adrenaline (1mg) every 3–5min. However, for patients in cardiac arrest due to a shockable rhythm, it is recommended that the first dose of adrenaline is deferred until after three shocks have failed to convert back to a perfusable rhythm. Considering this, it will be obvious that obtaining venous access and giving drugs to a patient in cardiac arrest in a custody setting is a relatively low priority. Given the limitations of the initial resuscitating team, attention should focus instead upon calling for paramedic assistance, providing good quality continuous basic life support, and (if appropriate and available) early defibrillation.

Pulseless electrical activity and asystole

In these rhythms, the focus is on maintaining good basic life support, providing O_2 and intravenous adrenaline. In addition, an underlying cause will be sought (remembered as 4 Hs and 4 Ts as follows: Hypoxia, Hypovolaemia, Hypothermia, Hypo/hyperkalaemia, Tension pneumothorax, cardiac Tamponade, Toxic disorders, Thrombosis).

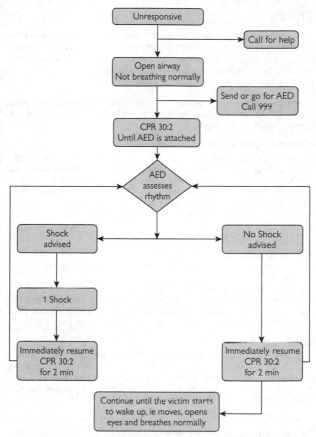

Fig. 7.10 Algorithm for use with the automated external defibrillator (Resuscitation Council guidelines, 2010). Reproduced with permission of the Resuscitation Council UK (🕮 http://www.resus.org.uk).

Shock

The common public interpretation of 'shock' refers to an emotional response to a sudden unpleasant experience. In the medical sense, 'shock' is quite simply inadequate delivery of O_2 to vital organs. Untreated, shock results in tissue damage, with acidosis and cell death.

Causes

Common causes are hypovolaemia, anaphylaxis, cardiogenic and septic shock. Other causes include neurogenic shock and cellular poisons (e.g. carbon monoxide, cyanide).

Hypovolaemic shock

Usually the result of haemorrhage from any cause (trauma, gastrointestinal bleeding, ruptured aortic aneurysm), but may also follow diarrhoea/vomiting, serious burns, and heat illness. The classical clinical picture is tachycardia combined with hypotension, but this is variable (especially in older patients and/or those on β-blockers). Look for cold extremities and a prolonged capillary refill time (>2s to pressure over the sternum, ≥4s peripherally).

Management
- Summon urgent paramedic assistance.
- Use swabs to provide direct pressure on any external bleeding wounds.
- Provide O_2 by face mask (if available).
- Occasionally, especially if the patient is moribund, it may be helpful to insert a venous cannula and commence rapid intravenous infusion of a litre of saline (resources, expertise, and time permitting).

Cardiogenic shock

May reflect arrhythmias, myocardial infarction, tension pneumothorax, or massive pulmonary embolus. Sit the patient up and summon urgent paramedic assistance and provide O_2 by face mask (if available). Check A, B, C—treat any obvious problems (e.g. tension pneumothorax—see p.227).

Septic shock

Typically, tachycardia and hypotension are associated with warm (vasodilated) peripheries. The source of sepsis may or may not be apparent. Aim to get the patient to hospital as rapidly as possible. Whilst awaiting paramedics, give O_2 (if available). It may be appropriate to consider insertion of a venous cannula and commence intravenous fluids. If there is any suspicion of meningitis/meningococcal disease, give an intravenous injection of 1.2g of benzylpenicillin (see p.240).

Neurogenic shock

High spinal cord injury interrupts sympathetic nerves, classically resulting in hypotension combined with bradycardia.

Anaphylaxis

This is the result of a generalized immunological reaction to a foreign material. Reactions may occur to drugs, stings, food (typically nuts), and other substances (e.g. latex).

Presenting features

There is a large variation in the types of reactions seen, but common features include: local skin reactions, swelling of lips, tongue or upper airway, peripheral vasodilatation (tachycardia and hypotension). Sometimes the first manifestation may be more unusual (e.g. vomiting, abdominal pain, diarrhoea). The principal *life-threatening presentations* are airway compromise, respiratory difficulty, and shock.

Management

See the Resuscitation Council guidelines (♒ http://www.resus.org.uk).

- Remove any obvious allergen.
- Summon urgent paramedic assistance.
- Provide O_2 (if available).
- Open and maintain the airway.
- Life-threatening features are an indication for intramuscular 0.5mg adrenaline (0.5mL of 1:1000 solution). This is available in many custody units and also carried by paramedics. Some patients with known previous anaphylactic reactions carry adrenaline autoinjectors (e.g. the Epipen®) which typically deliver 0.3mg (300 micrograms)—it is sensible to allow them to use their own 'pen' in the event of a serious reaction.
- If there is no response to the initial dose of intramuscular adrenaline within 5min, repeat it.
- Some patients may benefit from intravenous fluids and/or nebulized salbutamol (typically carried by paramedics).
- Note that administration of intravenous adrenaline carries significant potential risks and is certainly not appropriate outside of a hospital environment (unless given as part of the treatment for ensuing cardiac arrest).
- H_1 blockers (e.g. chlorphenamine), H_2 blockers (e.g. ranitidine), and steroids (e.g. hydrocortisone) are second-line agents which tend to take some time to work and do not affect the initial reaction.
- Occasionally, patients make a very rapid response to the first intramuscular injection of adrenaline. These patients are at risk of later deterioration as part of a biphasic response—they still require transfer to hospital for assessment, observation, and further treatment.

Epileptic fit

Many of the individuals who are detained in police custody are known to have epilepsy, and many others have alcohol-related fits. As a result, it is not unusual for patients to have fits in custody. Some fits are short-lived and followed by a rapid recovery, whilst others persist for longer and are not associated with full and quick recovery. Note that seizures which persist for >30min (status epilepticus) carry a significant mortality.

The fitting patient

- Protect the patient from further injury—consider the recovery position (see 📖 p.229), although this may prove impossible.
- Secure the airway. If the fit continues a nasopharyngeal airway (see 📖 p.222) may assist—provided that there is no head or facial injury present.
- Provide O$_2$ by mask (if available).
- If the fit persists for >2min, call for emergency paramedic assistance.
- If the fit persists for >5–10min, attempt to terminate the fit by pharmacological means. Give either 10mg rectal diazepam solution *or* if it is possible to obtain venous access, give 4mg lorazepam intravenously (now preferred to previous traditional choice of intravenous diazepam). Within the custody setting it can be tricky to secure venous access, particularly in a fitting patient. Given this, and the fact that rectal diazepam has unpredictable absorption, considerable attention has been given to the potential value of buccal liquid midazolam (10mg) in terminating fits. However, at the time of writing, this remains an unlicensed indication.
- Check blood glucose (BMG) and correct hypoglycaemia if present with 50mL of 20% glucose intravenous solution via a large cannula (intramuscular glucagon 1mg may be an alternative—see 📖 p.247).
- If the fit continues for 10min after initial administration of rectal diazepam or intravenous lorazepam, further doses may be given.
- Once the fit has stopped, place in the recovery position and reassess Airway, Breathing, Circulation. Provide oxygen, secure the airway (using adjuncts and/or suction as required). If it has not already been done, check the BMG and treat hypoglycaemia if present (as outlined earlier).
- It may be reasonable to keep in custody those patients who are known epileptics, and who have a brief fit with rapid complete recovery. Allow paramedics to transport to hospital all patients who have a 'first fit', a fit lasting more than a few minutes, or where drugs are used to terminate the fit or where rapid complete recovery does not occur.

The unconscious patient

Rapid assessment of conscious level ('responsiveness') involves categorization according to the AVPU scale:
- **A**lert, awake and conscious.
- Responds to **V**erbal stimuli.
- Responds only to **P**ainful stimuli.
- **U**nresponsive to any stimulus.

Inability to rouse a detainee in custody should prompt an immediate call for emergency paramedic assistance.

Causes

There are a large number of causes of reduced conscious level in custody, but the following occur relatively frequently:
- Hypoglycaemia.
- Drug overdose and/or alcohol intoxication.
- Epileptic fit (including post-ictal period).
- Head injury.

Other important causes are: subarachnoid haemorrhage (see 📖 p.266), stroke, encephalitis/meningitis (see 📖 p.240), any cause of shock or respiratory failure.

General approach

- Assess and open the airway (but avoid head tilt/chin lift if there is evidence of head/face injury—use a jaw thrust instead, as described on 📖 p.220).
- Call for O_2 (if available).
- Assess breathing, identifying the rate and listening to both lung fields. If breathing is absent or inadequate, consider the need to commence rescue breaths with self-inflating bag/mask or pocket mask (see 📖 p.228).
- Check pulse, blood pressure, and SaO_2 using pulse oximeter.
- Check BMG and treat hypoglycaemia if present. Intramuscular glucagon (1mg) can be used in insulin-dependent diabetics, otherwise give 50mL of 10% glucose intravenous solution via a large cannula (see 📖 p.247). Recheck BMG after treatment and consider need for further glucose.
- Perform a quick general examination, looking specifically for injuries, recent injection marks, evidence of meningitis/skin rash (see 📖 Suspected meningitis, p.240) and treat specific illnesses accordingly.
- Check pupils: large pupils are features of tricyclic overdose, sympathomimetic drugs, hypothermia. Small pupils are seen in opioid overdose, pontine haemorrhage. Note that small pupils and reduced conscious level in a custody setting is very suggestive of opioid overdose—support airway/breathing and give 0.8mg of naloxone intramuscularly (see 📖 p.228).
- Consider whether to place the patient in the recovery position (see 📖 p.229).
- Call for emergency paramedic assistance and continue to monitor the patient.

Suspected meningitis

Meningitis can be caused by a variety of different organisms. Amongst the bacterial causes, *Neisseria meningiditis* (the 'meningococcus') is understandably the most feared, being capable of rapid progression and carrying a high mortality. Note that the meningococcus can cause meningitis and/or septicaemic disease associated with a maculopapular rash becoming a characteristic non-blanching petechial rash.

Presentation

Bacterial meningitis typically causes headache, fever, neck stiffness, photophobia, vomiting, and reduced conscious level ± a non-blanching rash and clinical features of shock. This classical presentation sounds difficult to misdiagnose, but it is worth remembering that in the early stages there may be nothing more than non-specific 'flu-like' symptoms.

Management

See guidelines at http://www.meningitis.org
- Time is of the essence: call for an emergency paramedic transfer to hospital and *immediately* give a slow intravenous injection of 1.2g of benzylpenicillin (penicillin G). If venous access cannot be accessed within a few minutes, give the 1.2g benzylpenicillin by intramuscular injection, using a proximal limb site (aiming to inject into the part of the limb which is still perfused). Note that if the patient is allergic to penicillin, a third-generation cephalosporin is a suitable alternative (see BNF).
- Whilst awaiting arrival of paramedics, provide O$_2$ (if available) and ensure that the airway is patent (use opening manoeuvres and/or adjuncts) if conscious level is reduced.
- If the patient is clinically shocked, resuscitate with a rapid intravenous infusion of 1L of 0.9% saline.
- Document the treatment which has been given in a referral letter. Also, once the patient has left custody, contact the receiving hospital staff by telephone.

Prophylaxis for close contacts

The consultant in communicable disease control or consultant in public health medicine will notify the local health authority about any case of meningitis. He/she will also be able to advise on the need for prophylaxis for close contacts of patients with meningococcal disease. Prophylaxis typically takes the form of oral rifampicin (unless allergic, pregnant, or otherwise contraindicated), but is usually reserved for close family contacts or clinical staff who have provided mouth-to-mouth or other resuscitation at close quarters.

Assessing and managing illness in custody

Assessment of illness

Background to illness in custody

Many detainees are suffering from the effects of acute and/or chronic ill-nesses at the time of their detention. These illnesses are often either not treated at all or only partially treated, reflecting a chaotic lifestyle and inattention to personal health. Pre-existing illness may worsen during the period of detention. In addition, detainees may develop new ill-nesses during detention. Sometimes, individuals become unwell as the direct result of being detained (e.g. no access to usual medication, drugs, or alcohol). A cell or police custody suite is not the most appropriate place to observe changes in clinical condition. Forensic practitioners need to adopt a lower threshold of referral for more detailed observation or assessment than they would in a non-coercive setting in the community.

Difficulties in assessment

A variety of factors may individually or collectively render assessment of illness in a detainee very difficult. These factors include:

- Lack of knowledge about detainees and their medical conditions.
- An inability of detainees to provide information about their medical conditions/medications/allergies due to the effects of alcohol and/or drug ingestion.
- An unwillingness by the detainee to cooperate or provide accurate information (sometimes with the intention of being deemed unfit for detention due to illness).
- Lack of independent information about illnesses, medications, and drug allergies.
- A relatively difficult clinical environment.

Sources of information

There are a number of potential sources of information about a detained person's medical history, in addition to the account provided by the detainee. These sources include the following:

- Verbal information provided by arresting officers (e.g. from friends/ relatives that an individual is epileptic or diabetic, or that certain drugs or alcohol may have been consumed).
- Written information in the property of the detainee at the time of arrest (including list of medications, hospital letters, etc.).
- Information from the time of previous periods of detention in custody.
- information available by making telephone calls (with appropriate consent) to healthcare organizations (GP surgeries, local hospitals) and/or relatives/friends—forensic practitioners need to take care to comply with the wishes of the detainee in terms of confidentiality.
- Medalert bracelets or necklaces.

Medical history from the patient

As a minimum, a detained person needs to be asked about their regular medications/drugs consumed, together with chronic illnesses. In some cases it is not possible to obtain an accurate history. It is important to establish if there is a history of alcoholism, drug dependence, diabetes, heart disease, epilepsy, chronic respiratory disease (e.g. asthma). It is also important to record any drug allergies.

Examination

Information gathered at the time of initial consultation will be used to guide decisions about whether an individual is fit to be detained and/or interviewed (see ⬚ p.204), as well as being directed at the general and specific assessment of illness. Clinical examination will usually include the following basic information:

• Pulse rate
• Blood pressure
• Respiratory rate
• Breath sounds and heart sounds
• Conscious level (Glasgow Coma Scale)
• Pupil reactions
• Limb movement
• Signs of drug misuse (e.g. needle track marks).

Management of chronic illness

General approach

Many individuals who are detained in custody have underlying chronic illness for which they take regular medication. The aim of the forensic practitioner is to continue regular medication and to quickly identify and treat any acute problems as they arise. Often, the period of detention is so short that no regular medication needs to be prescribed/administered. When a longer period of detention (e.g. overnight) is planned, it is usually appropriate to arrange for usual medication to be continued. In many instances, detainees bring their own medication to the police station and this can be prescribed and administered at the usual times. On occasions when detainees do not have their usual medication with them, the best options are either to arrange for this medication to be brought to custody or for alternative medication to be provided from custody. In order to achieve the latter option, depending upon local arrangements and the contents of the custody medicines cabinet, it may be necessary to obtain drugs via a private prescription from a local pharmacy. Many detainees may be non-compliant or not have access to medication. Common chronic illnesses encountered in everyday custody practice include chronic heart disease, hypertension, asthma, epilepsy, diabetes, epilepsy, alcoholism, drug misuse, and mental health issues.

Heart disease

Ischaemic heart disease and atrial fibrillation are common in middle-aged and elderly detainees. Taking into account the stress of being arrested and detained, the forensic practitioner should strive to continue regular medications. Glyceryl trinitrate spray should be prescribed as appropriate and active consideration should be given to allowing the detainee to keep this with him/her in the cell during detention.

Hypertension

The aim should be to continue usual antihypertensive treatment whilst in custody. The stress of being detained may result in an increase in blood pressure. Very occasionally, a detainee will present with malignant hypertension (very elevated diastolic blood pressure, headache, fits, retinopathy) and require emergency referral to hospital.

Diabetes—see 📖 p.246.

Asthma

Asthma is common, but many detainees who report suffering from it do not use a regular inhaler, but rather use it only when required. Most asthmatics in custody do not experience any symptoms attributable to asthma, but should be prescribed their usual inhalers. Those who have symptoms (wheeze, breathlessness) require evaluation and treatment (see 📖 p.252). Asthmatics should be allowed to keep their usual inhalers with them in the cell provided that it is considered safe to do so.

Epilepsy

Although a significant proportion of detainees will admit to suffering from 'fits', some are alcohol withdrawal-related and not all have a diagnosis of epilepsy. Alcohol withdrawal is under-diagnosed in police custody. Those who are taking anticonvulsants should be prescribed their usual medication. Withdrawal fits are also a risk amongst those who are dependent upon benzodiazepines.

Depression

Many detainees report a diagnosis of depression, with some also reporting that they take medication for this. Although many antidepressants have a relatively long half-life, it is best practice to try to continue treatment—suddenly stopping antidepressants can cause problems.

Medicines in custody

Different systems exist in different regions, but detainees need to have the more commonly prescribed drugs easily available to them (see 📖 p.201). These drugs may be kept in a locked unit in custody or a locked doctor's bag. The process of prescribing and administering drugs needs to be safe and robust (see 📖 FFLM guidelines at www.fflm.ac.uk, and p.201).

Diabetes

Background

Given the prevalence in the general population, it is no surprise that diabetes is often encountered in detainees in custody. Patients with diabetes range from those who are diet controlled only, to those who are on oral medication to those who require insulin. As with patients with other chronic conditions, the diabetic detainee is likely to have a good understanding of his/her diabetes and its management.

History

The key points in the history are establishing the nature and extent of the diabetes and, most particularly, its treatment. It is important to identify the following information in relation to the diabetes:

- How long the patient has been diabetic.
- What control problems and/or complications the patient has experienced.
- The nature of usual medication (name and dose) and whether the detainee has brought this with him/her or has access to it (i.e. could someone bring it from home?)

Information/corroboration regarding the patient's diabetes may be available by contacting the GP.

Examination

Derangements in vital signs and conscious level may indicate a serious metabolic abnormality, but many individuals with low or high blood glucose may not exhibit any obvious signs.

Bedside measurement of blood glucose

Custody units and forensic practitioners (and some diabetics) have the means to easily measure blood glucose level at the bedside. Measurements using a meter are more reliable than those using visual assessment by comparing against a colour strip. It is best to consider checking the blood glucose level in every diabetic on initial assessment at custody, although on occasions, particularly, for example, when the patient is diet controlled only, it may not be necessary. However, in those whose fitness to interview is being determined, or who are symptomatic, use insulin, and/or have poorly controlled diabetes, it is sensible to obtain an initial baseline blood glucose measurement.

Blood glucose levels are usually maintained in non-diabetics in the range 3.6–5.8mmol/L, although diabetics may experience and tolerate much wider swings in blood glucose levels without reporting any symptoms.

Administering regular medication

The administration of excessive amounts of insulin or the administration of usual dose of insulin without usual food may result in hypoglycaemia. Occasionally, diabetic detainees may attempt (for various reasons) to develop hypoglycaemia. For these reasons, some advise all regular injections of insulin in custody to be given after food and supervised by a forensic practitioner.

Hypoglycaemia

This is a significant risk in diabetic detainees. It can be aggravated by alcohol intake. It may be manifest by irritability, sweating, irrational or aggressive behaviour, reduced conscious level, and even fits. Hypoglycaemia may mimic alcohol intoxication. If a diabetic has been arrested for public order or aggressive behaviour, it is important to exclude hypoglycaemia. If the detainee is symptomatic, conscious, cooperative, and has a blood glucose level of <4mmol/L, give oral glucose in the form of sugar lumps, a sugary drink, and/or biscuits. A detainee who fails to recover completely, suffers continuing effects, and/or low blood glucose levels may require urgent transfer to hospital.

Unconscious hypoglycaemic patients and those who are uncooperative require emergency treatment. Whilst awaiting arrival of an emergency ambulance, the options are:
- Administration of 50mL of 10% dextrose solution intravenously repeated if necessary.
- Glucagon 1mg intramuscularly (note that this is not likely to work in patients who have chronic alcoholism, liver failure, or whose hypoglycaemia is the result of sulphonylurea drugs as there may be little glycogen in the liver available for mobilization).

Hyperglycaemia

Some diabetics usually 'run' with higher than normal blood glucose levels and in the evidence of symptoms/signs, may be managed satisfactorily in custody. Blood glucose levels in excess of 18mmol/L in association with physical symptoms may reflect hyperglycaemic crisis in the form of either diabetic ketoacidosis or hyperosmolar non-ketotic hyperglycaemia. In the former, ketones will be apparent on testing the urine.

Clinical features are variable, but include evidence of dehydration, chest infection, abdominal pain, shock, and altered conscious level.

Management

Patients with suspected ketoacidosis or hyperosmolar non-ketotic hyperglycaemia require emergency transfer to hospital. Whilst awaiting the arrival of emergency paramedics, it may be appropriate to start treatment:
- High-flow O_2 by mask.
- The commencement of 1L of intravenous 0.9% saline.
- It is usually best to leave administration of insulin until hospital, where blood glucose levels can be more closely monitored.

Chest pain

Background

The symptom of chest pain is taken seriously as it may reflect serious (potentially fatal) underlying pathology. This includes myocardial infarction/acute coronary syndrome, dissecting aortic aneurysm, pulmonary embolism, pneumonia, pneumothorax. Amongst these, chest pain due to ischaemic heart disease is the most commonly encountered. For this reason, from a custody perspective, if a detainee reports chest pain, a low threshold should be adopted for calling an emergency ambulance.

History and examination

The nature, site, severity, character, relieving factors, and duration of chest pain will provide important clues to its origin. Useful comparison may be made to previously experienced chest pain. This may particularly help to positively diagnose chest pain due to ischaemic heart disease. Detainees who have underlying pneumonia or pneumothorax may exhibit obvious signs, but pulmonary embolism is notoriously difficult to diagnose on clinical grounds.

Approach to chest pain

Angina

If a detainee with known angina suffers an episode of chest pain typical of previously experienced angina, lasting for a few minutes, before resolving (with or without use of glyceryl trinitrate spray sublingually), then it may be reasonable to continue detention without transfer to hospital. Before this decision is made, however, it would be appropriate for the forensic practitioner to establish that the detainee is symptom-free, with normal examination findings.

Other chest pain of apparent cardiac origin

Chest pain which appears to be of cardiac origin and lasts for >10min should be treated as being of cardiac origin. If the forensic practitioner is not present, initial treatment may have to be given by telephone advice. Treatment approach comprises:
• Call for an emergency ambulance.
• Provide 1–2 puffs of glyceryl trinitrate sublingually.
• Administer 300mg aspirin orally.
• Give high-flow O_2 by mask (if available).
• Remain with the patient until the ambulance arrives.

Atypical chest pain

The bewildering array of potential differential diagnoses in a patient who complains of atypical chest pain is likely to result in referral to hospital. Without specialist investigations (e.g. ECG, chest X-ray, CT scan), it is impossible to exclude many important differential diagnoses.

Palpitations

Arrhythmias may present with palpitations and/or collapse (sometimes with chest pain or breathlessness). In the custody setting, in the absence of the ability to record an ECG or use a cardiac monitor, the forensic practitioner is limited to determining the heart rate and whether it is regular or not. The management of very fast and very slow heart rhythms (the so called 'periarrest arrhythmias') is hospital based and follows Resuscitation Council guidelines (see 🕮 http://www.resus.org.uk).

Tachyarrhythmias

Treatment depends upon making an ECG diagnosis, which is not usually available at custody. The underlying rhythms include:
- Atrial/supraventricular tachycardia.
- Ventricular tachycardia.
- Atrial fibrillation.
- Atrial flutter (typically with 2:1 block, giving a rate of 150 beats per minute).
- Sinus tachycardia (usually in response to significant underlying illness).

Bradyarrhythmias

The normal resting adult heart rate is 60–100 beats per minute. Fit healthy athletes may (normally) have much lower heart rates and individuals who take β-blockers may also have (pharmacologically induced) lower rates.

Slow heart rhythms include: sinus bradycardia, second- or third-degree heart block, and slow atrial fibrillation—clearly, an ECG/monitor is required to determine the rhythm.

Bradyarrhythmias can present in a number of ways, including collapse/loss of consciousness, palpitations, chest pain, or heart failure. Resuscitation Council guidelines (see 🕮 http://www.resus.org.uk) indicate that first-line treatment for symptomatic bradyarrhythmias is O_2, followed by intravenous atropine 500 micrograms with ECG monitoring—this is likely to be provided by emergency paramedics.

Breathlessness

Approach

The complaint of breathlessness needs to be considered within the context of the past medical history and any associated symptoms. Assessment of a detainee with breathlessness can prove to be difficult in the custody setting—deranged vital signs (pulse rate, blood pressure, and oxygen saturation level) may indicate a potentially serious underlying condition. Note that a variety of battery-operated matchbox-sized pulse oximeters are now widely available and ideal for custody use. Management of specific conditions is considered as follows.

Asthma—see 📖 p.252

Pulmonary oedema

Acute breathlessness in middle-aged or elderly individuals due to pulmonary oedema mostly reflects left ventricular failure (sometimes due to myocardial infarction), although there are other causes at younger ages (e.g. heroin overdose). Management involves sitting the patient up, providing O_2 by face mask (if available), and emergency ambulance transfer to hospital.

Pulmonary embolism

The clinical presentation of pulmonary embolus is highly variable and often non-specific. A high index of suspicion is required in order not to miss this sometimes elusive diagnosis, which requires specialist investigation at hospital.

Pneumonia

Many patients with a lower respiratory tract (chest) infection are satisfactorily managed in the community with amoxicillin 0.5–1g orally 3 times a day (🕉 http://www.brit-thoracic.org.uk). In the custody setting, abnormal vital signs (especially with reduced O_2 saturation on pulse oximetry) ± abnormal clinical findings (e.g. chest crackles, bronchial breathing) may indicate the need for chest X-ray and assessment at hospital.

Pneumothorax

This may or may not follow trauma. Tension pneumothorax is a life-threatening emergency and is considered on 📖 p.227. Small pneumothoraces can be difficult to detect clinically and may require an X-ray to make the diagnosis.

Hyperventilation

Primary ('psychogenic' or 'inappropriate' hyperventilation) is classically associated with circumoral paraesthesia and carpopedal spasm. It may be treated with reassurance and simple breathing exercises (breathe in through nose—count of 8, out through mouth—count of 8, hold for count of 4 and repeat).

Other causes of breathlessness

These include: anaphylaxis (📖 p.237), arrhythmias (📖 p.249), diabetic ketoacidosis (📖 p.247), acute exacerbation of COPD, and choking (📖 p.224). Usually, there will be additional clinical features to assist the forensic practitioner in reaching the correct diagnosis.

Asthma

Detainees who complain of breathlessness and/or wheeze require urgent assessment and treatment (generally involving hospital). Asthmatics should usually be allowed to keep their salbutamol (or equivalent) inhalers with them and use them if they develop symptoms. Initial assessment of the severity of the asthma may be guided by vital signs and other observations, together with the expiratory peak flow (see the British Thoracic Society guidelines, ℘ http://www.brit-thoracic.org.uk). Most asthmatics are aware of their own normal best peak flow rate. The peak flow may be used as an initial triage tool (flow rates in normal adults are shown in Fig. 8.1).

Acute severe or life-threatening asthma

The following are pointers of acute severe or life-threatening asthma requiring emergency transfer to hospital by ambulance:

- Peak flow ≤50% predicted or best.
- Respiratory rate ≥25/min.
- Heart rate ≥110/min.
- Inability to complete sentences in one breath.
- O_2 saturation level <92%.
- Silent chest, cyanosis, feeble respiratory effort.
- Bradycardia, arrhythmia, hypotension.
- Exhaustion, confusion, coma.

If a patient has any one of the listed features, then an emergency ambulance should be called and the patient given salbutamol inhalers and O_2 by mask (if available at custody). Note that it may be necessary for a forensic practitioner who is not present at custody to advise that an emergency ambulance be called for the detainee, based upon the information provided over the telephone.

Moderately severe asthma

Detainees who have none of the earlier listed criteria of severe or life-threatening asthma, but have increasing symptoms and/or peak flow 50–75% normal/best are likely to require hospital treatment for nebulizers, steroids ± admission.

Mild asthma

Detainees with relatively mild symptoms may be satisfactorily managed in custody. Clinical review after β_2-agonist treatment (e.g. salbutamol inhaler is advised).

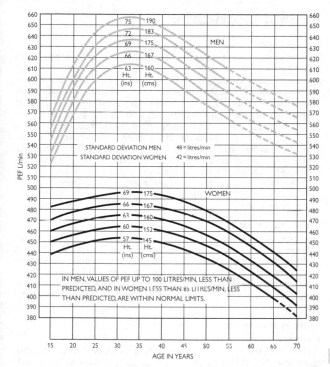

Fig. 8.1 Peak expiratory flow rates in normal adults. Reproduced from Nunn AJ and Gregg I (1989). New regression equations for predicting peak expiratory flow in adults. *BMJ* **298**:1068–70, with permission from BMJ Publishing Group Ltd.

Alcohol intoxication

Background

Unsurprisingly, perhaps, most forensic practitioners are only too aware of the acute effects of alcohol! The clinical effects and related toxicological aspects of alcohol excess are detailed on 📖 pp.460–5. Although the clinical effects of alcohol on an individual tend to become more pronounced as blood alcohol levels increase, there is a staggering variation in overt effects between different individuals who have similar levels. In addition to being capable of metabolizing alcohol much more rapidly, some chronic alcoholics are able to tolerate relatively large amounts of alcohol without appearing to be 'drunk'. Measuring the breath alcohol level (with consent) in detainees can provide useful information for custody staff who are tasked with safely managing detainees. Some custody units employ a system whereby all detainees whose breath alcohol levels exceed a certain value are automatically taken to hospital for assessment. Polydrug use combined with alcohol misuse is common and carries significant risks.

Clearance of alcohol

The rate of clearance of alcohol from the blood varies enormously between individuals, with typical quoted values of 10–20mg/dL/h in most adults, although higher values occur in some chronic alcoholics. Depending upon whether the detainee is in the absorptive or elimination phase, it is quite possible for blood alcohol levels to initially rise after arrival at custody. Every year, individuals die in police custody due to alcohol intoxication.

Clinical assessment

History

A history relating to alcohol consumption is notoriously unreliable when taken from heavy drinkers and chronic alcoholics, who may significantly under-report the extent of their drinking and its effect upon various aspects of their lives. Nevertheless, it is worth trying to establish:

• What, when and how much alcohol has been consumed in the past 24h?
• What is the usual daily consumption?
• What withdrawal symptoms/effects have occurred previously?

Referral to alcohol agencies is often appropriate.

Examination

The typical presentation of slurred speech, incoordination, unsteady gait and balance, nystagmus, and lethargy may present unmistakably as acute alcohol intoxication. However, in addition to performing a standard examination, it is important to specifically consider and look for possible alternative diagnoses. The differential diagnosis includes: hypoglycaemia, head injury, postictal confusional states, hepatic encephalopathy, meningitis, encephalitis, hypothermia, or intoxication with other drugs.

Fitness to detain

The decision as to whether or not a detainee is fit to be detained in custody is usually a clinical one, rather than one based purely upon breath alcohol measurements. The potential risks of detaining individuals who appear to be heavily under the influence of alcohol include the following possibilities:

- Hypoxic damage/death from vomiting/aspiration or succumbing to acute alcohol poisoning.
- Incorrectly attributing acute medical conditions (e.g. hypoglycaemia, hypothermia) to alcohol.
- Incorrectly attributing the effects of a head injury to alcohol.

Detainees who are not fully conscious or who cannot be roused to be fully conscious are not fit to be detained in custody. It should be remembered that reduced conscious level/altered mental state may reflect hypoglycaemia—this can be easily excluded by bedside measurement of glucose (see ☐ p.246).

Safe detention

Detainees who are under the influence of alcohol, but appear to be safe to detain at the time of assessment, do have the potential to deteriorate if blood alcohol levels continue to rise after detention. For this and other reasons, detainees who are under the influence of alcohol at the time of assessment usually require regular (initially 30-min) checks by custody staff, with rousals to appropriate response (see ☐ p.206). Custody staff should be advised to seek urgent medical assistance if the detainee deteriorates and/or has a reduced conscious level. They should encourage detainees to sleep on their side, which better protects the airway (see ☐ The recovery position, p.229). If it is not possible to obtain a comprehensible response (i.e. structured words), the detainee must be transferred immediately to hospital. It may be also worth reminding staff that 'snoring' can reflect obstruction of the upper airway, requiring urgent intervention. If a detainee who has consumed drugs, alcohol, and/or has a head injury is snoring, he/she should be immediately roused. Any detainee should be able to walk to the cell and say a few words—an inability to do this mandates transfer to hospital.

Fitness to interview

Issues relating to fitness to interview are considered on ☐ p.428. Breath alcohol levels may provide some useful information, but clinical assessment is more important.

Alcohol withdrawal

Regular users of alcohol may develop withdrawal symptoms when denied usual access to it. Many detainees who develop withdrawal symptoms may not at first appear to be chronic alcoholics. A variety of withdrawal symptoms may occur, from as early as 6h after the last alcoholic drink. A missed diagnosis of alcohol withdrawal is a relatively common cause of death in police custody.

Simple alcohol withdrawal

Uncomplicated ('simple') alcohol withdrawal is very common, usually starting within 12h of stopping (or reducing) alcohol intake. Withdrawal symptoms often commence before alcohol is completely cleared from the bloodstream. Features include anxiety, restlessness, tremor, insomnia, sweating, tachycardia, and ataxia.

Treatment

Most detainees are satisfactorily managed by a combination of oral benzo-diazepines and thiamine:

- Diazepam 10mg orally every 8h (additional doses may be required, if symptoms are not controlled, following careful reassessment). Chlordiazepoxide is an alternative.
- Thiamine 100mg orally every 6h.

Note that the Clinical Institute Withdrawal Assessment for Alcohol (CIWA) Score which is used in hospital practice, might also prove to be useful in custody (see http://www.agingincanada.ca/CIWA.htm).

Alcohol withdrawal fits

A proportion of alcoholics experience epileptic fits during withdrawal from alcohol, although the risk of this occurring may be reduced by regular administration of benzodiazepines to treat withdrawal (as described for 'simple alcohol withdrawal'). Treatment of fits follows standard lines, as outlined on p.238.

Delirium tremens

A true medical emergency, with a significant mortality, delirium tremens only occurs in a small minority of alcoholics who undergo withdrawal. It typically occurs at a time of >48h after stopping drinking. In addition to the features of withdrawal outlined earlier, there may be significant autonomic hyperactivity, with tachycardia, hyper-reflexia, hypertension, fever, visual or tactile hallucinations, sinister delusions, disorientation, and confusion. Delirium tremens may be complicated by fits and/or tachyarrhythmias.

Treatment

Urgent (emergency) transfer to hospital by ambulance is required. Some features may improve with oral diazepam 10mg (which may need to be repeated if there is any delay in transfer). It is also important to search for (and treat) any hypoglycaemia.

Alcoholic ketoacidosis
Although uncommon, this is a serious condition which can occur when an alcoholic individual stops drinking, vomits repeatedly, and does not eat. The ketoacidosis reflects breakdown of fatty acids, complicated by the dehydration associated with the vomiting. Alcoholic ketoacidosis typically develops 24–72h after a recent drinking binge. Gastrointestinal symptoms (vomiting and abdominal pain) may be associated with increased respiratory rate, clinical evidence of dehydration, and ketonuria. Suspicion of alcoholic ketoacidosis requires urgent referral to hospital.

Other problems of alcoholics

The extent of alcohol problems amongst the general population is quite considerable. The range of individuals with alcohol problems varies from those who appear to manage to work and have a stable family life to those who are unemployed with a chaotic lifestyle and little social support. Those at the latter end of the scale include individuals who are of no fixed abode—many of these do not have regular access to good medical care and neglect their health problems. This can result in them having significant health problems at the time of their detention in custody, including:

- Soft tissue infections
- Chest infections (including TB)
- Chronic skin problems
- Lice, fleas, etc.
- Dental problems including abscesses.

Although the forensic practitioner is only directly responsible for the care of detainees for the period that they detained, there is a professional and ethical duty which extends for longer than this. In other words, the forensic practitioner should take steps to try to ensure that detainees are able to complete a course of treatment after leaving custody (e.g. providing a full course of antibiotics or advising detainees specifically where/how to receive continuing treatment). Many custody units already use links to try to direct detainees with alcohol (or drug) problems to appropriate help (e.g. see ◌ http://www.addaction.org.uk). The 'CAGE' questionnaire (see later in this section) may help identify chronic alcohol dependence.

Chronic alcoholics may experience a range of medical problems, which are not specifically linked to withdrawal states, as detailed in the rest of this section.

Wernicke's encephalopathy

Acute thiamine deficiency in a malnourished chronic alcoholic may cause some or all of the following: acute confusional state, nystagmus/ocular palsies, ataxia, and polyneuropathy. Refer urgently to hospital for parenteral thiamine treatment—oral thiamine may be given in the meantime.

Korsakoff's psychosis

Untreated, Wernicke's encephalopathy may progress to Korsakoff's psychosis, which is characterized by short-term memory impairment, confabulation, and apathy.

Gastrointestinal haemorrhage

Upper gastrointestinal bleeding may result from a number of different sources, most notably Mallory–Weiss tears, gastritis, peptic ulceration, and oesophageal varices (usually due to cirrhosis and portal hypertension).

Liver problems

As the principal organ which metabolizes alcohol, the liver is perhaps the natural target of damage from chronic alcohol use. Liver problems range from fatty infiltration, through alcoholic hepatitis to cirrhosis.

CAGE questionnaire

Four simple screening questions may provide an indication that an individual has a chronic alcohol problem:
- Have you ever felt you should *cut down* your drinking?
- Have people ever *annoyed* you by criticizing your drinking?
- Have you ever felt *guilty* about your drinking?
- Have you ever had a drink first thing in the morning to steady your nerves or to get rid of a hangover (*eye opener*)?

Any single positive answer is significant and more than one positive answer is probably diagnostic of chronic alcohol dependence.

Detainees under the influence of drugs

A significant proportion of those who are arrested and taken into custody have taken drugs of abuse in the hours prior to arrest. The potential problems associated with the detention of individuals who have taken drugs include:

- Acute intoxication/deterioration (and/or overdosage) with damage or even death—every year detainees die in police custody because of drug intake.
- Intoxication masking underlying disease.
- Not being properly fit to interview due to the effects of drugs (see 🕮 p.431).
- Drug withdrawal syndromes (see 🕮 p.262).
- Unwanted interaction between drugs taken prior to arrest and medication prescribed after arrival at custody.

The forensic practitioner needs to be mindful of all of these potential problems in order to safely manage detainees in custody.

Assessment of those under influence of drugs

History

It is standard practice for the forensic practitioner to ask detainees questions about illicit drug use. A detailed history is particularly pertinent when arresting police officers and/or custody staff provide information or raise concerns about drug use. The forensic practitioner needs to try to establish what drug(s) has been taken, when/how it was taken, and how use in the past 24h compares with usual use of this drug.

Detainees provide accurate information about their drug use more often than might be imagined.

Examination

Relevant information relating to possible use and effects of drugs includes: assessment of vital signs (pulse, blood pressure, respiratory rate, and ideally, O_2 saturation by pulse oximetry), conscious level (Glasgow Coma Scale), pupil size and reactions, identification of needle track marks, speech, and coordination tests.

Specific syndromes due to drugs

Clinical effects of drugs of abuse are considered on 🕮 pp.466–79. Although some drugs result in characteristic signs, it is often not possible to identify the exact drug(s) taken from the clinical picture alone. Perhaps the most characteristic presentation is that of opioid poisoning: pinpoint pupils, depressed respiration, reduced conscious level, needle track injection marks, and, in extremis, respiratory arrest (see 🕮 p.466).

Management of those under influence of drugs

Fitness to detain

The first decision facing the forensic practitioner is whether or not a detainee is fit to be detained in custody or whether he/she requires immediate transfer to hospital. Detainees who are under the influence of drugs and have altered vital signs (in particular, reduced conscious level) are likely to need urgent hospitalization (± resuscitation/treatment).

Suspected opioid overdose usually responds to the following measures:
- Intravenous or intramuscular naloxone (0.4–0.8mg, repeated as necessary).
- Provision of O_2 by face mask (if available).
- Ventilation if apnoeic by bag, valve, mask (if available), or pocket mask.
- Emergency ambulance transfer to hospital. Note that once naloxone has been administered, the detainee needs to go to hospital even if they appear to recover fully (there is still a significant risk of deterioration as naloxone has a shorter half-life than many opioids).

Another group of individuals who are often taken directly to hospital are suspected body stuffers (see 📖 p.264), who may be at significant risk of drug overdose.

Observations in custody
Detainees who are under the influence of drugs (± alcohol) need to be carefully monitored, in order to identify any deterioration in their condition. The most important period is likely to be the first 6h after detention, although deterioration can occur after this time. Custody staff need to be advised to check detainees initially every 30min (see 📖 p.208) and to call for urgent medical assistance if the detainee deteriorates and/or is difficult to rouse and/or exhibits behavioural change.

Fitness to interview
Although fit to detain, many detainees may not be fit to interview. This can be a difficult decision for the forensic practitioner and will depend upon the exact circumstances (see 📖 p.428). In general terms, detainees who exhibit overt clinical effects from drug (or alcohol) use (e.g. slurred speech, impaired coordination, drowsiness, abnormal pupils) are unlikely to be fit to interview—they may require reassessment to confirm fitness for interview after a period of a number of hours.

Drug withdrawal

Chronic users of some illicit and prescribed drugs may develop withdrawal symptoms whilst they are in custody if they do not take these drugs as usual. When considering how to manage a detainee who has possible drug withdrawal, the forensic practitioner should consider the following:

- Detainees in police custody are entitled to the same standard of medical care as any other member of the public and this includes the right to have prescribed medication continued whilst in custody, as long as it is safe to do so.
- Detainees may not provide a reliable history about their regular and recent drug use.
- It is unusual for an individual to be already experiencing withdrawal symptoms at the time of arrest.
- Most forensic practitioners choose to wait for a number of hours before contemplating the initiation of symptomatic or drug substitution treatment—this is in case the detainee consumed a significant quantity of drugs immediately prior to being detained (giving rise to the potential risk of adding to or even inadvertently precipitating an overdose). Once intoxication has been excluded, it may be safe to consider starting treatment of withdrawal symptoms. The practice of never giving any replacement therapy for the first 6h in custody is inappropriate—decisions must be based upon an appropriate clinical assessment.
- Depending upon the time of day and the day of the week, it may be possible to obtain useful corroborative information from other healthcare professionals (e.g. GP, chemist, hospital specialist) about prescribed medication.
- Many detainees do not remain in custody for a significant period of time and may not therefore require symptomatic or substitution therapy whilst detained.
- Withdrawal from alcohol is usually (but not always) more 'dangerous' than withdrawal from opioid drugs. However, detainees who suffer opioid withdrawal are often much more vocal in their requests for medical treatment than those who are withdrawing from alcohol.
- It is usually not possible to ascertain with any certainty the exact drug from which an individual is withdrawing simply from an analysis of the clinical features of withdrawal. This situation is complicated by the fact that many detainees who are drug users take more than one drug of misuse, which may include sedatives and stimulants.

Effects of withdrawal

Opioid withdrawal

Symptoms include: sweating, agitation, insomnia, feeling 'hot and cold', nausea, abdominal cramps, yawning. Typical signs are: sweating, dilated pupils, tachycardia, 'goose flesh', lacrimation, hypertension.

Benzodiazepine withdrawal

This may cause anxiety, sweating, insomnia, headache, and altered perceptions. Withdrawal fits and psychosis can occur.

Cannabis withdrawal

Symptoms (if any) tend to be mild: sleep disturbance and irritability.

Stimulants

Amphetamines, ecstasy, and cocaine do not cause significant physical withdrawal syndromes, although insomnia and depression may require assessment, including for the risk of self-harm.

Management of withdrawal symptoms

Useful guidelines for the management of drug withdrawal have been published jointly by the Faculty of Forensic and Legal Medicine (previously Association of Forensic Physicians) and the Royal College of Psychiatrists (see ♒ http://www.fflm.ac.uk).

Opioid withdrawal treatment

A number of different approaches have been used. One approach which carries relatively little risk is to use a combination of substitution and symptomatic treatment as necessary:
• Substitution therapy with dihydrocodeine 60–90mg, 3 or 4 times a day, tailored to effect; ±
• Symptomatic treatment with diazepam 10mg orally 3 times a day.

Additionally, simple analgesics (e.g. paracetamol, ibuprofen) may be useful for treating minor symptoms and loperamide (4mg orally initially, then 2mg with each loose stool) may reduce gut spasm and help treat diarrhoea.

A number of other drugs have been used (e.g. methadone, lofexidine, buprenorphine), but are not without risks.

Benzodiazepine withdrawal treatment

Standard treatment is to use diazepam 10mg orally 3 times a day, although additional doses may be required (following reassessment).

The pregnant drug user

Drug users who are pregnant often present a considerable challenge in order to ensure that they are managed safely. There is a particular risk to the fetus if opioids are abruptly stopped—special attention needs to be given to continuing medication in pregnant drug users whilst they are in custody. The forensic practitioner may obtain expert advice from specialist community and hospital teams.

Body packers, pushers, and stuffers

Individuals who ingest or conceal relatively large quantities of drugs within their bodies have an obvious potential risk of drug overdose. For this reason, most detainees who are suspected of having swallowed drugs immediately prior to arrest are taken to the nearest hospital Emergency Department.

Body packers

Individuals who swallow drugs in packages in an attempt to transport (smuggle) them from one country to another without being detected are called 'body packers'. Usually, the packaging is composed of rubber or latex and the contents either heroin or cocaine. The quantity of drug within each package is typically far in excess of fatal dose.

Body pushers

Individuals who insert drugs into the rectum and/or vagina in order to smuggle them across international borders may be known as 'body pushers', although some experts prefer to include this group under the heading of 'body packers'.

Body stuffers

Some individuals swallow drugs immediately prior to arrest, usually in an attempt to conceal the drugs from police. Drugs ingested in this way may be wrapped, but the packaging is likely to be much less robust than that used by body packers or pushers. Considering risks of drug overdose, police usually take individuals who appear to have ingested or stuffed drugs immediately prior to arrest to hospital for assessment. When an individual appears to try to swallow a package in the presence of police officers and/or forensic practitioner, it is recommended that no attempts are made to put pressure around the face or neck in order to try to prevent the object being swallowed, as this can cause or exacerbate choking on the object. If an individual appears to be choking on a drug package, then Faculty of Forensic and Legal Medicine (℘ http://www.fflm.ac.uk) and Resuscitation Council guidelines on choking should be followed (see 🕮 p.224).

Drugs Act 2005

The Drugs Act 2005 amended the Criminal Justice Act and the Police and Criminal Evidence Acts of England and Wales and Northern Ireland. Key features of the Act are:
- It enables an intimate search to be authorized by a senior police officer (rank inspector or above)—see 🕮 p.194. An intimate search is defined as an examination of any body orifice other than the mouth. A forensic practitioner will, however, only undertake such a search with the detainee's consent.
- It enables a police inspector (superintendent in Northern Ireland) to authorize an X-ray or ultrasound to search for a drug package. Again, however, these tests will only be performed by a doctor when the detainee gives consent.

Risk of deterioration

Most individuals who have concealed drugs can be managed conservatively, although there is a risk of deterioration (and even death) from drug toxicity. The evidence suggests that the following are risk factors for complications occurring when an individual has concealed drugs:[1]

- Abdominal pain, vomiting, abnormal vital signs, or clinical evidence of poisoning.
- Home-made or improvised packaging.
- Large size and/or number (>50) packets.
- Delayed passage of packets (beyond 48h).
- Fragments of packets in stool.
- Poisoning in a cotransporter.
- Previous abdominal surgery (when there is a greater risk of obstruction secondary to adhesions).
- Concomitant drug use (especially constipating agents).
- Positive urine drug test following previous negative test (may herald packet breakdown or rupture).

Reference

1 Booker RJ, Smith JE, and Rodger MP (2009). Packers, pushers and stuffers—managing patients with concealed drugs in UK emergency departments: a clinical and medicolegal review. *Emerg Med J* **26**:316–20.

Other presentations and problems

Headache

A common symptom, most headaches do not reflect serious underlying illness and are easily treated with simple analgesics (starting with paracetamol 1g orally 4 times a day). Serious underlying pathology often presents in characteristic fashion:
- *Subarachnoid haemorrhage*—classically presents with sudden onset 'worst ever' occipital headache, possibly with photophobia and neck stiffness.
- *Meningitis*—one or more of: fever, rash, neck stiffness, photophobia (see 🕮 p.240).
- *Encephalitis*—fever, irritability, reduced conscious level.
- *Subdural haemorrhage*—elderly or middle aged (particularly alcoholics), there may or may not be an obvious history of trauma in the past two weeks.

Abdominal pain

The differential diagnosis of abdominal pain is very wide and includes some 'chest' causes (e.g. myocardial infarction, pneumonia) and in some patients at least, gynaecological causes too. Associated back pain may reflect ruptured aortic aneurysm, pancreatitis, or ureteric colic. Patients with evidence of peritonitis and/or abnormal vital signs (temperature, pulse rate, blood pressure) require urgent referral to hospital.

Gastrointestinal haemorrhage

Bleeding from the upper or lower gastrointestinal tract is reported relatively frequently in custody. It can be difficult to corroborate the extent of any bleeding and indeed, if there was any haemorrhage at all. It takes a large amount of bleeding to cause derangement of vital signs, which should not be relied upon to decide about referral. Most patients with acute gastrointestinal haemorrhage will require some investigation at hospital.

Haemoptysis

This is a relatively unusual symptom, but if corroborated and is apparently a new symptom, it warrants investigation at hospital.

Pregnancy related problems

The custody setting is not the ideal environment to assess and manage individuals with acute problems in pregnancy. Sometimes it is not entirely clear as to whether or not a detainee is pregnant, although a urine pregnancy test may clarify this.

Ruptured ectopic pregnancy is the most worrying potential diagnosis and should be considered in any woman of child bearing age who presents with a combination of abdominal pain and vaginal bleeding. Urgent transfer to hospital by emergency ambulance is required.

Assessing and managing injury in custody

Approach to assessment of injury

Forensic practitioners are asked to see a variety of different individuals with injuries, including victims, alleged perpetrators, and police/related staff. Depending on circumstances and the patient, the underlying reason for the requested examination may be one or more of the following:

- To assess the need for treatment.
- To provide treatment.
- To determine if injury has affected fitness to detain and/or interview.
- To assess and record for forensic purposes.

It is important for the forensic practitioner to establish at the outset exactly what the reason(s) for the assessment is.

Injured detainees

Injuries to detained persons may have been caused prior to, during, or after arrest. Injuries may have been deliberately inflicted by others, inflicted unintentionally ('accidentally'), or be self-inflicted. Not infrequently, detainees have injuries of different ages which were acquired in different ways.

Handling a telephone request from custody

When called by a custody unit with a request to attend to see an injured detainee, having initially established the reason for the request, the forensic practitioner needs to ascertain the urgency of the situation. In particular, it needs to be established if any serious or life-threatening features are present. In the presence of such features, advise the custody staff to dial (999) for an emergency ambulance to take the detainee to hospital, then aim to attend the custody unit to render additional assistance as quickly as possible. Even if no serious features are present, it is still worthwhile asking some questions, as it may be quickly apparent that the detainee requires hospital attention anyway. For example, a detainee with a (full thickness) skin wound caused by broken glass will inevitably require an X-ray to exclude retained glass. Similarly, a detainee who has sustained a recent needlestick injury will almost certainly require blood tests and possibly urgent postexposure prophylaxis.

Assessment of injury at custody

Having established the name and details of the detainee to be examined, ascertain the relevant background information and in particular, the reason(s) for the examination as outlined earlier. Ensure that the examination takes place in the best possible circumstances—in most instances, the best lighting and facilities will be the medical room.

Consent

Prior to any examination, the forensic practitioner needs to obtain the patient's consent. It is particularly important to explain the potential legal implications of an examination and to document that such an explanation was provided. Note that if for whatever reason, a detainee refuses to allow an examination to be performed, the forensic practitioner can still record observations of external injuries.

Clinical assessment of injury

Assessment of specific injuries is covered on 📖 pp.280–300. The general approach to clinical assessment and treatment is summarized here.

History

Record the following information:
- When and how the injury occurred.
- What symptoms have resulted.
- What treatment has already been administered.
- Relevant past medical history.
- Drug history and allergies (paying particular attention to any history of bleeding tendency and/or ongoing anticoagulant therapy, e.g. warfarin).
- In the case of skin wounds or burns, whether or not there is adequate cover against tetanus.

Examination

Follow the general basic examination of a detainee in custody, to include basic observations (pulse rate, blood pressure, conscious level, pupil reactions). Look carefully for injuries other than the most obvious one and, in particular, examine for (and document) the presence or absence of any hand injuries as these may have great legal significance depending upon the various accounts of exactly what happened in cases of alleged assault. For each injury, consider the following details (as appropriate): the nature, position, size, colour, associated swelling, and tenderness. Document the injuries using charts and as set out on 📖 p.122. Look for possible secondary effects of the injury (e.g. nerve damage or infection after limb injury). Consider what mechanism might have been responsible for causing each injury.

Management of injury

For any injury, the following questions are relevant:
- Does the detainee need to go to hospital for assessment and/or treatment?
- If he/she does require hospital attention, is emergency treatment needed before transfer?
- If transfer is required, is an emergency ambulance required to effect this, or can he/she be safely transported by the police alone?
- If he/she does not need to go to hospital, what treatment is needed in custody and what treatment/follow-up/advice following release from custody is needed?

In general terms, if the detainee is identified as having potentially serious injuries and requires immediate transfer by emergency ambulance, then the forensic practitioner should remain with him/her until the paramedics arrive. Bear in mind the fact that having identified an injury which requires treatment and/or follow-up, the forensic practitioner needs to ensure that appropriate care is continued following release/transfer from custody.

Documenting injuries

Background

It is crucial that the forensic practitioner ensures accurate and complete documentation of injuries, not least because there is a high chance that this documentation will be required to be produced in court as evidence. With this in mind, it is important to avoid any pressure to provide a 'quick check' of a detainee, police officer, or other individual in an informal or semi-formal fashion.

Procedure

Records of all injuries need to be clear and complete. It is worth trying to develop and follow a standard approach, in order to ensure that nothing is missed. As with other forms of documentation, notes need to be legible, written in black ink, and retained/stored safely and securely. It is worth taking time to accurately measure injuries and to record their exact positions by reference to distances from fixed landmarks (e.g. 'anteromedial aspect of the right shin, 10cm distal to the tibial tuberosity').

Diagrams

Diagrams with injuries marked are very useful. In all but the most straight-forward cases, use a diagram to record the injuries. Standard anatomical charts (such as those recommended by the Faculty of Forensic and Legal Medicine) are very useful to accurately convey the pattern and extent of the injuries. If the injuries are very numerous, consider marking them with a number on the chart and writing the details of the injury in full underneath—an example of this is shown in 📖 Fig. 5.1, p.122.

Photographs

In cases involving serious allegations and/or multiple injuries, photographs may prove to be important evidence. Photographs are usually taken by specialist police staff using standardized equipment. Typically an L-shaped ruler is included in the photograph adjacent to the injuries in order that the size of the injuries can be assessed from the photograph (allowing for distortion in both vertical and horizontal dimensions). Photographs are particularly useful when the individual has what is suspected to be a human bite—the photograph can be analysed at a later date by an appropriate expert (forensic odontologist).

Restraint techniques and injuries

Police are frequently faced with individuals who are agitated or violent or both. Restraint techniques employed to deal with this situation may or may not involve specialized equipment and can result in injuries. The police officer's duty is to employ reasonable force, taking into account the seriousness of the situation and the extent of the threat faced.

Arm holds

The simplest form of restraint involves a restrained person's arms being grabbed and held firmly. This may result in fingertip imprint bruising to the arms—bruising to the medial aspect of the upper arm is a classic injury. Note that soft tissue injuries to the shoulder can occur when an individual's wrist is grasped firmly behind his/her back and raised up in an attempt to gain control, possibly in the process of applying handcuffs.

Neck holds

Holds involving compression of the neck are dangerous and not recommended. The *'chokehold'* refers to placement of the forearm flat across the neck, resulting in airway compression, with or without associated damage to the larynx. When the elbow is placed more to the front in the *'carotid sleeper hold'*, resulting compression of the carotid arteries on either side of the neck (by the forearm on one side and biceps on the other) can impair circulation and cause loss of consciousness within a matter of seconds. Petechial haemorrhages to the eyes and face may be a pointer to the recent use of this technique.

Body holds

When a number of individuals are involved in restraint of an agitated person who is standing, it is traditional for him/her to be grasped from behind and taken down in a controlled trip. There is a significant risk of asphyxia when a person is held on the ground for any length of time, particularly when lying prone with force applied to the back. The simultaneous application of handcuffs and leg restraints (*'hog-tying'*) is associated with particular risks of positional asphyxia (see 📖 p.108) and death.

Physical restraint in a medical setting

Metal rails (cotsides) are frequently used to prevent patients falling off a bed or trolley, but do carry a (small but definite) risk of positional asphyxia (see 📖 p.108). *Straitjackets* were traditionally used to restrain patients with psychiatric problems who were judged to be at risk of injuring themselves or others. Very tight application may cause mechanical asphyxia. They are no longer in widespread use. *Restraint belt and straps* may be effective in temporarily restraining agitated patients and preventing them from moving out of a chair or bed.

Modern medical approach to the violent patient

Emergency tranquillization is regarded as a 'last resort'. See National Institute for Health and Clinical Excellence (NICE) guidance (⌕ http://www.nice.org.uk) (📖 p.423).

Chemical restraint agents

Also known as 'crowd control agents', there is a long history of chemicals being used against individuals as well as crowds. Agents used by modern law enforcement agencies differ from traditional chemicals used in warfare (e.g. mustard gas, chlorine, phosgene) in that they are not primarily designed to inflict long-term damage.

CS spray ('tear gas')

Available as an aerosol spray, the active constituent of CS is orthochloro-benzylidene malononitrile. It is used by police in riot/crowd control, for self-protection and to assist apprehension of suspected offenders. The spray is used within close range (a few metres) and aimed at the face.

Effects

CS spray has an immediate effect upon the exposed mucous membranes, causing blepharospasm (blinking), painful lacrimation (eye watering), rhin-orrhoea (runny nose), coughing, sneezing, burning in the throat. Blurred vision and photophobia (sensitivity to light) usually resolve within an hour. Less frequently reported effects include: skin burns with blistering, iritis, laryngospasm, pulmonary oedema.

Treatment

Most symptoms resolve quickly, helped by being in a well-ventilated area, but all detainees who have been exposed to CS should be assessed medically. Forensic practitioners should wear gloves (and ideally, goggles) when treating someone who has been exposed to CS spray.
- Place the patient in a well-ventilated environment.
- Remove contaminated clothes and place them in a sealed plastic bag.
- Consider using a fan to blow dry air onto the eyes to enhance vapourization of any remaining CS material. Irrigating the eyes with saline is an alternative, although accompanied by a transient worsening of symptoms.
- Wash affected skin thoroughly.
- Give simple oral analgesics as required.
- Provide salbutamol inhaler for clinical bronchospasm.
- Arrange to review patients with severe or persisting effects.

CN spray

Chloroacetophenone (CN) gas was developed prior to CS spray and has similar effects.

Pepper spray (OC spray)

Oleum capsicum (OC) or 'pepper spray' has many similar effects to CS and CN. It causes pain at the site of exposure and can produce significant skin problems, including blistering. Occasional severe effects can occur and it is believed by some that it may have played a role in some deaths in custody.

Treatment of those exposed to OC follows similar lines to that described following CS and CN.

Handcuffs

History

Handcuffs are the most commonly employed physical restraint. The use of handcuffs can be traced back thousands of years to ancient times, when they played an important role in controlling large numbers of prisoners taken in battle. The word 'handcuff' derives from the Anglo-Saxon 'hand-cop' (something which 'cops' or 'catches' the hands).

Design

Handcuffs come in a variety of materials and designs. Most are metal, in the form of either steel or aluminium. Modern handcuffs have the two cuffs connected by a metal block or bar ('rigid handcuff'). These have replaced the older flexible styles in which the cuffs were connected with a small chain. Handcuffs are locked around the wrists and can still be tightened until the double locks are engaged—a lock spring prevents further tightening of the cuffs. Release requires a key (the custody sergeant will usually first confirm that they were correctly applied).

Disposable thin self-locking plastic ties

These are sometimes used as a temporary measure in operations which involve the detention of many individuals. They can be tightened as required, but do have the disadvantage that they can be over-tightened. Typically, at least two interlocking ties are used on each prisoner. They require to be cut through in order to be removed.

Application

In the past, handcuffs were 'worn' at the front, but they are now typically applied with the arms behind the back. The rigid handcuff has the advantage of enabling further control and restraint once one hand is cuffed. The application of handcuffs behind the back renders individuals more unstable on their feet (particularly in the context of alcohol and/or drug ingestion) and less able to protect themselves in the event of a fall. Once applied, handcuffs are tightened until there is a reasonable fit, when they are double locked to prevent further (excessive) tightening.

Handcuff-related injuries

The use of handcuffs is relatively frequently associated with erythema (redness) and superficial abrasions to the wrists, particularly when the restrained individual has struggled. Fractures of the wrist have been reported, but appear to be quite rare, unless there is some additional trauma, such as a fall. Neuropraxia (closed nerve compression with the nerve in continuity) occurs relatively frequently and deserves careful assessment (see Fig. 9.1).

Nerve compression damage

This occurs to some extent in >5% of individuals who have handcuffs applied. The most frequently affected nerve is the (purely sensory) superficial radial nerve, damage to which causes reduced sensation over the dorsum of the thumb and webspace between it and the index finger (see box). Sensory and motor damage to other nerves can occur. Although most individuals experience only temporary effects, all patients

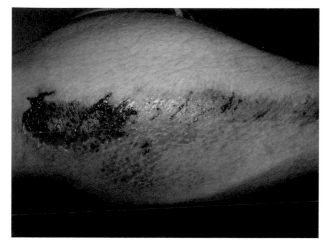

Plate 1 Abrasion.

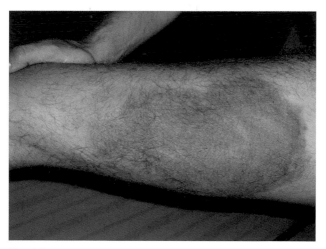

Plate 2 Bruising.

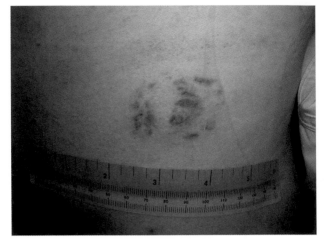

Plate 3 Human bite.

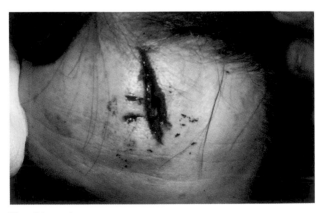

Plate 4 Laceration.

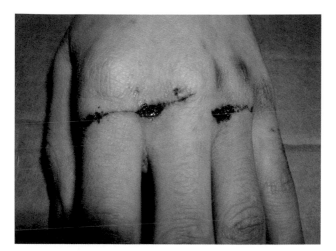

Plate 5 Incised wounds.

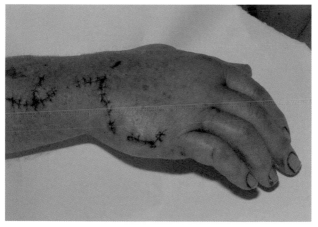

Plate 6 Sutured knife defence wounds.

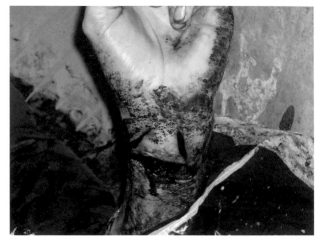

Plate 7 Deliberate self-harm incised wounds.

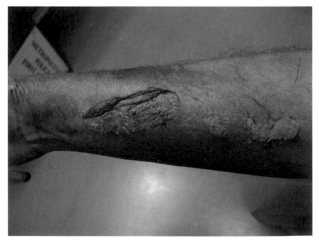

Plate 8 Partial thickness burns with blistering.

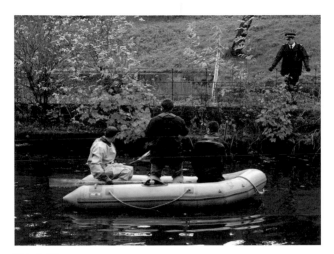

Plate 9 Crime scene.

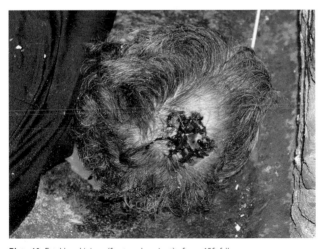

Plate 10 Fatal head injury (fractured occiput) after a 15ft fall.

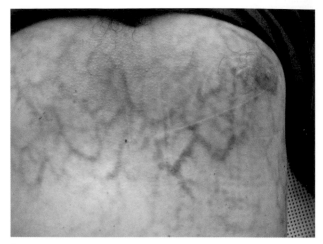

Plate 11 Marbling of skin after death.

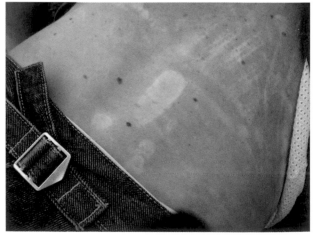

Plate 12 Lividity.

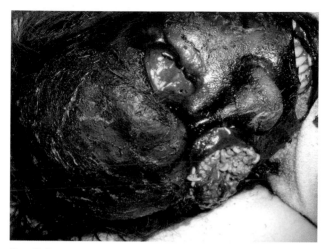

Plate 13 Decomposition.

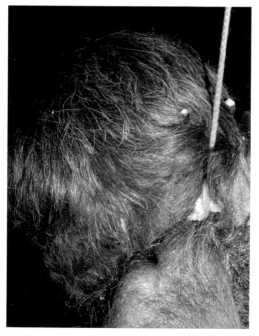

Plate 14 Neck suspension.

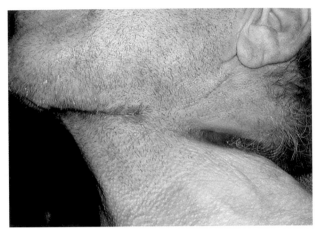

Plate 15 Ligature impression and parchmenting after hanging.

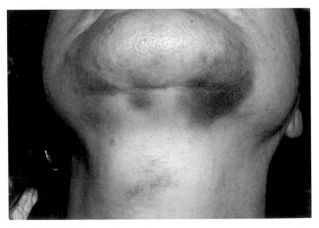

Plate 16 Neck/chin injury after manual strangulation.

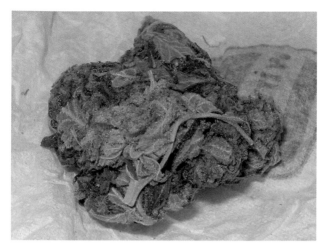

Plate 17 Cannabis leaf.

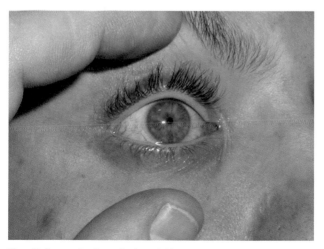

Plate 18 Drugs—pinpoint pupils after opioid use.

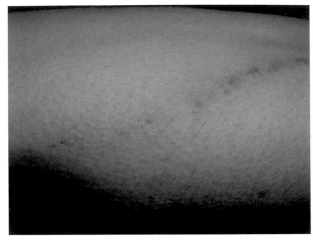

Plate 19 Trackmarks and gooseflesh—intravenous heroin misuse and withdrawal.

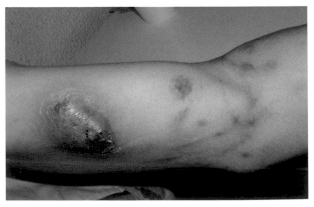

Plate 20 Multiple intravenous injection sites and abscess.

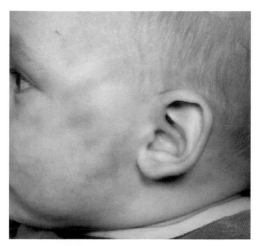

Plate 21 Hand slap mark to face.

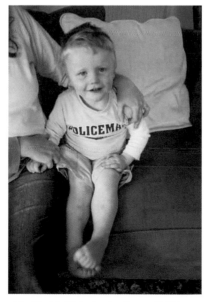

Plate 22 Normal (accidental) shin bruises in a 2-year-old child.

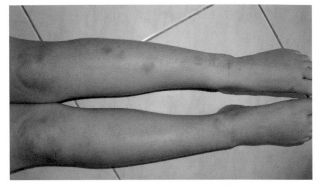

Plate 23 Accidental shin bruising in a 6-year-old child.

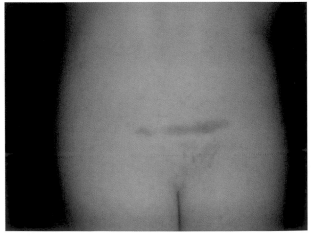

Plate 24 10-year-old hit by a hockey stick the previous day.

need careful assessment and documentation of their injuries. Patients can be reassured that pain at the site of application of the handcuffs with distal tingling and reduced sensation usually settle quite rapidly (within a few days). However, they need to be advised of the need for follow-up and if there are any motor effects, to passively put the fingers and wrist through full range of movement several times each hour. In some instances, this advice may need to be reiterated once an initially agitated and intoxicated detained person becomes sober. In severe cases, nerve damage may persist and be demonstrated by nerve conduction studies.

Nerve damage at the wrist
- *Superficial radial nerve injury*— reduced sensation to the dorsum of the thumb and index finger. (No motor branches at the wrist.)
- *Median nerve injury*—reduced sensation to the radial half of the palm and difficulty abducting thumb against resistance.
- *Ulnar nerve injury*—reduced sensation ulnar 1½ fingers (front and back) and reduced ability to abduct/adduct fingers or cross index and middle fingers.

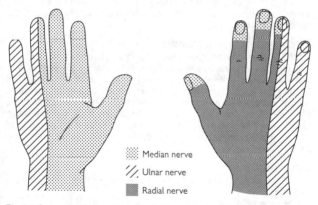

Median nerve
Ulnar nerve
Radial nerve

Fig. 9.1 Sensory hand innervation. Adapted from Wardrope J and Edhouse JA (1999). *The Management of Wounds and Burns*, 2nd edn, with permission of Oxford University Press.

Injury from police weapons

Police officers are equipped with different weapons according to the country/jurisdiction, the situation, and their training. Injuries which result from the deployment of police weapons vary according to the type of weapon used.

Batons and truncheons ('nightstick' in the USA)

Traditionally, police officers in the UK have carried a wooden truncheon. This has now been replaced by several different types and design of baton, including some collapsible versions. They are constructed of materials ranging from metal to plastic. Batons can cause classic tramline bruising to the skin (see 🕮 p.124) and underlying fractures and/or serious internal damage depending upon the area affected. Strikes against the abdomen, head, and neck are acknowledged to have a relatively high risk of serious injury. It is important to carefully consider the possibility of significant intra-abdominal injury in any detainee who has abdominal bruising after use of a baton. It can be particularly difficult to assess individuals who under the influence of alcohol and/or drugs. Pay particular attention to any altered vital signs and adopt a low threshold for referral to the Emergency Department.

In addition to causing linear bruising, the use of a baton in a thrusting fashion can cause smaller oval or circular bruising reflecting impact of the end of the weapon.

Plastic bullets (baton rounds)

In the UK, baton rounds (previously known as 'plastic bullets') were initially introduced to replace the rubber bullets which were used to help deal with public order disturbances in Northern Ireland in the 1970s. Although they typically produce bruises and abrasions, they can also cause internal damage and have been responsible for deaths. The latter are often associated with direct hits to the head. The current acrylic baton round in use in the UK (the L21A1) is considered to be safer, as a result of allowing more accuracy. The target is the belt buckle area (i.e. away from the head).

Other rounds

In other countries, a variety of other rounds are employed, including the following:
• Rubber baton rounds
• Wood baton rounds
• Beanbag or 'sock' rounds.

Taser

Thomas **A S**wift's **E**lectrical **R**ifle (Taser) was first developed in 1974 by NASA researcher Jack Cover. The device fires two dart-like electrodes with barbs in the end which lodge in skin or clothing and then impart a series of (high voltage, low amp) electric shocks for 5s. The shocks are delivered by each of the darts trailing a 6-m long wire (thereby defining the range of the weapon). The two wires complete an electrical circuit through the skin, with the shocks resulting in painful, uncontrollable muscular contractions. As a result of this, the victim falls and is temporarily incapacitated, allowing subsequent restraint and detention. The devices may be fitted with an integral video camera to capture a record of what happens as it is deployed.

Stun capacity

Some models also have the ability to 'stun' a subject without completely causing complete incapacity. The 'Drive Stun' mode is achieved by holding the device directly against the skin of the target causing localized pain, which may assist with his/her detention.

Uses

The Taser is designed to cause a person to be incapacitated for a short period of time during which he/she can be safely apprehended. The device is suited for use against (often armed) individuals who appear to pose a significant risk of harm to others. The advantage of the Taser over other weapons (such as firearms) is that it has the potential to allow an individual to be detained without sustaining long-term injury and without injury to the person using it. It has received considerable attention in the context of being able to subdue and detain a would-be suicide bomber before deployment of any terrorist device.

Medical effects

The two barbs in the end of the darts are able to penetrate the skin by approximately 0.5cm and can be removed relatively easily, unless the eye is involved. There have been reports of deaths following deployment of the Taser, although it is not entirely established what mechanism was responsible. Proponents of Tasers have taken extreme measures to demonstrate their confidence in the safety profile of the device—in May 2007, Michael Todd, Chief Constable of Greater Manchester Police, allowed himself to be 'shot' by a Taser, which created the intended considerable media attention.

There is a theoretical risk to individuals who have a pacemaker or pre-existing heart disease. Detained individuals who have had a Taser deployed on them do not necessarily require to attend hospital, but they should be seen and assessed by a forensic practitioner. The following individuals should be referred to hospital for further assessment: those who have heart disease, a pacemaker, are agitated, pregnant, tachycardic, or appear to be unwell.

Head injury from a custody perspective

Background

Signs of recent head injury are relatively common in the population of individuals who are arrested and taken into custody—in some cases, the head injury occurred during the arrest, in others, during some previous event which may or not be related to the arrest (e.g. violent altercation, fall, road traffic collision). When faced with a detainee who has sustained a head injury the forensic practitioner has the following tasks:

- To identify and document the nature and extent of the injury (including for forensic purposes).
- To assess what treatment is required and if the patient needs to be transferred to hospital for this.
- To assess whether there is a significant risk of deterioration, requiring transfer to hospital for investigation/observation.
- To provide treatment and advice, both for the patient and custody staff/others who will be caring for him/her during the subsequent 24h.

The problem with head injuries in custody

Custody staff have historically been concerned about accepting detainees with head injuries, and not without reason. There is a risk of deterioration in anyone with a head injury. Patients have died from a head injury in custody. Patients may develop intracranial haemorrhage, infection, brain swelling, or other secondary complications. One particular concern is that the combination of a head injury with drug and/or alcohol consumption may impair the usual airway protective reflexes, thereby increasing the potential for aspiration of stomach contents. It is particularly difficult to assess the head injury in a person who is intoxicated, hence the following rule:

Never attribute reduced conscious level to alcohol or drugs in a patient with a head injury (instead, treat as if the head injury was responsible).

When accepting patients into custody, forensic practitioners should regard the custody unit of only being able to provide a level of observation equivalent to that which they might expect from a close relative at home. Hospital doctors sometimes make the mistake of considering the custody unit to be a sort of 'mini-hospital'. Patients who have been seen and treated at hospital should only be accepted back to a custody unit if they would have otherwise been deemed fit to discharge home into the care of a relative.

Risk of intracranial haematoma

A key role of the forensic practitioner is to identify those detainees who are at risk of developing an intracranial complication (especially a haematoma) and having identified this risk, to transfer them urgently and safely to hospital. Data from Emergency Departments suggests that patients with a head injury who present to hospital fully conscious and with no 'worrying features' have quite a low risk (<1 in 6000) of developing an intracranial haematoma requiring surgical intervention. For this reason, such patients are often discharged with advice to a carer. Patients who have a reduced conscious level and/or other 'worrying factors' (such as taking oral anticoagulants) are at a greatly increased risk of developing an intracranial haematomas—they require hospital attention (and usually CT scan as well).

Alcoholics and subdural haematomas

The group of 'frequent attenders' at custody includes a group of middle-aged alcoholics who are at a greatly increased risk of attending custody with a developing subdural haematoma. This increased risk reflects a combination of a number of factors, including:

• Increased risk of head injury due to falls whilst intoxicated.
• Increased risk of head injury due to chronic instability as a result of chronic alcohol abuse (peripheral neuropathy etc.).
• Enhanced bleeding tendency due to alcohol related liver damage.
• Cerebral atrophy due to age and alcohol.
• Reduced opportunities to receive standard medical attention via usual channels (especially GP) due to chaotic lifestyle.

The forensic practitioner needs to be aware of the possibility of a slowly developing (chronic) subdural haematoma in an alcoholic who does not seem 'quite right' or fails to 'sober up' as expected, even in the absence of any previous head injury.

Head injury assessment

NICE has produced well-referenced guidelines on the assessment and management of head injury (see ℗ http://www.nice.org.uk). Injuries to the face are often incorrectly disregarded as not being head injuries. A head injury may be considered to be any trauma to the head, except superficial injuries to the face.

History

It can be difficult to obtain an accurate history from a patient in custody who has a head injury. Detainees who sustain a head injury whilst committing an alleged offence need to be reminded that they are not obliged to reveal information about the incident and how the head injury occurred. The forensic practitioner should ideally attempt to ascertain (and document) the following:
• Time (and in some cases, date) of injury.
• Mechanism of injury (especially considering the possibility of a medical collapse as cause of the injury, or glass being implicated in causing the injury—this mandates X-ray at hospital).
• Whether there was any loss of consciousness.
• If there is any amnesia.
• Past history and drug history (particularly: any bleeding tendency and/or warfarin ingestion).
• Alcohol and/or drug ingestion.
• Tetanus status (if there are wounds present).
• Subsequent symptoms: headache, vomiting, limb weakness, fits, neck pain, rhinorrhoea, otorrhoea, diplopia.

Examination

The assessment and documentation of any injury is covered on 📖 p.120 and should be followed for head injuries. It can be particularly important from a medicolegal perspective to try to decide if a wound is incised or a laceration. In addition to the standard documentation of an injury, consider the following:
• Conscious level, as measured by the Glasgow Coma Scale (see box).
• Evidence of neck injury: midline tenderness and/or inability to rotate the neck by 45° to left and right after recent injury implies the need for immobilization, transfer to hospital, and X-ray.
• Pulse rate, blood pressure, and ideally, respiratory rate/oxygen saturation level.
• Pupillary reactions.
• Limb weakness.
• Other injuries.
• Blood glucose.

Special considerations apply to examination of facial injuries—see 📖 p.286.

Glasgow Coma Scale

Eye response		
	Open spontaneously	4
	Open to voice	3
	Open to pain	2
	No response	1
Verbal response	Talking and orientated	5
	Confused/disorientated	4
	Inappropriate words	3
	Incomprehensible sounds	2
	No response	1
Motor response	Obeys commands	6
	Localizes pain	5
	Flexion/withdrawal	4
	Abnormal flexion	3
	Extension	2
	No response	1
Total (GCS)	**Range**	**3–15**

Referral of head injury to hospital

In addition to NICE guidance on the management of head injury (℘ http://www.nice.org.uk), the Faculty of Forensic and Legal Medicine have produced guidelines specifically aimed at forensic practitioners (℘ http://www.fflm.ac.uk).

Criteria for referral to hospital

The following criteria mandate referral of any head-injured patient to hospital:

- Reduced conscious level (GCS $<^{15}/_{15}$) at any time since injury.
- Focal neurological symptoms or signs (e.g. problems understanding, speaking, reading, or writing; decreased sensation; loss of balance; general weakness; visual changes; abnormal reflexes; problems walking).
- Any suspicion of a skull fracture or penetrating injury (e.g. cerebrospinal fluid leak; 'black eye' with no associated damage around the eyes; bleeding from or new deafness in one or both ears; mastoid haematoma; signs of penetrating injury; visible trauma to the scalp or skull of concern to the forensic practitioner).
- Pre- or post-traumatic amnesia.
- Persistent headache since the injury.
- Any vomiting since the injury.
- Any seizures since the injury.
- Medical comorbidity (e.g. previous cranial surgery, anticoagulant therapy, bleeding or clotting disorder).
- High energy head injury (e.g. fall from a height of >1m or 5 stairs).
- Current drug or alcohol intoxication.
- Continuing uncertainty about the diagnosis after first assessment.
- Age greater than 65 years.

Transfer to hospital

Prior to transfer, the forensic practitioner may need to consider the following supportive measures for a patient with head injury:

- Airway opening techniques (see 📖 p.220).
- Manual stabilization of the cervical spine and minimizing neck movement.
- Application of direct pressure to stop bleeding from a head wound.

Usually, patients should be transferred from the custody unit to the Emergency Department by emergency ambulance. Paramedics with specialist training and equipment are better placed to manage deterioration in a patient's clinical condition and/or associated airway problems during transfer.

Transfer letter

The letter to hospital should include at least the following information: the history/mechanism of injury, the injuries sustained, GCS, pulse rate, blood pressure, pupil size and reactions, limb weakness, blood glucose measurement.

Patients with head injury transferred back from hospital

It is to some extent reassuring that a patient has been assessed at hospital. However, patients in custody who arrive at the custody unit after having been seen at an Emergency Department (or following overnight observation) are still at some risk of developing serious problems. Some patients may deteriorate during the transfer to custody. For these reasons, it is essential to ensure that the forensic practitioner promptly reviews each patient who returns from hospital with a head injury.

Custody management of head injury

Some patients with minor head injury can be safely managed within the custody unit.

Wound management

Some minor wounds not requiring formal cleaning and/or exploration for foreign body (the possibility of glass mandates X-ray) may be cleaned and dressed by the forensic practitioner.

Analgesia

Patients with even minor head injuries can be expected to experience a headache. The best treatment in the first instance is oral paracetamol (1g every 6h as required is the standard adult dose). Patients who report severe or worsening headache despite analgesia should be reassessed, as this can be a sign of a developing intracranial haematoma.

Advice to custody staff

The Faculty of Forensic and Legal Medicine (see ℘ http://www.fflm.ac.uk) has published guidelines on the advice which should be given to custody staff as follows:

Custody staff should **rouse and speak** with the detained person (obtaining a comprehensible verbal response) every 30min (in accordance with Annex H to Code C of PACE Codes of Practice).

If the detained person:

- Becomes **unconscious**.
- Becomes **increasingly sleepy** or **drowsy**.
- Complains of **persistent or increasingly severe headache**.
- Complains of **any visual disturbance such as blurred or double vision**.
- **Vomits**.
- Has a **fit**.
- Exhibits behaviour that is of any concern.

Then the Forensic Physician must be contacted urgently. If an immediate response from the doctor is not obtained, the detained person **must be at once transported**, via an ambulance, to the nearest Emergency Department. When released from custody the detained person should be released to the care of a responsible adult and both should be given appropriate guidance.

Fitness to interview

In general terms, if a detainee is not fit to interview due to the effects of a head injury, then he/she is unlikely to be fit to detain without having been assessed at hospital.

Advice following release from custody

It is the responsibility of the forensic practitioner to ensure that detainees who are released from custody are given appropriate advice regarding continuing care and that advice is also given to their carers. Suggested written head injury warning advice has been published by the Faculty of Forensic and Legal Medicine (see ℘ http://www.fflm.ac.uk). The head injury warning advice to the patient is as follows:

Faculty of Forensic and Legal Medicine: advice to patient

Head injury warning

The following advice must be followed after you have sustained a head injury to ensure your safe recovery and to minimize the risk of complications safely:

- ***Do*** make sure you stay within easy reach of a telephone and medical help.
- ***Do*** have plenty of rest and avoid stressful situations.
- ***Do not*** take any alcohol or drugs.
- ***Do not*** take sleeping tablets, sedatives, or tranquillizers unless they are given by a doctor.
- ***Do not*** play any contact sport (e.g. football) for at least 3 weeks without taking advice from your doctor first.
- ***Do not*** return to your normal school, college, or work activity until you feel you have completely recovered.
- ***Do not*** drive a car, motorbike, or bicycle or operate machinery unless you feel you have completely recovered.

Complications are not always immediately obvious following a ***head injury***. Therefore (although you have been examined by a doctor) you are advised to stay with a ***responsible*** adult for the next ***48h*** and that person should be shown the guidance on the *Advice to responsible adult* card, see www.fflm.ac.uk.

Facial injury

Except for very minor injuries, facial wounds also need to be regarded as being head injuries (with potential for intracranial complication). Facial injuries are often of great forensic significance and so accurate documentation is very important.

Facial abrasions

These assume special importance, given the cosmetic implications. Abrasions which have ingrained dirt require to be scrubbed clean to remove the risk of 'tattooing'. Often, proper cleaning can only be achieved with local anaesthetic in a good light, possibly requiring hospital.

Facial lacerations and incisions

These need careful attention, with only accurate opposition and closure of the wound edges resulting in the best scarring. This is particularly true of wounds which cross the vermilion border (junction of lip with facial skin). Full thickness facial wounds requiring interrupted sutures under local anaesthetic are usually closed in the Emergency Department, not the custody unit. Size 6/0 nylon sutures (removed at 5 days) are appropriate to close facial skin wounds, with non-absorbable (e.g. vicryl) inside the mouth.

Nose injury

The nasal bones are delicate and relatively exposed. Although it can often be demonstrated on X-ray, the diagnosis of nasal fracture is a clinical one. It is based upon a history of trauma, with accompanying epistaxis and tenderness (± swelling and asymmetry). An important, albeit unusual, complication is septal haematoma—apparent as a tense bulging swelling which may obstruct the nostril.

Management

- If the nose is swollen, but straight and not actively bleeding, the detainee requires oral analgesia and advice to attend their GP for follow-up if there are any concerns (especially if the nose appears 'bent' after about 5 days).
- If the nose is obviously deviated to one side, it is likely to need to be straightened under general anaesthetic (within 10 days when the fractures start to unite). Either refer to the Emergency Department or liaise with the department to arrange follow-up for this to occur.
- Detainees with a septal haematoma or continuing epistaxis need to be seen by the local Ear, Nose, and Throat team as an emergency.

Mandible injuries

Fractures to the mandible not infrequently result from punches. A blow landed on the chin may cause fractures at the mandibular neck, with relatively little evidence of the fracture. The report of an 'abnormal bite' (feeling that the teeth do not meet properly) is an indication of possible fracture. It is important to carefully check for tenderness around the mandibular neck/temporomandibular joint. Any suspicion of mandibular fracture requires X-ray at hospital (orthopantomogram).

Maxillary fracture

Punch injuries and other forms of blunt trauma (including falls) can result in isolated fractures of the maxilla (cheek bone). The combination of swelling and bony tenderness should prompt suspicion of a fracture and the need for transfer to hospital for X-ray. Other occasional features of maxillary fracture are: reduced sensation over the cheek (implying damage to the infraorbital nerve) and diplopia/reduced range of eye movement.

Periorbital haematoma (often referred to colloquially as a 'black eye') is the term applied to bruising with swelling around the eye. Swelling which is so dramatic that the eye cannot be opened may reflect an underlying fracture to the maxilla and/or orbit (eye socket).

Spinal injury

Blunt injury to the spine may follow direct trauma (e.g. fall, kick) or be indirect (e.g. 'whiplash' injury after car crash). In general, patients with the following should be referred to hospital for assessment (and likely X-ray):
- A high-energy mechanism of injury with subsequent reported spinal pain.
- Tenderness (± swelling) over the spine in the midline.
- Neurological signs which may be attributed to the injury.

Cervical spinal injury

Experience has taught hospital staff to adopt a relatively low threshold for cervical spine imaging following injury. In the context of neck pain following a road traffic collision, X-rays are not routinely requested in a fully conscious patient who has no midline tenderness, no neurological signs, and is able to rotate the neck by 45° to both right and left. Pain and stiffness from 'whiplash' injury tends to worsen during the first 24h. Symptoms may be helped by use of painkillers (e.g. ibuprofen and/or co-dydramol).

Thoracic and lumbar spine injury

The thoracolumbar junction is particularly prone to fractures as a result of high falls or high-energy impacts in road traffic collisions. There may be associated haematuria.

Dermatomes

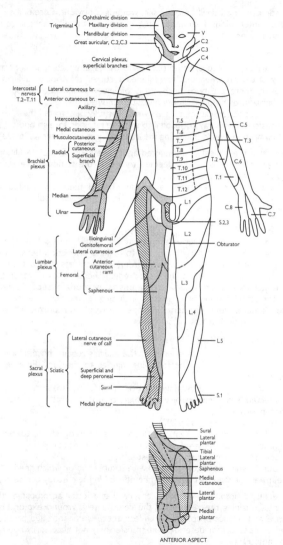

Fig. 9.2 Dermatomes. Reproduced from Wyatt JP I. (2006). *Oxford Handbook of Emergency Medicine* 3rd edn, with permission of Oxford University Press.

Skin wounds

The potential legal significance of skin wounds is obvious. Careful assessment and meticulous documentation may make all the difference in court at a much later date.

History

For a variety of reasons, some relating to the legal process, an accurate history of exactly when and how injuries occurred may not be available. However, there are two mechanisms of injury which deserve special consideration, as hospital attention will be required:

- A wound possibly caused by glass which has fully penetrated the dermis requires X-ray at hospital to exclude retained foreign body.
- A human bite wound (including the 'reverse fight bite'—see 📖 p.293).

Ascertain if the patient is immunized against tetanus. Complete lifelong cover against tetanus is now deemed to follow the standard five active immunizations given in childhood.

Take a past medical history to include whether there is any need for prophylactic antibiotics: immunosuppression (e.g. previous splenectomy) or prosthetic heart valve.

Examination

Take time to examine injuries and carefully consider the exact nature of each injury. It is particularly important to make a distinction between an incised wound and a laceration, recording relevant associated features such as bruising adjacent to the wound edge (see 📖 p.116). Document injuries accurately, using ruler and diagrams as appropriate (see 📖 p.120). Look for associated and other injuries, including related nerve, tendon, or vessel damage. Note that nerve damage can result in reported 'altered' sensation, rather than 'absent' sensation.

Custody or hospital?

The first decision to make is whether the injuries require hospital attention. Refer patients with the following injuries to the local Emergency Department:

- Wounds with possible retained glass or other foreign material.
- Suspected nerve, tendon, or vessel injury or possible fracture and/or joint involvement.
- Human bite wounds (📖 p.292).
- Need for tetanus immunization (<5 previous doses of tetanus toxoid).
- Significantly contaminated or dirty wounds (including abrasions) requiring cleaning under local anaesthetic.
- Wounds which need to be closed with sutures and/or which need treatment beyond that which can be offered in the custody centre.

If referral to hospital is required, ensure that a letter accompanies the patient explaining the reason for the referral (e.g. wound exploration/closure and tetanus prophylaxis). Unless, there is uncontrolled haemorrhage or potential for deterioration, transfer may not necessarily need to be by ambulance.

Wound management in custody

Incised wounds and lacerations

Some smaller wounds can be satisfactorily managed at the custody unit. Thorough cleaning is most important in order to reduce the chance of infection developing. For some wounds, it is appropriate to initially wash under running tap water. Follow this with irrigation using 0.9% saline. Many wounds of <4cm length can be closed with the application of tissue glue externally to the skin edges and/or adhesive paper strips. However, if there is any doubt regarding closure, it may be better to send the patient to hospital—wound suturing is generally easier to undertake in an Emergency Department.

Puncture wounds to the foot

A detainee who reports treading on a nail, usually requires hospital referral for an X-ray to exclude a retained foreign body (rusty nails can break!), antiseptic foot bath, tetanus, and antibiotic (e.g. co-amoxiclav) prophylaxis.

Abrasions

Extensive abrasions, especially those significantly ingrained with dirt, require hospital attention for cleaning under local (or even general) anaesthetic. Smaller superficial abrasions can be managed in custody (with or without use of local anaesthetic injection) by cleaning with saline and application of a dressing with adherent edges. It is worth remembering that on occasions the ingrained material can have significant forensic implications and so needs to be collected and retained formally as a sample for analysis.

Notes

• Any wound can become infected and the patient needs to be told about this risk and the warning signs to look out for.
• Avoid the use of bandages in custody as these can be used as ligatures.

Infected wounds

Not infrequently, individuals have established infection in older wounds at the time of their arrest and detention. Consider tetanus prophylaxis in addition to starting appropriate antibiotic treatment, unless infection has spread ± systemic upset and/or collection of pus, in which case refer to hospital.

Bite wounds

Bite injuries can result from humans or animals. They can take a variety of different forms, including erythema, abrasions, bruising, crushing to soft tissues, lacerations, and tissue loss. In addition to treatment considerations, there are often significant clinical forensic issues.

Analysis of bite marks

A bite mark can, on occasion, act as the equivalent to a fingerprint in being able to identify an individual responsible for biting. In order to achieve this, a forensic odontologist needs to be able to 'match' an individual's dentition with the bite mark(s) and so it is critically important that good quality photographs (using a standard L-shaped ruler) are obtained at an early stage. A forensic odontologist will be able to compare photographic images with dental imprints and/or records, including X-rays in order to make a 'match'.

DNA analysis

Saliva left behind on the bitten skin may contain enough DNA to provide a useful match. Avoid washing the skin of the bitten area before taking swabs for DNA analysis—preferably, pairs of dry swabs, damp swabs (dampened with sterile saline), and control swabs.

Clinical assessment

Risks from human bites

Human bites can result in physical injury (e.g. tendon damage, retained foreign body), bacterial infection (including tetanus and other bacteria), viral infection (hepatitis B/C and HIV). Assessment needs to address each of these issues. On occasions, it may be impossible to establish exactly who was responsible for the bite and what the risk profile of that individual is.

Treatment

Many detainees with bite injuries which penetrate the skin and cause bleeding require hospital attention for one or more of the following:
• Wound exploration, cleaning, and possible closure.
• X-ray for possible retained foreign body (tooth) or fracture.
• Tetanus prophylaxis.
• Antibiotic prophylaxis (traditionally co-amoxiclav 375mg, 3 times a day).
• Hepatitis B prophylaxis (accelerated active immunization ± passive immunization also, according to the likely risks involved).
• Storage of serum for later testing for hepatitis/HIV as required.
• HIV prophylaxis (unusually required).

Reverse fight bites

A punch injury delivered to the face of an individual can result in a 'reverse bite' injury to the closed fist. This typically affects the skin over the 2nd–5th metacarpophalangeal joints, where in the situation of a closed fist, the distance between the skin and underlying tendon and joint space is relatively small. Skin wounds in this region can appear to be innocuous, but hide considerable underlying damage. Not infrequently, the history of injury is not clear, so adopt a high index of suspicion of possible reverse fight bites when treating wounds in this region.

Closed limb injury

Assessment of limb injuries amongst detained persons can be rendered difficult by several factors, including: alcohol and drug intoxication/withdrawal, detainees' preoccupation with the legal process, and/or a desire to leave custody. In particular, the exact history (and mechanism) of injury may be difficult to establish with any certainty. Significant injuries, however, are usually readily apparent upon examination. Detainees with dislocations or angulated fractures require urgent transfer to the local Emergency Department. However, in the absence of these, it may be reasonable to rest, elevate, wait a few hours, and reassess once the effects of alcohol/drugs or withdrawal symptoms have subsided.

Signs of a fracture

The classic signs of a fracture are swelling, tenderness, deformity, and reduced neighbouring joint movement. Fractures of certain bones, however, may not exhibit all of these features. For example, fracture of the scaphoid may result in no swelling or deformity, but simply swelling in the anatomical snuffbox alone.

Dislocations

Most dislocations are clinically obvious. It is not usually appropriate to try to reduce dislocations prior to X-ray. The exceptions, for those with appropriate training, include patellar dislocations, ankle fracture/dislocations where skin is under tension and/or there is neurovascular deficit, but there is rarely a reason to attempt reduction in custody.

Soft tissue injuries

These include bruising, muscle strains, and ligament sprains. Traditional treatment measures include the following:
- Initial rest.
- Elevation to reduce swelling.
- Analgesia: typically paracetamol (1g orally, 4 times a day) and/or ibuprofen 400mg orally, 3 times a day taken with food. For more significant/painful injuries, paracetamol may be replaced with co-dydramol, 2 tablets, 4 times a day.
- Later movement/mobilization, possibly with formal physiotherapy (usually arranged via GP).

The use of compression bandages is traditional, but of no proven benefit. Bandages are best avoided in custody, especially considering the potential risk of self-harm (ligature).

Upper limb injury

Thumb injuries

The thumb is at particular risk of injury during scuffles which involve grappling. Tenderness at the ulnar aspect of the metacarpophalangeal joint implies damage to the ulnar collateral ligament ('gamekeeper thumb')—complete rupture is a serious injury requiring early surgical repair.

Hand injuries

Fractures of the 5th metacarpal neck typically follow a punch—most simply need 'buddy strapping' after X-ray confirmation. Swelling and tenderness at the base of the 5th metacarpal may indicate dislocation at the carpometacarpal joint, requiring urgent reduction and fixation.

Wrist injuries

Fractures of the distal radius typically result in visible swelling. Always check for (and document) the presence of tenderness in the anatomical snuffbox—patients who are tender here require a series of X-rays to exclude scaphoid fracture.

Elbow injuries

A fracture is very unlikely if the patient is able to fully extend the elbow and flex it so that the hand touches the shoulder tip.

Shoulder injuries

Dislocations are usually anterior and clinically obvious, with characteristic deformity and grossly reduced movement. Posterior dislocations can be more easily missed—the patient has an internally rotated shoulder with grossly reduced movement. There may be a history of an epileptic fit.

Fractures around the shoulder can result in little obvious swelling, but there is usually tenderness and significantly reduced shoulder movement.

Clavicle fractures

Clavicle fractures are relatively easily missed if not looked for. It is important to check for tenderness over the clavicle in any patient with shoulder injury.

Lower limb injury

Hip injuries

Neck of femur fractures are unlikely to be seen in custody, but pain, tenderness, reduced hip movement, and difficulty weight bearing may reflect a fractured greater tuberosity.

Knee injuries

It can be difficult to assess knee injuries in custody. Some useful tips are:
• Dramatic swelling within minutes of injury implies haemarthrosis, reflecting an intra-articular fracture or cruciate ligament rupture.
• Cruciate rupture may cause an audible snap.
• Inability to straight leg raise or extend the knee implies damage to the extensor mechanism (patellar tendon, patella, quadriceps tendon).

The Ottawa knee rules have been developed to assist staff in the Emergency Department to decide which patients to X-ray after knee injuries. These rules are useful indicators for custody staff. Patients requiring X-ray include those with the following:
• Isolated tenderness over the patella.
• Tenderness over the fibula head.
• Inability to flex the knee to 90°.
• Inability to weight bear both immediately and when assessed (at hospital).

The rules have been validated for patients aged 18–55 years. It is prudent to adopt a more cautious approach to patients outside this age range.

Calf muscle tears

A history of a sudden injury with pain in the mid-calf characterizes tears of calf muscles. Treatment is conservative, comprising rest, elevation, and analgesia, followed by physiotherapy accessed via GP. The differential diagnoses are Achilles tendon rupture and deep venous thrombosis, both of which require hospital attention.

Achilles tendon ruptures

Classic signs of a complete rupture are a palpable gap in the Achilles tendon, combined with an abnormal calf squeeze (Simmonds) test, where squeezing the mid-calf on the injured side fails to result in (normal) plantar flexion. Suspicion of (even partial) rupture mandates a visit to hospital for assessment and equinus cast.

Ankle and foot injuries

Inversion injuries to the ankle frequently result in lateral ligament sprains. The Ottawa ankle rules were developed to try to ascertain the need for X-ray—these can be usefully employed by custody staff to determine the need to attend the Emergency Department. Bony tenderness on palpation over the areas shaded in the Fig. 9.3 indicates the need for X-ray (hospital assessment).

In addition, patients who were unable to weight bear for four steps both immediately after injury and at the time of examination, require X-ray, as do patients with tenderness of the metatarsal or other foot bones.

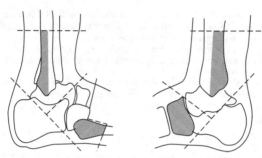

Fig. 9.3 Ottawa ankle rules – bony tenderness over any of the shaded areas indicates the need for X-ray (hospital assessment). Reproduced from Wyatt JP l. (2006). *Oxford Handbook of Emergency Medicine* 3rd edn, with permission of Oxford University Press.

Blunt chest injury

Blunt injury to the chest not infrequently precedes detention in custody. The causes of chest injury are varied and include road traffic collisions, falls, and interpersonal violence (e.g. punches and kicks). In view of the potential for serious internal damage, careful assessment is required. The key role for the forensic practitioner is to distinguish between chest wall trauma which can be managed in the custody centre and more significant internal damage, particularly pneumothorax.

Clinical assessment

History

As with injuries to other regions, there may not be a reliable history of injury available from the patient. The police may have relevant details of events prior to arrest (e.g. high-speed car crash).

Relevant symptoms to enquire about following any chest injury are: site, nature, and severity of pain; analgesia taken and its effect; breathlessness (at rest or on exertion).

On occasions, patients report symptoms after chest injury which occurred several days previously—in this instance, enquiry should be made about symptoms relating to possible infection (fever, cough, sputum).

Examination

In any patient with chest trauma, it is relevant to examine for the following:
- External evidence of bruising consistent with restraint by a seat belt (the orientation of the 'diagonal' component of the belt across the chest may provide an indication of which side of a vehicle an individual was sitting at the time of the crash).
- Pulse rate, blood pressure, and capillary refill time.
- Respiratory rate.
- Oxygen saturation level on air using a pulse oximeter.
- Area of chest tenderness on palpation.
- Resonance on percussion over lung fields.
- Air entry over both lungs.
- Evidence of injury to the abdomen, spine, and/or loins—it is particularly important to check for hypochondrial tenderness in any lower lateral chest injury.

Diagnosis

- Tenderness over a single rib with no other abnormal findings implies an isolated chest wall injury which may comprise an isolated rib fracture.
- Tenderness over the sternum implies sternal fracture.
- Tenderness over more than one rib, abnormal observations (e.g. reduced air entry on the affected side, reduced oxygen saturation level) implies more serious injury requiring urgent transfer to hospital by emergency ambulance.

Isolated rib fracture

Patients need to be advised that this is a clinical diagnosis (rather than requiring an X-ray). They require treatment with regular oral analgesia (e.g. co-dydramol) and need to be warned about the possible risk of chest infection and to see their GP after release from custody if symptoms worsen or continue.

Fractured sternum

Usually seen in the context of restraint by a seat belt in a high-speed car crash, suspicion of sternal fracture should prompt hospital referral for ECG and X-rays. Emergency ambulance transfer is appropriate.

Suspected pneumothorax

Although descriptions of clinical features of traumatic pneumothorax make it sound a straightforward clinical diagnosis, the truth is rather different! Objective evidence (in the form, for example, of reduced oxygen saturations) should be taken seriously. An emergency ambulance should be called for any detainee who is suspected of having a pneumothorax. In the meantime, the forensic practitioner should reassess and provide O_2 by face mask (if available).

Abdominal injury

The principles which underpin the approach to the detainee with a chest injury (see 📖 p.298) may also be applied to those who sustain blunt injury to the abdomen. The following specific points may be usefully added:

- Unlike the chest, the anterior abdominal wall is relatively soft, offering little protection to underlying organs in the event of external blunt trauma being applied.
- Bruising or imprinting (including from a seat belt) implies a significant amount of force having been applied.
- Serious internal injuries can occur in the absence of significant external evidence of abdominal wall injury.
- Some of the intra-abdominal organs lie under cover of the lower chest wall. Tenderness in the left hypochondrium and over the left lower lateral ribs may reflect splenic injury—a contained haematoma has the potential for sudden deterioration and intra-abdominal haemorrhage. Referral for imaging and observation at hospital is the safest course.
- Vital observations (pulse rate, blood pressure, and capillary refill time) may be preserved relatively near normal until later stages of hypovolaemia in some fit healthy adults.
- It can be very difficult in the custody unit to distinguish what some have curiously termed 'voluntary guarding' from objective evidence of peritonitis.
- Serial measurements of abdominal girth cannot be used as a reliable indicator of intra-abdominal bleeding.
- It is important to remember that the custody unit is not a safe place in which to observe someone with potentially serious injury.

Traffic law and medicine

Road traffic accidents in perspective

Road accident statistics

The large-scale, production-line manufacturing of affordable automobiles began more than a century ago and the numbers of automobiles on the roads continues to increase rapidly, especially in China and India. In 2007, there were estimated to be about 806 million cars and light trucks on the world's roads, burning over 260 billion gallons of gasoline and diesel fuel yearly. While the invention of the automobile has been liberating, changing both the way we live and where we live, it has also caused immeasurable grief. Since what is believed to have been the first recorded motor vehicle accident fatality (see box), more than 25 million people have died on the roads worldwide. The World Health Organization estimates that road incidents result in the deaths of about 1.2 million people worldwide each year and injure about 40x this number.

In the UK, about 3000 people are killed on the roads each year with a further 320 000 injured (38 000 seriously). The economic costs to the community are estimated to be in excess of £12 billion per year.

The first automobile fatality

Mary Ward became what is believed to be the first documented auto-mobile fatality in 1869 in Parsonstown, Ireland. Born in Ballylin, near Ferbane, Co. Offaly in April 1827 to an aristocratic family, she was a first cousin of the famous astronomer Lord William Rosse and was a frequent visitor to his home at Birr Castle where she developed her fascination for microscopes. She subsequently became one of the best known 19th-century writers on the use of the microscope. Unfortunately, just as Mary was well known in life, she is also well known in death. On 31 August 1869, while travelling with her husband in an experimental steam car invented by her cousin Parsons, she was thrown from the carriage when it hit a bump and was crushed by one of the wheels, dying instantly and thus becoming the victim of the world's first automobile accident.

Accidents or collisions? (see 📖 p.56)

The dictionary definition of accident is 'an unforeseen event or one without an apparent cause'. Given that an estimated 95% of traffic accidents are the result of driver error, it has been suggested that the term 'accident' is a misnomer implying, as it does, that no blame is attached to such incidents and that they are just one of those things that happen. There is a view that society treats road traffic accidents too lightly simply because of the name given to them and, as a result, police forces now use the term 'crash' or 'collision' in preference to 'accident'.

Road traffic safety

Road traffic safety aims to reduce the harm (deaths, injuries, and property damage) resulting from crashes of road vehicles. Harm from road traffic crashes is greater than that from all other transportation modes (air, sea, rail, etc.) combined and given the scale of the problem, road traffic crashes are one of the world's largest public health and injury prevention problems. The problem is all the more poignant because the victims are overwhelmingly healthy prior to their crashes.

Road safety interventions

Factors that contribute to road traffic collisions may be related to the driver, the vehicle, or the road itself. Road safety interventions seek to reduce or compensate for these factors, or reduce the severity of crashes that do occur.

Interventions aimed at the driver

Safety can be improved by measures that encourage safe behaviour, or reduce the chances of driver error. Some of these include:
- Compulsory training and licensing.
- Restrictions on driving while drunk or impaired by drugs.
- Restrictions on mobile phone use while on the move.
- Restrictions on commercial vehicle driver hours and fitting of tachographs.
- Conventional and automated enforcement of traffic laws, such as speed cameras.
- Road safety advertising campaigns to convince drivers to operate vehicles safely.
- Special policies for novice drivers who are more likely to crash because of inexperience, possibly combined with over-confidence, peer pressure, a desire to show off, and incomplete neurological development. Novice drivers are more likely to be involved in serious collisions occurring at night, when the car has multiple occupants, and when seat belt use is less. This has led some to call for:
  - Curfews being imposed on young drivers to prevent them driving at night.
  - Experienced supervisors to chaperone the less experienced driver.
  - Banning the carrying of passengers.
  - A zero alcohol tolerance.
  - Vehicle restrictions (e.g. restricting access to 'high-performance' vehicles).
  - A sign placed on the back of the vehicle (an N- or P-plate) to notify other drivers of a novice driver.

Vehicle design

Road safety can be improved by designing vehicles that reduce the severity of crashes that do occur. Most countries have comprehensive requirements and specifications for safety-related vehicle devices, systems, design, and construction. These may include:
- Seat belts (often in conjunction with laws requiring their use).
- Airbags.

- Lights and reflectors to improve visibility.
- Driver assistance systems such as electronic stability control and automated braking systems.
- Crash survivability design features such as fire-retardant interior materials, standards for fuel system integrity, and the use of safety glass.
- Annual inspections to ensure a vehicle's roadworthiness.
- Sobriety detectors which prevent the ignition key from working if the driver breathes into one and it detects significant quantities of alcohol.

Road design

Measures to improve road safety vary depending on the type of road concerned. Motorways (called *'freeways'* in North America) have the highest design standards for speed, safety, and fuel efficiency and deliver lower fatalities per vehicle-kilometre of travel than other roadways by:

- Prohibiting more vulnerable road users (e.g. learner drivers).
- Segregating opposing traffic flows with crash barriers, thus reducing potential for head-on collisions.
- Separating crossing traffic by replacing intersections with interchanges, thus reducing the risk of side impacts (the most vulnerable vehicle section).
- Removing roadside obstacles and surrounding the carriageways with energy attenuation devices (e.g. guardrails, wide grassy areas, sand barrels).
- Improved road engineering (e.g. banking on curves, in order to reduce the need for tyre-traction and increase stability for vehicles with high centres of gravity; cambering to reduce standing water and ice and to increase traction in poor weather; surfacing some sections of road with porous bitumen to enhance drainage).

On neighbourhood roads, where many vulnerable road users, such as pedestrians and bicyclists can be found, traffic calming has been an effective tool to improve road safety.

Risk compensation theory

An interesting theory suggests that as activities (e.g. driving a car) are made safer (e.g. by antilocking brakes), so the driver 'compensates' for these improvements by taking more risks (e.g. by driving faster).

Investigating road traffic collisions

Up until the mid-1970s, road collision investigations relied primarily on assessing a vehicle's speed by measuring the length of skid marks it left and referencing this against the *Highway Code* stopping distances. For example, the *Highway Code* indicates that a car travelling at 40mph (64km/h) needs 36m (116 feet) to stop. So, if a car involved in a collision leaves skid marks that are 96m (315 feet) long, it can be concluded that it was travelling well in excess of 40mph. This fairly unscientific method of calculating a car's speed is no longer admissible in court and the whole science of road traffic collision investigation has moved on considerably since then.

Police collision investigators

The police service has a duty to conduct a thorough investigation to establish the circumstances that lead to deaths or serious injury on the roads. Most importantly, the investigation will enable the police to provide an explanation of what happened to the family and friends of the injured party. In addition, the outcome of investigations can be used to learn lessons which may assist in the prevention of further deaths and serious injuries on the road. In the UK, every police force has collision investigators who are specially trained to undertake this work.

The role of the collision investigator is to:
- Identify the full extent of the scene(s).
- Ensure that all scenes are secured to prevent, as far as possible, the loss of evidence.
- Identify, preserve, and record all physical material which could be relevant to the circumstances of the collision.
- In conjunction with other staff as required, ensuring that such material is photographed (supplemented by video recording if appropriate), along with the surrounding topography in order to give context. In addition, the scene should be surveyed to enable the subsequent production of a scale plan showing the position of the material identified.
- Conduct, or make arrangements for, any tests or forensic examinations in relation to reconstruction.
- Review any witness evidence in line with known or established facts.
- Ensuring the SIO is kept informed in respect of findings and ultimately preparing a comprehensive written report.

Vehicle examiners

Working alongside collision investigations are specially trained vehicle examiners. This role may be undertaken by police officers (e.g. the collision investigator or a dedicated vehicle examiner). It may also be undertaken by civilians employed as vehicle examiners. Regardless of who performs it, the key requirements of vehicle examination include:
- Establishing the precollision mechanical condition of the vehicle, in so far as the consequences of the collision allow; and
- Considering the likelihood of a vehicle-related factor having caused or contributed to the collision.

In addition to these requirements, the vehicle examiner may also undertake a number of extra tasks:

- Obtaining forensic material from the vehicles involved.
- Establishing the precollision position of controls, switches, and other components which may have had an influence on the position or movement of the vehicle prior to the collision.
- Recording details of the position and extent of any damage in order to ascertain the immediate preimpact positions of vehicles and objects relative to each other.
- Identifying whether any devices have been fitted to the vehicle, for example, engine management systems, satellite navigation systems, airbags or antilock braking systems (ABS), and whether they contributed to the collision or hold material that would be useful to the investigation.
- Identifying any vehicle design implications and ascertaining if any defects may have caused the collision or have a potential to affect the overall safety of similar vehicle models. This may require checking vehicle maintenance records for vehicles involved in a fatal collision and, if necessary, reviewing records for vehicle fleets in cases of potential corporate manslaughter, in order to identify any system failures.

Protocol for the investigation of road deaths

In 2007, the Association of Chief Police Officers (ACPO) produced an updated edition of the *Road Death Investigation Manual*, designed to ensure that police forces conduct effective and professional investigations into fatal collisions. One of the key investigative principles of the manual is that all fatal collisions should be investigated as 'unlawful killings' until the contrary is proved. While acknowledging that fatal collisions may include a wide range of circumstances, for example, investigating an incident involving one vehicle which results in the death of the single-occupant driver, through to a full-scale murder investigation, the manual emphasizes that whatever the initial circumstances appear to be, all fatal collisions must be investigated to the highest standard. As there can be no prescriptive response to cover all types of fatal collision investigation, the manual provides investigators with a suitable framework to ensure that the most thorough and appropriate investigation is conducted.

Further reading

ACPO (2007). *Road Death Investigation Manual.* Available at: ☞ http://www.acpo.police.uk/asp/
policies/Data/road_death_investigation_manual_18x12x07.pdf

Patterns of injury in fatal road trauma

Road deaths may involve pedestrians, cyclists, motorcycle riders, car drivers, and/or passengers. The patterns of injury which result vary depending on the activity of the deceased and the circumstances of the crash. Although no two road traffic collisions will share exactly the same circumstances, characteristic injury patterns are seen in the different types of road user—these are discussed in this section and the following two topics.

Temporal distribution of death from trauma

Traditionally, deaths resulting from trauma were reported to have followed a 'trimodal distribution', with three large 'peaks' of death occurring immediately (within minutes of injury), soon after ('early'—within hours of injury), and much later (days afterwards). The causes of these deaths vary according to the time that they occurred:

Immediate deaths

Deaths occurring rapidly at the scene reflect an overwhelming catastrophic insult. They include those injuries which are coded as '6' by the Abbreviated Injury Scale (see 🕮 p.64):

- Brainstem laceration, massive crush destruction, transection or penetrating injury.
- Decapitation.
- Complete cord transection at level of third cervical vertebra or higher.
- Bilateral destruction of skeletal, vascular, organ, and tissue systems ('crush' injury) of the chest.
- Major laceration to the thoracic aorta with haemorrhage not confined to the mediastinum.
- Complex, multiple, or ventricular heart rupture.
- Avulsion of the heart.
- Avulsion of the liver.
- Second- or third-degree burns to ≥90% body surface area (including incineration).

Early deaths

Deaths occurring within hours of injury are traditionally those which are potentially treatable, including blood loss and the development of intracranial haematomas (e.g. extradural haemorrhage—see 🕮 p.149).

Late deaths

Deaths which occur late after trauma often result from multiorgan failure, adult respiratory distress syndrome (ARDS), chest, and/or generalized infection and pulmonary embolism.

The impact of improved treatment

Recent research suggests that deaths from all forms of trauma no longer follow a trimodal pattern, but instead there is a very large initial peak of individuals who die quickly or are found dead at the scene, followed by a smaller peak of late deaths. It is suggested that the 'disappearance' of the second peak of 'early' deaths reflects dramatic improvements in treatment.

Patterns of fatal pedestrian injury

Pedestrians form a significant proportion of deaths from fatal road collisions, partly reflecting the fact that they have virtually no protection against injury. Many pedestrians who succumb to injuries on the roads are under the influence of alcohol and/or elderly (with visual, hearing, mobility, and other impairments).

Injuries may be classified as primary, secondary, or tertiary.

Primary injuries

These are caused by the first impact of the vehicle with the pedestrian. The commonest site of primary injury is to the legs: injuries include abrasions and lacerations to the shin and knees from bumper contact and fractures, particularly to the tibia and fibula. Injuries may appear too low for normal bumper contact, due to severe braking prior to impact lowering the point of contact as the car pitches forward. When larger vehicles are involved (e.g. buses, lorries), impact may be higher, leading to primary damage to pelvis, abdomen, arms, or head.

Secondary injuries

These are caused by the person being thrown against the bonnet, windscreen, and door pillars. The head is the most frequently injured site in secondary impact with skull fractures and consequent brain damage being the commonest cause of death. Secondary injuries may also include fractures to ribs, arms, and pelvis and other internal abdominal damage.

Tertiary injuries

These occur when the car decelerates faster than the pedestrian, causing the person to be thrown to the ground. Broad 'brush' abrasions may result, most commonly on the trunk and limbs—these may have forensic importance as they can indicate the direction of travel across the road surface (see 📖 p.128). Tertiary impact may also lead to head injuries, limb fractures, bruises, and lacerations.

Patterns of injury in fatal crashes: vehicle occupants

The pattern of injuries sustained by occupants of vehicles involved in fatal road traffic collisions depends on their position in the vehicle (e.g. usually only the driver sustains injury from impact against the steering wheel). Furthermore, injuries depend on the direction of impact (frontal, rear, or side impact) and on whether the occupant was wearing a seat belt and/or was protected by an air bag. Injuries may be caused as a result of:

- Impact against the fascia, causing abrasions, lacerations, and fractures around knee and upper shin level.
- Impact against steering wheel causing severe internal injuries of chest and/or abdomen.
- Impact from intrusion into cabin (e.g. engine) resulting in lower limb fractures and/or posterior or central hip dislocation.
- Impact against and ejection through windscreen causing multiple facial lacerations and abrasions ± head injury.
- Whiplash injury resulting in fractures or dislocation of the neck.
- Internal deceleration injuries causing rupture of the thoracic aorta.

Seatbelt injuries

Introduction of legislation making the wearing of front and rear seatbelts compulsory is estimated to have reduced deaths and serious injury by about 25%. Nonetheless, seatbelts can cause injuries themselves. Impact against the restraining belt can cause bruising and fractures to clavicle, sternum, or ribs. More seriously, internal injuries may occur, including rupture of the mesentery, intestine, aorta, and bladder. The belt may act as a garrotte around the neck when occupants who are too small for the harness slip underneath it at impact. Occasionally, the wearing of a seatbelt may impede or delay escape from a burning vehicle.

Airbag injuries

When airbags deploy, injury to vehicle occupants may be caused by impact with either the bag itself or the casing overlying it. Minor injuries (abrasions, contusions, and lacerations) are most common, mainly on face, neck, chest, and upper extremities. However, more serious (occasionally fatal) injuries, such as head injuries, finger amputation, and fractures to the arms and cervical spine have been reported.

Airbag deployment also causes superficial burns to the upper extremities, face, and neck. Even full thickness burns can occur. These include both thermal burns from the hot gases released during inflation and chemical burns from the alkaline corrosives, especially sodium hydroxide in the aerosol.

Airbag-related eye injuries are well documented. Injuries include corneal abrasions, hyphaema, lens dislocation, vitreous haemorrhage, retinal tears and haemorrhage, and scleral rupture. The alkaline aerosol may produce chemical keratitis and orbital bone fractures can also be sustained from the deploying airbag.

Fatal injury patterns: motorcyclists and cyclists

Injuries to motorcyclists

The rate of injury and death amongst motorcyclists is much higher than for car drivers (see 📖 p.56). Particular injuries that may be seen include:
- Head (and neck) injuries—often severe and accounting for about 80% of deaths.
- Lower limb injuries—lacerations, brush abrasions, and fractures as a result of impact with other vehicles or objects, or by the legs becoming trapped by part of the motorcycle itself.
- Tail-gating injuries—severe head (and/or neck) injury and even decapitation can occur when the motorcyclist drives into the back of a lorry, the motorcycle passes under the lorry but the rider's head hits the tail-board.
- Injuries to other bodily parts—injuries to the head and lower limbs predominate, but any part of the body may suffer injury.

Injuries to cyclists

Bicyclists are similar to motorcyclists in being relatively unprotected, but have the additional potential vulnerability of being unable to keep up with fast moving traffic. The patterns of injury which occur are similar to motorcycle injuries:
- Head injuries are common.
- Primary injury, particularly at thigh, hip, or chest level, can be caused by impact from a striking vehicle.
- Secondary injury may also occur as the rider falls and strikes the ground, often injuring the shoulder, arms, and chest.

Medical conditions and fitness to drive

Ordinary driving licences issued by the Driving and Vehicle Licensing Agency (DVLA) in the UK are inscribed with: 'You are required by law to inform Drivers Medical Branch, DVLA, Swansea SA99 1AT, at once if you have any disability (either physical or medical condition) which is, or may become likely to affect your fitness as a driver, unless you do not expect it to last more than three months.'

- It is the responsibility of the driver to inform the DVLA (and their insurance company of any condition disclosed to the DVLA).
- It is the responsibility of their doctor to advise patients that medical conditions (and drugs) may affect their ability to drive and for which conditions patients should inform the DVLA.

Conditions that make driving illegal

- Severe mental disorder (including severe mental impairment).
- Severe behavioural disorders.
- Alcohol dependency (including inability to stop drink-driving).
- Drug abuse and dependency.
- Psychotic medication taken in quantities to impair driving ability.
- Vision acuity (± spectacles) should be sufficient to read a 79.4-mm high number plate at 20.5m.
- Monocular vision is allowed only if the visual field is full.
- Binocular field of vision must be ≥120°.
- Diplopia is not allowable unless mild and correctable (e.g. by an eye patch).

Conditions requiring notification to the DVLA

- An epileptic event (seizure or fit).
- Sudden attacks or disabling giddiness, fainting, or blackouts.
- Severe mental handicap.
- A pacemaker, defibrillator, or antiventricular tachycardia device fitted.
- Diabetes controlled by insulin.
- Angina while driving.
- Parkinson disease.
- Any other chronic neurological condition.
- A serious problem with memory.
- A major or minor cerebrovascular event.
- Any type of brain surgery, brain tumour, or severe head injury involving inpatient treatment at hospital.
- Any severe psychiatric illness or mental disorder.
- Continuing/permanent difficulty in the use of arms or legs which affects the ability to control a vehicle.
- Dependence on or misuse of alcohol, illicit drugs, or chemical substances in the past 3 years (not including drink/driving offences).
- Any visual disability which affects *both* eyes (do not declare short/long sight or colour blindness).

Vision

For new drivers, vision should reach the following standards:
- 6/9 on the Snellen scale in the better eye and 6/12 on the Snellen scale in the other eye (wearing glasses or contact lenses, if needed).
- 3/60 in each eye without glasses or contact lenses.

Cardiovascular disorders

Driving must cease for at least 1 week after:
- Angioplasty.
- Non-ST elevation myocardial infarction (MI) with successful angioplasty.
- Pacemaker implantation.

Driving must cease for at least 4 weeks after:
- Coronary artery bypass graft.
- ST elevation MI.
- Non-ST elevation MI (not followed by successful angioplasty).

Diabetes

Diabetics must inform the DVLA if:
- They need treatment with insulin.
- They need laser treatment to both eyes or in the remaining eye if they have sight in one eye only.
- They have problems with vision in both eyes, or in the remaining eye if they have sight in one eye only. Vision must conform to the required standard (see 'Vision' section).
- They develop any problems with the circulation or sensation in their legs or feet which make it necessary for them to drive certain types of vehicles only (e.g. automatic vehicles or vehicles with a hand-operated accelerator or brake).

Drivers do not need to tell the DVLA if their diabetes is treated by tablets, diet, or both and they are free of the complications previously listed.

Epilepsy

- A person who has suffered an epileptic attack whilst awake must not drive for 1 year from the date of the attack. There must be a medical review before restarting to drive.
- A person who has suffered an attack whilst asleep must also refrain from driving for 1 year from the date of the attack, unless they have had an attack whilst asleep >3 years ago and have not had any awake attacks since that asleep attack.
- In any event, they should not drive if they are likely to cause danger to the public or themselves.

Other neurological disorders

The DVLA needs to know about unexplained blackouts, multiple sclerosis, Parkinson's disease, motor neuron disease, recurrent transient ischaemic attacks, and cerebrovascular events, dementia (unless mild).

Further reading

DVLA (2009). *At A Glance Guide for Medical Practitioners to the Current Medical Standards of Fitness to Drive.* Available at ℜ http://www.dvla.gov.uk/medical/ataglance.aspx

Alcohol and driving performance

In 2007, the number of crashes in the UK involving a driver over the legal limit rose to one crash in six, accounting for 460 deaths and 1800 serious injuries. The specific effects of alcohol on driving performance have been studied primarily in the following ways:
- By extrapolation from the general effects of alcohol.
- From clinical examination of alcohol-impaired drivers.
- From tests in vehicle simulators.
- From epidemiological studies.

General effects of alcohol

Much research has been conducted on how the general effects of alcohol may affect driving performance. Those general effects of alcohol that are thought to have a direct adverse impact on driving performance include:
- Increased risk taking.
- Loss of self-control.
- Diminished faculty for self-criticism.
- Impaired concentration.
- Impaired coordination.
- Impaired sensory perception.
- Delayed reaction time.

Examination of alcohol-impaired drivers

Prior to the introduction of a prescribed limit offence in the UK, prosecutions for drink-driving relied on establishing impairment, often by means of a clinical examination of the driver by a doctor. Whilst a number of recommended schemes for examination were published in the 1950s and 1960s, the discriminatory powers of the tests were poor. Indeed, in the 1950s, the *average* blood alcohol level of motorists charged with drink-driving was 220mg/100mL and only about 10% of drivers charged had a blood alcohol concentration <150mg/100mL.

Vehicle simulator tests

Studying the effects of alcohol on driving performance through use of vehicle simulators has the advantage that the tests can be accurately standardized and controlled, but the disadvantage that the subjects know they are being tested and may not behave in exactly the same way as they would whilst driving on normal roads. One of the most quoted pieces of such research was the *Coldwell Study*, from the late 1950s, which set out to determine the blood alcohol level at which impairment became evident. 50 male drivers were grouped into 'light', 'medium', and 'heavy' drinkers based on their normal weekly consumption of alcohol. Their driving performance was studied in slow-speed closed-course driving tests before and after they were given whisky designed to produce blood alcohol concentrations (BACs) within the range of 40–160mg/100mL. Although heavy drinkers performed better than light drinkers at similar blood alcohol levels, 8 out of 10 were impaired at levels of 51–120mg/100mL. The overall probability of impairment is shown in Table 10.1.

Table 10.1 Probability of impairment

Blood alcohol concentration (mg/100mL)	Probability (%)
85	50
100	64
150	91

Epidemiological studies

The Grand Rapids Study (1964)

This was the most extensive and authoritative epidemiological study ever conducted and the survey's results had a strong influence on the drafting of the Road Safety Act 1967 and the introduction of the prescribed limit of 80mg alcohol per 100mL of blood in the UK. Researchers compared the BAC of drivers involved in a random sample of all crashes in Grand Rapids with a control group of drivers selected from the city's traffic at the same locations and times as the crashes. It was found that the crash risk increased with increasing BAC, the risk curve steepening as higher alcohol levels were reached (Table 10.2).

Although different interpretations have been placed on some of the data in the years since the survey was conducted, it is widely accepted that the results show that as blood alcohol levels increase, so does the risk of being involved in a collision.

Table 10.2 Relative risk of Crash Involvement (Grand Rapids Study)

Blood alcohol concentration (mg/100mL)	Relative risk
0	1.0
20–50	0.8–1.1
50 80	1.0–1.8
80–120	2.5–4.5
120–150	4.0–9.0
150–180	5.0–40
180–200	10–40

Drink-driving legislation

Legislation governing driving after the consumption of alcohol is considered one of the most successful harm-reduction programmes, having led to a reduction in the number of deaths and serious injuries from road traffic collisions and having had a positive impact on the social and economic cost of alcohol misuse.

Legislation

In the UK, 'drink-driving' is governed by the Road Traffic Act 1988 (RTA). The relevant sections are s4 and s5:

> **4.**—(1) A person who, when driving or attempting to drive a mechanically propelled vehicle on a road or other public place, is unfit to drive through drink or drugs is guilty of an offence.
>
> **5.**—(1) If a **person**—
> (a) drives or **attempts** to drive a motor vehicle on a road or other public place, or
> (b) is in **charge** of a motor vehicle on a road or other public place, after consuming **so** much alcohol that the proportion of it in his breath, blood or urine exceeds the prescribed limit he is guilty of an offence.

Note that section 4 makes no reference to any objective measure for assessing 'unfit to drive'. This is a judgement that is eventually made by the court after hearing evidence, including from police officers, forensic physicians, forensic scientists, and bystanders who may have witnessed the manner of driving (see 🔲 p.330).

The prescribed limits

The current prescribed alcohol limits relevant to the s5 offence are:
• Breath—35 microgrammes/100mL.
• Blood—80mg/100mL (sometimes quoted as 80mg/dL).
• Urine—107mg/100mL.

There is no universal agreement as to what the limits should be. The UK blood limit is amongst the highest (80mg/100mL is also adopted by, for example, USA, Canada, Ireland, and New Zealand). European countries such as France, Germany, Italy, Belgium, and the Netherlands have set a limit of 50mg/100mL, the limit in Norway is 20mg/100mL, while some jurisdictions have adopted a zero limit. Following a recent review, it seems likely that the UK limit will be reduced to 50mg/100mL.

Roadside breath testing

In the UK 'random testing' is not permitted (c.f. Australia, a jurisdiction in which randomized testing is allowed). However, the UK legislation does permit roadside breath testing of drivers suspected of drink driving according to the provisions of section 6 of the RTA:

6.—(1) Where a constable in uniform has reasonable cause to suspect—

    (a) that a person driving or attempting to drive or in charge of a motor vehicle on a road or other public place has alcohol in his body or has committed a traffic offence whilst the vehicle was in motion, or

    (b) that a person has been driving or attempting to drive or been in charge of a motor vehicle on a road or other public place with alcohol in his body and that that person still has alcohol in his body, or

    (c) that a person has been driving or attempting to drive or been in charge of a motor vehicle on a road or other public place and has committed a traffic offence whilst the vehicle was in motion, he may, subject to section 9 of this Act, require him to provide a specimen of breath for a breath test.

(2) If an accident occurs owing to the presence of a motor vehicle on a road or other public place, a constable may, subject to section 9 of this Act, require any person who he has reasonable cause to believe was driving or attempting to drive or in charge of the vehicle at the time of the accident to provide a specimen of breath for a breath test.

Section 11(2) of the Act defines a breath test as:

'A preliminary test for the purpose of obtaining, by means of a device of a type approved by the Secretary of State, an indication whether the proportion of alcohol in a person's breath or blood is likely to exceed the prescribed limit.'

A number of breath testing devices are approved for use in the UK. If the device indicates that the driver has a blood alcohol level that is likely to be over the prescribed limit, he/she can be arrested and taken to a police station to provide a sample of breath for evidential analysis or a sample of blood or urine for laboratory analysis.

Provision of specimens for analysis

A specimen of breath, blood, or urine for analysis can be requested under the provisions of section 7 of the RTA.

> **7.**—(1) In the course of an investigation into whether a person has committed an offence under section 4 or 5 of this Act a constable may, subject to the following provisions of this section and section 9 of this Act, require him—
>
>   (a) to provide two specimens of breath for analysis by means of a device of a type approved by the Secretary of State, or
>   (b) to provide a specimen of blood or urine for a laboratory test.
>
> (2) A requirement under this section to provide specimens of breath can only be made at a police station.

The default position is that a police officer must request a sample of breath for analysis. Requests for blood or urine samples can be made in the circumstances outlined in s7(3):]

> **7.**—(3) A requirement under this section to provide a specimen of blood or urine can only be made at a police station or at a hospital; and it cannot be made at a police station unless—
>
>   (a) the constable making the requirement has reasonable cause to believe that for medical reasons a specimen of breath cannot be provided or should not be required, or
>   (b) at the time the requirement is made a device or a reliable device of the type mentioned in subsection (1)(a) above is not available at the police station or it is then for any other reason not practicable to use such a device there, or
>   (c) the suspected offence is one under section 4 of this Act and the constable making the requirement has been advised by a medical practitioner that the condition of the person required to provide the specimen might be due to some drug;
>   but may then be made notwithstanding that the person required to provide the specimen has already provided or been required to provide two specimens of breath.

If the provision of a specimen for laboratory analysis is required, the question whether it is to be a specimen of blood or a specimen of urine shall be decided by the constable making the requirement, unless a medical practitioner is of the opinion that for medical reasons a specimen of blood cannot or should not be taken, in which case a urine specimen will be required (s7(4)).

When urine is requested, drivers are required to provide a first specimen (which is destroyed) and then provide a second sample for testing within 1h of the requirement for its provision being made and after the provision of the previous specimen of urine (s7(5)).

When samples of breath are requested, s8 of the RTA lays down which sample should be used for evidence in court and provides a statutory option for drivers to ask for breath samples to be substituted with a sample of blood or urine for laboratory analysis:

8.—(1) Subject to subsection (2) below, of any two specimens of breath provided by any person in pursuance of section 7 of this Act that with the lower proportion of alcohol in the breath shall be used and the other shall be disregarded.

(2) If the specimen with the lower proportion of alcohol contains no more than 50 microgrammes of alcohol in 100mL of breath, the person who provided it may claim that it should be replaced by such specimen as may be required under section 7(4) of this Act and, if he then provides such a specimen, neither specimen of breath shall be used.

(3) The Secretary of State may by regulations substitute another proportion of alcohol in the breath for that specified in subsection (2) above.

Taking blood alcohol samples in a police station

Procedure when requested to take blood in a police station

When requested to take a sample of blood under the provisions of s7(1)(b) of the RTA, it is important that the forensic practitioner follow a standardized routine:

- The first step is to obtain an initial briefing from the custody sergeant/ arresting officer about the circumstances leading to the decision to request blood.
- The next is to witness the officer in charge obtaining consent from the driver, ensuring that he/she understands why the blood sample has been requested and what it will be tested for.
- A single sample of blood (approximately 10mL) is taken from the driver, dividing it equally into two separate RTA blood alcohol vials. (The choice of which vein to take the blood sample from is the forensic practitioner's and not the driver's. If unable to obtain sufficient blood at first attempt, that sample should be destroyed and a further sample obtained.) Note that alcohol-free swabs are used to clean the skin prior to sampling.
- Each vial is labelled, signed, and sealed appropriately and the time that the specimen was taken recorded carefully. Note that standard labels are usually included in the forensic 'pack' provided.
- The driver should be allowed to choose one of the two specimens and this should be given to him/her for later testing at an independent laboratory. This process needs to be explained to the driver and in particular, he/she be informed of which laboratories could provide the independent analysis for the driver (most forces have a booklet containing a list of laboratories which could be used).
- The other appropriately signed, sealed, and packaged blood specimen should be handed to the police officer in charge of the case (and a record made of the officer's name).
- A 'HO/RT 5' form is completed—this acts as the witness statement confirming when, where and from whom the forensic practitioner took the specimen.
- The forensic practitioner needs to ask the driver a few screening questions to ensure his/her well-being (e.g. Are you currently well? Are you on any medication? Have you suffered any injuries?).
- The forensic practitioner should check if the driver has any further questions about the procedure. Usually, the police officer in charge of the case will explain that it may take a few weeks for the laboratory to complete the analysis and return the result.

Hospital procedures

Drivers who are patients in hospital can be required to provide a sample of breath for 'roadside' testing or specimens of blood or urine for laboratory testing. However, provisions in s9 of the RTA provide protection in these circumstances.

9.—(1) While a person is at hospital as a patient he shall not be required to provide a specimen of breath for a breath test or to provide a specimen for a laboratory test unless the medical practitioner in immediate charge of his case has been notified of the proposal to make the requirement; and —
   (a) if the requirement is then made, it shall be for the provision of a specimen at hospital, but
   (b) if the medical practitioner objects on the ground specified in subsection (2) below, the requirement shall not be made.
(2) The ground on which the medical practitioner may object is that the requirement or the provision of a specimen or, in the case of a specimen of blood or urine, the warning required under section 7(7) of this Act, would be prejudicial to the proper care and treatment of the patient.

Practical advice

In practical terms, the doctor in charge of the patient's care at hospital is unlikely to object, other than temporarily, to a forensic practitioner taking blood from a hospital patient under s9. Access to the patient may be temporarily delayed for a variety of reasons (e.g. whilst X-rays are obtained, or wounds sutured under local anaesthetic).

Taking blood from incapacitated drivers

There is a belief that some hospitalized drivers may, in the past, have escaped appropriate prosecution for drink-driving offences, such as causing death by careless driving whilst under the influence of drugs or alcohol (which can carry a heavy penalty) owing to a lack of supporting evidence. The Police Reform Act 2002 and The Criminal Justice (Northern Ireland) Order 2005 permit the taking of blood from incapacitated drivers for future consensual testing, therefore putting them in the same position with respect to testing for drug and alcohol levels as drivers with capacity, while at the same time protecting doctors from actions for assault if they take a specimen without consent. Detailed guidance about these provisions has been issued by the British Medical Association and the Faculty of Forensic and Legal Medicine (see Further reading).

In summary, a blood specimen may be taken for future testing for alcohol or other drugs from a person who has been involved in an accident and is unable to give consent where:

• A police constable has assessed the person's capacity and found the person to be incapable of giving valid consent due to medical reasons; and

- The forensic physician taking the specimen is satisfied that the person is not able to give valid consent (for whatever reason); and
- The person does not object to or resist the specimen being taken; and
- In the view of the doctor in immediate charge of the patient's care, taking the specimen would not be prejudicial to the proper care and treatment of the patient.

The specimen is not tested until the person regains competence and gives valid consent for it to be tested. If doctors follow the advice in this summary they will fulfil both legal and ethical requirements.

Further reading

British Medical Association and the Faculty of Forensic and Legal Medicine (2007). *Taking blood samples from incapacitated drivers. Guidance for doctors from the British Medical Association and the Faculty of Forensic and Legal Medicine.* Available at http://www.fflm.ac.uk

Failure to provide samples under the Road Traffic Act

Background

It is relatively common for individuals who are suspected of having been drink-driving to fail to provide a sample (of blood, urine, or breath). There can be understandable reasons why an individual fails to provide a sample. Reasons for failure to provide are sometimes complex, are sometimes not entirely clear, and are sometimes the subject of much legal argument at a later date. For all these reasons, it is important that the forensic practitioner has a good understanding of the subject, in order to be able to make the most appropriate decisions.

Legislation

Section 6(4) of the RTA makes it an offence for a person, without reasonable excuse, to fail to provide a sample of breath for a breath test. Likewise, Section 7(6) of the RTA makes it an offence for a person, without reasonable excuse, to provide a sample of blood or urine when required to do so. However, there will be no conviction if the subject was not warned of the consequence of failing to provide, or did not understand the warning through a poor command of English.

'Reasonable excuse'

Once the defence of reasonable excuse is advanced, it is for the prosecution to negate the defence. It is a question of fact as to whether there is a 'reasonable excuse' and the court must be satisfied beyond reasonable doubt that the defendant had no reasonable excuse. It was said in R v Lennard that a reasonable excuse *'must arise out of a physical or mental inability to provide one or a substantial risk to health in its provision'*. For an excuse of reasonable excuse to succeed in law, the defence will need to show that:

• The driver did not deliberately fail to provide the specimen.
• The existence of any known relevant medical condition was made known to the constable at the time; and
• The test in Lennard (described earlier) is satisfied.

Failure to provide blood and/or urine

Blood samples

If a driver offers a potential medical reason for failing to provide a blood sample, the police officer should consult with a doctor or appropriate healthcare professional. No blood sample need be provided if:
- The medical practitioner who is asked to take it is of the opinion that for medical reasons it cannot or should not be taken; or
- The registered healthcare professional who is asked to take it is of that opinion and there is no contrary opinion from a medical practitioner.

Medical reasons for failing to provide a blood sample include poor venous access and needle phobia.

Assessment of needle phobia

When assessing a driver who claims to be unable to supply a blood sample because of needle phobia, it is necessary to distinguish between 'repugnance' and a genuine 'phobia' and to establish 'inability' rather than just 'unwillingness' to provide the sample. In doing so, the past medical history should be noted, paying particular attention to current or past psychiatric history, previous operations, vaccinations, body piercing, tattoos, or dental procedures with local anaesthetic. It is important to attempt to identify the criteria required to establish a diagnosis of needle phobia:
- A marked and persistent fear of needles.
- Exposure to needles almost invariably provokes an immediate anxiety response.
- A recognition that the fear of needles is unreasonable or excessive.
- Avoidance of needles.

Needle phobia is often characterized by a strong vasovagal response.

Urine samples

Medical reasons for failing to provide a urine sample include:
- Drugs such as opiates, which can affect the bladder sphincter and cause urinary retention.
- Neurological problems affecting the bladder.
- Bladder outflow obstruction (e.g. urethral stricture, bladder stone, prostatic hypertrophy).
- Embarrassment at having to provide a sample in front of a member of the opposite sex.

Failure to provide a breath sample

Under s7(3)(a) of the RTA, a constable can request a sample of blood or urine from a driver if he has *'reasonable cause to believe that for medical reasons a specimen of breath cannot be provided or should not be required'*. The constable is not required to obtain confirmation of the medical reason from a doctor or nurse in order to request a laboratory specimen. However, if the constable believes that there is no medical reason for failing to provide a sample of breath, he/she may ask the forensic practitioner to conduct an independent assessment of the driver.

Medical reasons for failing to provide a breath sample

These include:
• Injuries to the mouth, lip, or face.
• Rib or chest injury.
• Respiratory problems, such as asthma, acute infections, or COPD.
• Short stature (implying greatly reduced vital capacity).
• Neurological problems, such as facial palsy.
• Genuine phobia of catching AIDS from using intoximeter.
• Shock if it renders the driver physically or mentally unable to provide the specimen.
• Severe alcohol intoxication.

Assessment of failure to provide a breath sample

In making an assessment of this, the forensic practitioner should consider the following:
• Was a proper attempt made (as suggested by misting of the mouth piece, bars appearing on the display, and the sound of breath flowing)?
• Was the person able to complete a roadside screening test (which generally requires more respiratory effort than station machines)?
• Was the person able to provide the first of the two specimens required (or did so at another time)?
• Do respiratory function tests show low function (persons with an FEV_1 of <1L are unlikely to be able to provide a sample)?
• Do other medical reasons exist?

It can be difficult to be certain (and to argue with conviction) that there was no reasonable excuse for an individual failing to provide a breath specimen. Perhaps for this reason, if difficulty is encountered obtaining a breath sample, in practice, many police officers will ask simply for the breath sample to be replaced by a blood or urine sample.

Field impairment testing by police

In the UK, forensic physicians have traditionally performed the examination of drivers suspected of driving whilst under the influence of drugs. However, given the inevitable time delay between a driver being arrested and the actual medical examination being conducted, there is a strong chance that the effects of any drug intoxication will have worn off by the time the doctor sees the driver, particularly when the drug involved has a short duration of action.

In recognition of these difficulties, standardized preliminary impairment tests, introduced under the powers of the Railways and Transport Safety Act 2003, have been devised to enable specially trained police officers to test drivers at the roadside. These tests are based on 'standardized field sobriety tests' used in the USA.

Effectiveness of preliminary impairment testing

Research commissioned by the Department for Transport and published in 2006 set out to evaluate the effectiveness of preliminary impairment testing as applied by UK police officers. Overall, the roadside application of field impairment tests demonstrated a sensitivity of 65%, a specificity of 77%, and an accuracy of 66%. The authors concluded that preliminary impairment testing in its current form is useable for screening purposes (i.e. is not conclusive evidence of drug-impaired driving). In the UK, if, on the basis of preliminary impairment testing, a police officer considers that a driver may be unfit to drive through drugs, the driver will be arrested and taken to a police station where he/she will be examined by a forensic physician. This provides some safeguard against wrongful convictions for driving under the influence of drugs.

Preliminary impairment tests

The tests are performed using a national pro forma, MG DD/F. Several parameters are looked at for each test. It is generally accepted that a driver has to 'fail' at least two parameters for a test to be considered abnormal.

Pupillary examination

Pupil size and equality are assessed by comparing the size of the pupils against a 'pupillometer' on a card held up at the side of the face. The normal range for pupil size is said to be 3.0–6.5mm, given the lighting conditions during roadside testing. A note is made of whether the eyes are watering or reddened.

The 'Romberg test'

The Romberg test is used to evaluate the driver's internal clock and body sway. The driver is instructed to stand up straight with his feet together and arms by his sides. The driver is then asked to tilt his head back slightly and close his eyes while estimating to himself when 30s have elapsed. The test is considered abnormal if the body sways (Romberg's positive) and the timing is <25s or >35s.

The 'walk and turn' test

The driver is instructed to place his left foot on an imaginary line and then to place the right foot on the line in front of the left foot, with the heel of the right foot in contact with the toe of the left foot. He is then told to put his arms by his sides and take nine heel-to-toe steps along the line, turning around and take a further nine heel to-toe-steps back along the line. Signs of impairment include whether the individual (nine parameters):

- Starts too soon
- Stops walking
- Misses heel/toe
- Raises arms
- Starting balance impaired
- Turns improperly
- Steps off line
- Counts the steps incorrectly
- Fails to follow instructions.

The 'one leg stand' test

The driver is asked to stand with his feet together and arms by the side. In this position, he is then asked to raise his right foot 6–8 inches off the ground keeping his leg straight. The toes must be pointing forward and the foot parallel to ground. The driver is then asked to count out aloud '1001, 1002, 1003' and so on progressively until told to stop. The test is then repeated for the left foot. Signs of impairment include whether the individual (five parameters for each side):

- Sways
- Raises arms
- Hops
- Puts foot down
- Fails to follow instructions.

The 'finger and nose' test

This is performed with the driver's eyes closed. Standing with feet together and arms at the sides, he is asked to tilt his head back slightly. He then extends both hands, palm side up, out in front and makes a fist keeping the index finger of both hands extended. The police officer then says either left or right to indicate which hand should be moved and the driver is then expected to touch the tip of his nose with the tip of the finger of that hand. The hand is then lowered until the next is indicated. The hands are called out in the following order: left, right, left, right, right, left. Signs of impairment include whether the driver (four parameters):

- Misses tip of nose
- Uses incorrect hand
- Sways excessively
- Fails to follow instructions.

Further reading

Department of Transport (2004). *Code of Practice for Preliminary Impairment Tests*. Available at ✋ http://police.homeoffice.gov.uk/publications/road-traffic-documents/Code_of_practice_order.pdf

Oliver JS, Seymour A, Wylie FM, et al (2006). *Road Safety Research Report No. 63. Monitoring the Effectiveness of UK Field Impairment Tests*. London: Department for Transport.

Medical examination of drug-impaired drivers

Purpose of the examination

When a driver is arrested under suspicion of driving under the influence of alcohol and/or drugs (section 4 of the RTA) a forensic physician has traditionally been called to examine the driver in order to:

- Assess whether the person is fit to be detained in police custody and ensure their physical well-being.
- Exclude a condition that may mimic intoxication by alcohol or drugs.
- Determine whether a person's ability to drive is impaired.
- Determine whether there is a condition that might be due to drink or drugs.

Conditions that may mimic intoxication by drugs (or alcohol) and need to be excluded include:

- Head injury.
- Metabolic and endocrine disorders—hypo- or hyperglycaemia, uraemia, hyperthyroidism.
- Neurological disorders associated with dysarthria, ataxia, tremor, and drowsiness (such as multiple sclerosis, epilepsy, acute vertigo, Parkinson's disease, cerebrovascular events).
- Psychiatric disorders—hypomania, general paresis.
- High fever.
- Fatigue.
- Carbon monoxide poisoning.

The legal context

The police have the legal authority to require a specimen (blood or urine) for analysis from a driver as long as the doctor advises the police officer that the person has a condition present that might be due to a drug. The doctor does not have to establish impairment in order for a sample to be legally required.

There are no formal medical definitions of a 'condition' and 'impairment' and neither term is defined in the RTA. Impairment is ultimately a decision reached by the Court after hearing evidence from several sources, which may include bystanders, police officers, the FP, and the forensic scientist. Medical evidence of impairment is not essential in order to secure a conviction.

The examination

When conducting an examination of a driver suspected of driving under the influence of alcohol and/or drugs it may be advisable to choose to use a pro forma, such as the one prepared by the Faculty of Forensic and Legal Medicine (available at ℘ http://www.fflm.ac.uk). Before beginning the examination, the forensic practitioner should speak to the arresting officer to find out the circumstances of the arrest and why the officer felt that the driver's ability was impaired. The forensic practitioner is allowed to take into consideration the findings of the arresting officer in coming to a conclusion as to whether or not there is a 'condition'.

The history
A detailed history is taken with an emphasis on:
- A general medical history.
- Medication (prescribed or over the counter).
- Use of illicit drugs and/or alcohol.
- Last meal.
- Sleep pattern, last period, and length of sleep.
- Memory and account of events leading up to the arrest.

The physical examination
A general physical examination is conducted to identify coexisting medical problems and to document physical signs (physiological effects) of a drug (e.g. tachycardia, conjunctival reddening). Examination includes:
- Appearance.
- Dress/hygiene.
- Demeanour (mannerisms, activity, cooperation).
- Talking or gesturing to him/herself.
- Breath odour (alcohol, ketones).
- Signs of drug misuse, such as venous 'tracking'.
- Pulse rate.
- Temperature (if the history suggests this might be relevant).
- Blood pressure.
- Examination of heart and lungs.
- Examination of any significant injuries.

Impairment testing
The forensic practitioner will then normally conduct a number of tests designed to determine whether there is evidence of impairment. Whilst the precise scheme of examination is down to the individual, increasingly forensic practitioners are being advised to adopt similar divided attention tests to those used by police officers when undertaking preliminary impairment testing (see 📖 p.328). These include Romberg's, the 'walk and turn', 'finger and nose', and 'one leg stand' tests.

Outcome of the assessment
When assessing a person's ability to drive, the overall condition of the individual should be considered rather than relying on single signs. For example, it is accepted that the use of cannabis results in the presence of reddened eyes. However, if that is the only abnormal finding, the forensic practitioner should not certify impairment, but can advise that there is a condition present that *may* be due to drugs.

Drugs and driving performance

Legislation

In the UK, driving whilst under the influence of drugs is governed by the RTA section 4:

> **4.**—(1) A person who, when driving or attempting to drive a mechanically propelled vehicle on a road or other public place, is unfit to drive through drink or drugs is guilty of an offence.

'Drug' is defined in sections 11(2) of the Act as including *'any intoxicant other than alcohol'*. 'Intoxicant' means any substance that affects the self-control of the body and applies to prescribed medication as well as illicit drugs. (Thus, a diabetic, who suffered a hypoglycaemic attack whilst driving and crashed his car into trees following administration of his normal dose of insulin some 12h earlier, was convicted of 'drug-driving' because a stipendiary magistrate found his unfitness to drive was caused by the drug insulin.)

Specific drugs

The effects of specific drugs on driving performance are considered in detail in other sections:

- Cannabis: see 📖 p.333
- Opioids: see 📖 p.334
- Benzodiazepines: see 📖 p.335
- Stimulants: see 📖 p.336.

Drugs and driving: cannabis

Pharmacokinetics (see 📖 p.474)

Cannabis, or marijuana, is typically self-administered orally or by smoking. The acute effects of intoxication typically peak within 10–20min of smoking cannabis and last for 2–3h, depending on the amount used.

Once absorption has taken place, THC (tetrahydrocannabinol—the major psychoactive cannabinoid) is rapidly distributed to tissues resulting in a fast decline in blood plasma THC concentrations, with levels >10ng/mL being uncommon 1h after administration of even high doses.

Effects on driving

The effects of cannabis on driving are not clear-cut, although the drug does have a measurable effect on psychomotor performance, particularly tracking ability. Its effect on higher cognitive functions, for example, divided attention tasks associated with driving, appear not to be as critical. Drivers under the influence of cannabis seem aware that they are impaired and attempt to compensate by reducing the difficulty of the driving task, for example, by driving more slowly.

Signs of intoxication

- Dry mouth
- Euphoria or anxiety
- Disinhibition
- Concentration difficulties
- Sedation
- Slurred speech
- Tachycardia
- Increase in blood pressure
- Poor coordination
- Distortion of time sense
- Conjunctival injection
- Anisocoria
- Change in pupil size
- Nystagmus
- Flushing.

Results of impairment tests are shown in Table 10.3.

Table 10.3 Results of impairment testing—cannabis

Test	Result
Pupils	Possible dilatation
Romberg's	Impaired (body clock may be slow)
Walk and turn	Impaired
One leg stand	Impaired
Finger to nose	Impaired

Drugs and driving: opioids

Pharmacokinetics (see 📖 p.466)

Heroin is typically self-administered by intravenous or intramuscular injection and also by nasal insufflation (snorting) or smoking. Peak heroin concentrations are achieved 1–5min after intravenous and smoked administration and within 5min after intranasal and intramuscular injection. Heroin has a very short half-life of a few minutes and is rapidly converted to an active metabolite 6-acetylmorphine and then morphine.

Methadone is a synthetic opiate drug with a long duration of action that is used as a substitute to heroin in treatment programmes to prevent the onset of withdrawal symptoms. The half-life of methadone is 10–25h after a single dose and 13–55h after repeated doses.

Effects on driving

Opioids impair driving ability through CNS depressant effects, although the effect of a given dose depends on the individual's tolerance to opioids. Because of the variability in tolerance to the effects of opioids, the actual blood concentrations of these drugs are not useful in predicting the likely extent of any impairment. Patients on prescriptions of methadone should be advised by their treating doctor to inform the DVLA about the treatment as it is considered a '… disability likely to affect safe driving'. However, *'applicants or drivers complying fully with a Consultant supervised oral Methadone maintenance programme may be licensed, subject to favourable assessment and, normally, annual medical review'*. Part of favourable assessment involves the driver demonstrating, by means of a urine test, that he/she is not using other illicit drugs.

Signs of intoxication

- Sedation
- Euphoria
- Poor concentration
- Memory difficulties
- Pin-point pupils
- Slow pulse rate
- Sluggish pupil reaction to light
- Decreased blood pressure
- Decreased respiratory rate.

Results of impairment tests are shown in Table 10.4.

Table 10.4 Results of impairment testing—opioids

Test	Result
Pupils	Constricted
Romberg's	Impaired (body clock may be slow)
Walk and turn	Impaired
One leg stand	Impaired
Finger to nose	Impaired

Drugs and driving: benzodiazepines

Pharmacokinetics

When administered in tablet form, benzodiazepines are generally well absorbed reaching peak blood levels in about 1–2h. Their duration of action depends on their rate of elimination. Half-lives for commonly misused benzodiazepines are:

- Diazepam: 30 (20–50)h
- Nitrazepam: 26 (16–48)h
- Temazepam: 10 (5–15)h
- Lorazepam: 13 (8–25)h
- Chlordiazepoxide: 12 (5–30)h.

Effects on driving

Because of CNS depressant effects, benzodiazepine intoxication is incompatible with safe driving of a motor vehicle.

Signs of intoxication

- Somnolence
- Diplopia
- Slurred speech
- Dilated pupils
- Unsteady gait
- Intellectual impairment.

Results of impairment tests are shown in Table 10.5.

Table 10.5 Results of impairment testing—benzodiazepines

Test	Result
Pupils	Possibly dilated
Romberg's	Impaired (body clock may be slow)
Walk and turn	Impaired
One leg stand	Impaired
Finger to nose	Impaired

Drugs and driving: stimulants

Pharmacokinetics (see 📖 p.470)

Ecstasy (MDMA) is administered in tablet form and is rapidly absorbed from the intestinal tract, reaching its peak concentration in the plasma about 2h after ingestion. The half-life of ecstasy is about 8h.

Amphetamines are well absorbed and can be taken by a variety of means—smoking, snorting, orally, and intravenously. Peak concentrations after oral dosing occur within 1–2h after administration, with much faster peaks after the drug is smoked, snorted, or injected. The half-life of amphetamine is 4–24h; it is so variable because it is very dependent on the pH of the urine. Urinary excretion increases with increasing acidity of the urine, leading to faster elimination of the drug.

Effects on driving

Amphetamines do not cause central impairment of coordination. In moderate doses, at least, they improve performance in a number of psychomotor skills as well as the ability to sustain attention over prolonged periods of time, especially when performing monotonous tasks. These effects may explain why they have been used by long-distance lorry drivers and why they were given to US pilots as recently as the Gulf War (1991).

There has been very little published research considering the effect of amphetamines and amphetamine-related drugs on driving. Available data suggests that the drugs may both improve certain aspects of the driving task, such as road-tracking performance, while reducing performance in other aspects, such as accuracy of speed adaptation during car-following performance.

Signs of intoxication

• Dilated pupils
• Tachycardia
• Raised blood pressure
• Raised body temperature
• Increased reflexes
• Tremor
• Teeth grinding
• Restlessness
• Garrulousness
• Dry mouth
• Urinary retention.

Results of impairment tests are shown in Table 10.6.

Table 10.6 Results of impairment testing—benzodiazepines

Test	Result
Pupils	Dilated
Romberg's	Fast internal body clock
Walk and turn	Fast (but not impaired)
One leg stand	Fast (but not impaired)
Finger to nose	Fast (but not impaired)

Adult sexual assault

Definitions and law

Every jurisdiction has its own laws or statutes relating to sexual assault. In England and Wales, the Sexual Offences Act 2003 applies. This describes a number of offences related to actual, possible, or intended sexual contact. Examples of definitions and offences from this Act are provided in the rest of this section.

Definition of rape

Under s1 of the Act, 'rape' is defined as follows:

A person ('A') commits an offence [of rape] if:
• He intentionally penetrates the vagina, anus or mouth of another person ('B') with his penis and
• 'B' does not consent to the penetration, and
• 'A' does not reasonably believe that 'B' consents.

It further describes:

Whether a belief is *reasonable* is to be determined having regard to all the circumstances, including any steps 'A' has taken to ascertain whether 'B' consents.

The penalty for rape
A person found guilty of rape under this section is liable, on conviction on indictment, to imprisonment for life.

Assault by penetration

Under s2 of the Act, the offence of 'assault by penetration' is defined as:

A person ('A') commits an offence if:
• He intentionally penetrates the vagina or anus of another person ('B') with a part of his body or anything else, and
• The penetration is sexual, and
• 'B' does not consent to the penetration, and
• 'A' does not reasonably believe that 'B' consents.

Penalty for assault by penetration
A person guilty of an offence under this section is liable, on conviction on indictment, to imprisonment for life.

Sexual assault

Under s3 of the Act 'sexual assault' is defined as:

A person ('A') commits an offence if:
• He intentionally touches another person ('B')
• The touching is sexual
• 'B' does not consent to the touching, and
• 'A' does not reasonably believe that 'B' consents.

Penalty for sexual assault
A person guilty of an offence under this section is liable (a) on summary conviction, to imprisonment for a term not exceeding 6 months or a fine not exceeding the statutory maximum or both; (b) on conviction on indictment, to imprisonment for a term not exceeding 10 years.

Other offences

There are numerous other offences defined within the Act. These include 'causing a person to engage in sexual activity without consent' and 'rape and other offences against a child under 13' (see 📖 Chapter 12).

Background to adult sexual assault

Scale of the problem

Sexual assault takes place in every country and within every culture worldwide. Female victims predominate, but male victims form a very significant minority—up to 10% according to some data. Rape and other forms of sexual assault are often associated with crimes against humanity, war crimes, and genocide. Reporting and documentation of different types of assault varies. In the US, the National Crime Victimization Survey reported approximately 250 000 rapes and sexual assaults in 2006, of which about 60% were perpetrated by non-strangers. The British Crime Survey 2006/7 recorded approximately 44 000 serious sexual crimes (rapes, sexual assaults, and sexual offences against children). It is generally believed that all of these figures actually underestimate the true incidence of sexual crimes. Embarrassment, fear of re-victimization, and risk of social ostracism may be some of the reasons for under-reporting.

After the initial trauma, long-term effects of being sexually assaulted can be considerable. They include physical effects, depression, and post-traumatic stress disorder.

Forensic practitioners and sexual assault examinations

The assessment of individuals in connection with matters of sexual assault is a complex area. Ideally, any practitioner assessing a patient in connection with allegations of any form of sexual assault and/or advising relevant bodies, needs to be aware of:

- The range and frequency of normal sexual practices.
- Normal human anatomy, development, and physiology.
- How social, cultural, religious, ethnic, and sexual orientation issues may alter sexual behaviour.
- The legal issues.
- The reasons for the assessment.
- The reasons for sampling.
- The methods of sampling.

Sexual Assault Referral Centres (SARCs)

The best outcomes for victims result from a multidisciplinary approach provided by specialists. Increasing emphasis is now being placed upon developing SARCs. SARCs specifically focus upon the assessment of individuals complaining of rape or sexual assault. They provide specialist forensic, medical, and aftercare services for women, men, and children who have been sexually assaulted or raped. In addition to the initial assessment and forensic sampling, they offer follow-up care in the form of support clinics, sexual health check-ups, and psychotherapy counselling services. If complainants do not wish at the time of reporting to involve police, systems are in place to allow anonymous assessment and collection of samples, so that a complainant may report later if they choose to.

Purposes of medical assessment

Medical assessment of sexual assault *complainants* has a number of different purposes, which may include:

- To identify, record, and treat injuries (some injuries may need to be referred for treatment elsewhere).
- To collect evidence (e.g. forensic swabs) which may assist an investigation and/or the courts, depending upon medical and scientific interpretation.
- To identify potential for infection and provide prophylaxis as appropriate (e.g. against hepatitis B, HIV).
- To identify and treat infection.
- To provide treatment to prevent unwanted pregnancy.
- To provide psychological counselling and support.

The principal purpose of medical assessment of sexual assault *suspects* is to collect evidence which may assist the courts. Consideration of this evidence in the light of medical and scientific interpretation may help to establish the facts of the case. It needs to be remembered that suspects may also have other medical needs which need to be addressed (e.g. the treatment of injuries).

Interpretation of evidence

Medical and scientific evidence may help confirm or corroborate the account of either the complainant or suspect. In many cases, the medical and scientific evidence may be neutral, merely confirming that contact has taken place—the issue of consent being one that the courts have to make a determination on, in the light of all evidence presented in the case.

Examination suites

In the UK, the standards of equipment have been defined for the examination rooms of victim examination suites (VES). Examination suites may be located either within a SARC or within a police station.

Operational procedures

Standardization of operational procedures in the maintenance of examination suites is of paramount importance in order to avoid contamination. Key points are summarized as follows:

Security and documentation

- The suite should be locked when not in use.
- The suite should only be used for medical purposes.
- A log book should be kept indicating all persons who enter the suite and a note made of the date and time and reason for entering (e.g. cleaning, examination). There should be a book available containing relevant information (for example, how to call out a cleaner) and useful telephone numbers (e.g. local genitourinary clinics, social services).

Cleaning

- The suite needs to be cleaned after each use to prevent DNA contamination. The cleaning should cover all relevant areas, including the forensic waiting room, the medical examination room, together with the bathroom and toilet within the facility. In the medical examination room itself, the floor, couch (even if covered with a protector at the time of the medical), worktop, writing desk, sink, and taps need to be cleaned each time the room is used.
- An alcohol-based wipe with organic content should be used to wipe down vinyl chairs in the waiting room area and for the medical examination couch. A virusolve disinfectant should be used as a general cleaning reagent for all hard work surfaces, such as counter tops and sinks. Virusolve disinfectants are required to be in contact for at least 10min to be effective.
- Disposable white paper towels should be used for cleaning surfaces with the disinfectant (the coloured varieties can cause fluorescence problems in the DNA process). Surfaces that could potentially collect dust (e.g. exposed storage shelves) should be cleaned at least once a week.
- After disinfectant has been used to clean the sinks, they should be wiped with 'J cloth®' type wipes. Each cleaning cloth should be used once and its use restricted to one room only.

Gloves

- The medical examiners and chaperones present must wear disposable powder-free gloves.

Drugs

- The medical room in the suite should have a lockable drug cupboard.

Stocking up, waste disposal, and storing samples
- A named person should have responsibility for checking and re-stocking the suite on a regular basis (at least once a week). Unopened, in date, kits from medical examination kits can be retained for use in subsequent cases. A cupboard should be available with appropriately labelled shelves to facilitate this process. All unused items from opened kits must be appropriately disposed of. There should be a wall-mounted clinical waste bin with foot lever to open. This must be emptied at least once a week, regardless of how full it is.
- Sharps disposal bins should be replaced when three-quarters full.
- Used towels and gowns should be placed in a linen basket.
- There should be access to a refrigerator and freezer for storage of samples.

Further reading

Fellow of the Faculty of Forensic and Legal Medicine (latest update 2007). *Operational procedures and equipment for medical rooms in police stations and victim examination suites.* Available at ℘ https://fflm.ac.uk/upload/documents/1193757602.pdf

Principles of assessment

Attitude of examining doctor

Examination of cases of sexual assault can involve a complainant or a suspect. The terms 'victim' and 'perpetrator' should not be used until a case has completed through a court system, as the terms are overtly judgemental.

Complainant sensitive examination

The role of the forensic practitioner is to undertake a sympathetic and appropriate assessment without being judgemental. The forensic practitioner needs to make a special effort to remain sensitive to the needs of the complainant throughout the examination. Positive evaluations from complainants of sexual assault examinations are associated with:

• The doctor taking care to explain procedures.
• Being called by one's name.
• Being talked to throughout the process.
• Having their feelings monitored.
• Being asked if anything hurts.
• The presence of a sympathetic third party.

Unsurprisingly, negative evaluations from complainants are associated with a doctor appearing to 'cross-examine', having a brusque manner, and performing examinations that are humiliating, degrading, and unnecessarily painful.

Skills of examining doctor

Primary clinical assessment of complainants and suspects follow the same general principles, although the structure and content of the assessments varies. A doctor's duties of consent and confidentiality apply in such assessments. Wherever possible, assessments should be undertaken by those with specific training, experience, and knowledge as forensic physicians or sexual offence examiners. The skills required (in addition to those mentioned previously) include a good knowledge of:

• Appropriate history taking and examination.
• Relevant medical care and need for referral.
• Retrieval of evidence.
• Preservation of evidence.
• Presentation of evidence.
• Principles of forensic analysis.

Location of examination

Wherever possible, the examinee should have the opportunity to determine the gender of the examining doctor (although this may prove to be difficult in remote areas). The location of the assessment for a complainant may be a SARC or a VES within a police facility. Most suspects are examined within medical examination rooms in police custody suites.

Assessment procedure

Initial priorities

Having been made aware of the need to examine a complainant or suspect, the primary task is to determine whether any need for urgent medical attention/treatment over-rides the immediate need for a sexual assault examination. In some instances, it may be appropriate for a forensic physician to join a treating doctor (e.g. gynaecologist) to undertake (with consent) an examination under anaesthetic to assess and treat vaginal or anal tears. Healthcare considerations take priority. In the absence of any need for medical treatment, examination should be undertaken at the earliest opportunity in order to ensure best opportunities for evidential sampling.

Documentation

It is important to follow a standardized system of recording information when undertaking a sexual assault examination. The information documented is likely to become part of court proceedings. As such, it will be scrutinized by others, including prosecution teams, defence lawyers, expert witnesses, and judges, so it is essential to ensure that it is complete and legible. The most appropriate way to record and to ensure that relevant data are not omitted is to use standardized pro formas.

Preliminary information that must be documented includes:
- Time and date of examination.
- Location.
- Referral details (reasons, name of referrer).
- Time introduced to complainant.
- The examining doctor's name and contact details must be recorded, as must the names, contact details, and roles of all those present (e.g. specialist police officer, crisis worker).

Complainant details that should be documented are:
- Name
- Date of birth and age
- Gender
- Ethnicity
- Partnership status (if any)
- Occupation
- Residence status.

Chaperones

Consideration must be given to the appropriate use of chaperones once written informed consent for the examination, sample taking, and provision of a report for police and legal purposes has been obtained. Sometimes, complainants ask for a relative/friend to remain with them during the examination for support. A police officer (of the same sex) may be present in the room to receive samples taken.

Consent

It is essential that the examining doctor explains the nature, purpose, and process of the assessment in order that consent is fully informed. In particular, explanation must be made that the doctor will observe their duty of confidentiality with regard to irrelevant medical issues, but that in most jurisdictions (including England and Wales), the court has the power to order disclosure of confidential information. Note that on certain occasions, a distressed complainant may agree/consent to only part of the usual full examination.

In certain circumstances, adults may lack capacity to provide consent. This may be for a variety of reasons (e.g. head injury, drug or alcohol intoxication, age, mental health issues, being on a ventilator). Such incapacity may be permanent or temporary (see 📖 Mental Capacity Act—p.434). The determination of whether examination and sample taking is appropriate and lawful may require legal advice and advice from a medical defence organization. Recommendations have been published to address certain specific scenarios (e.g. guidance from the Faculty of Forensic and Legal Medicine, March 2008, *Consent from patients who may have been seriously assaulted*. Available at 🔗 https://fflm.ac.uk/library).

Faculty of Forensic and Legal Medicine

Pro forma

Sample consent form for Forensic Physicians

Consent

Verbal consent obtained YES ☐ NO ☐	Signed
Special features	Date
	Witnessed (if appropriate)
I consent to a medical examination, including the taking of notes and samples if appropriate on myself or my _____ as explained to me by Dr_____	Date
	Name of Witness
	Relationship of witness

I understand that Dr_____ may have to produce a report based on the history and examination and that details of the examination may have to be revealed in court.

Prepared and updated by Dr Guy A Norfolic, on behalf of the Academic Committee of the Faculty of Forensic and Legal Medicine, May 2008 ©

Fig. 11.1 Example consent form. Reproduced with permission of the Faculty of Forensic and Legal Medicine.

History of assault: the complainant

The information discussed in this section relates predominantly to the examination of the complainant of sexual assault.

Context

A detailed history of the alleged assault is usually obtained by the police from the complainant (taking the form of a statement or interview). However, on occasion, this history may not be complete at the time of the medical assessment.

The doctor should ensure that he/she records the briefing details from the referring police team and then confirms the basic details of what happened with the complainant. If the police have already obtained a detailed account, it is unnecessary for the doctor to go through all of the detail again. However, the doctor should record verbatim the account given by the complainant—discrepancies may become very significant at a later stage of any legal proceedings.

Specific questions

Essential questions to be determined from the briefing account or/and the history given by the complainant and by direct questioning are:

Full history of events
- Specific physical contacts (Yes or No responses):
  - Penis to mouth
  - Mouth to genitalia
  - Penis to anus
  - Penis to vulva/vagina
  - Ejaculation (if Yes—site?)
  - Object/implement penetration of mouth/vulva/vagina/anus (if Yes—which and what object/implement?).
- Kissing/licking/biting/sucking/spitting (if Yes –sites?)
- Any known injuries?
- Bleeding—any orifice?
- Clothing damage?
- Last contact with assailant (and any contact prior to the current event—if so, give details).

Previous drug or alcohol use
This needs to be determined in detail:
- Last use of alcohol (times, amounts in 24h prior to incident).
- Illicit drugs (times, amounts in 4 days prior to incident).
- Prescribed medications (times, amounts).
- Any drug or alcohol dependencies—if Yes, elicit full history.

Post-assault events

Post-assault events need to be described, as they may influence the nature and potential recovery of evidence, which may identify a suspect from DNA traces. Some investigators may use Early Evidence Recovery Kits which provide samples of saliva and urine, prior to medical examination. These may be used to identify drugs administered that may be rapidly metabolized and eliminated from the body (e.g. gamma-hydroxybutyrate) and provide foreign DNA where oral sexual assault is alleged. Establish when the samples were retained and where they are. The following information may be relevant and require a Yes/No response which may then require elaboration:

Since the assault have you:
- Noted pain?
- Noted soreness?
- Noted bleeding?
- Eaten?
- Drunk anything?
- Brushed teeth/gums/dentures (is toothbrush recoverable)?
- Used a mouthwash or spray?
- Passed urine?
- Opened bowels?
- Wiped/washed genitalia (is cloth or towel recoverable)?
- Removed or inserted tampon/pad/sponge/diaphragm
  (is it recoverable)?
- Changed clothes?

Further medical history: complainant

The relevant points of the history of sexual assault having been documented, attention should turn to other elements of the medical history. These include symptoms post-assault, the past medical history, and perhaps controversially, the past sexual history.

Symptoms post-assault

Essential elements of this part of the history necessitate establishing the responses to the following questions on symptomatology, pre- and post-assault (if relevant to the assault description):

- Urinary tract infection
- Urinary incontinence
- Vaginal discharge or bleeding
- Diarrhoea
- Constipation
- Faecal incontinence
- Genital/anal injury
- Anal bleeding/itching
- Threadworm infection
- Genital or anal surgery.

Past medical history

The relevant past medical history includes standard questions about previous surgery, major and chronic illnesses. It may be particularly relevant to ask about chronic skin conditions (which may mask or be mistaken for evidence of injury).

Drug history

As outlined earlier, the drug history should include prescribed drugs as well as over-the-counter medication. In particular, this should identify drugs that might affect the appearance, evolution, and speed of healing of injuries (e.g. anticoagulants and steroids).

Past gynaecological history

Relevant details include:

- Menstrual history
- Last menstrual period
- Use of tampons/towels
- Pregnancies and delivery mode
- Contraceptive history.

Past psychiatric history

It is important to establish if there is a history of psychiatric illness, including previous deliberate self-harm. On occasions, it may be appropriate to perform a mental state examination.

Social and educational history

Aspects of the social history which may affect interpretation of clinical findings includes engaging in contact sports (which may result in 'normal' bruising). The history provided by the complainant may be placed in context by establishing educational attainment.

Previous sexual history

It may be understandably difficult for the complainant to understand the relevance and appropriateness of enquiring about previous sexual history. The forensic practitioner may need to take time to explain the potential importance of this information within the context of the alleged assault (e.g. intimate samples may reveal DNA which requires explanation). The way that the practitioner approaches this part of the history may indicate the extent to which he/she adopts a 'complainant-centred approach'. It is important to sensitively enquire about sexual activity within the 10 days prior to assessment:

- Recent sexual activity prior to the alleged assault (with whom, nature, time, use of condom/lubricant).
- Any sexual activity post-assault (with whom, nature, time, use of condom/lubricant).

Examination for adult sexual assault

The nature of the examination of the adult in sexual assault cases is determined in part by the history elicited, in that certain points may direct an examiner to areas of particular interest. There are some differences in the examination of complainants and suspects and in the examination of males and females—these will be identified later in this section.

Basic information

There are key elements to document in all examinations, although not all the information will be relevant. The following general points should be documented:
- Weight
- Height
- General appearance (±demeanour)
- Skin appearance (scars, tattoos, injection sites, piercing)
- Hair appearance (scalp and elsewhere—e.g. dyed, shaved).

General physical examination

A standard general physical examination should be performed of the cardiovascular, respiratory, gastrointestinal, neurological, and musculoskeletal systems, recording relevant positive and negative findings.

Injuries and abnormalities

A detailed physical external examination is required in all cases, identifying injury or abnormality. It is also important to record the absence of injury and abnormality. This examination should be documented on body diagrams (see 📖 p.122).

Often what appear to be trivial or insignificant marks or injuries may have substantial evidential value, corroborating accounts or allowing swabs to be taken to identify contact. For each mark seen (if possible), the following information should be elicited and related to the history previously obtained:
- Location of injury/abnormality
- Pain, tenderness, stiffness
- Type of injury (e.g. bruise, laceration, superficial scratch abrasion)
- Size (use metric values)
- Shape, colour, appearance (e.g. fading)
- Orientation
- Causation (is it consistent with history?)
- Time.

Detailed external examination

Following a 'routine' for detailed external examination helps to ensure that it is thorough and complete. The exact order of the routine is less important than ensuring that everything is looked at. In order to be complainant sensitive, it may be best to start with examination of the hands (usually the least 'threatening' area to examine), work up the upper limbs to the head and then down the body to the feet. The following summarizes this approach (examples of specific features to be looked for are given):

• Hands (note handedness).
• Fingernails (note condition: length, bitten, false, broken).
• Upper and lower limbs—all surfaces (look for grip or restraint marks).
• Scalp/hair (note debris/dried semen, hair pulled, hair loss, petechiae).
• Ears—externally and internally.
• Eyes, including conjunctiva at extremes of movement (note petechiae).
• Face.
• Lips (check for bruising, torn frenulum).
• Mouth—buccal and lingual surfaces (for bruising and/or petechiae).
• Palate.
• Teeth, including dentures and braces.
• Neck (look for grip marks, scratches, tenderness, petechiae).
• Torso—both anterior posterior surfaces.

Specific focused examination

The detailed external examination should focus particularly on those areas which were described in the history as having been injured (e.g. gripped, squeezed, bitten, scratched) or subjected to contact which might have left DNA or other trace material (e.g. rubbed against, licked, kissed, sucked, ejaculated on).

On completion of the external examination, genito-anal examination is undertaken (if indicated).

Female genital examination

Approach

Genital examination needs to be approached with considerable sensitivity. Complainants should be given as much time as needed. They should be aware that they are able to change their mind about consenting to any aspect of the examination at any time.

Positioning

Female genito-anal examination may be undertaken by naked eye, or with the assistance of specialist lighting, magnification, or colposcopes. Such examinations aim to maximize the possibility of identifying injury and securing trace evidence. The position(s) of the examinee for the examination should be documented (e.g. left lateral, lithotomy, supine), as should any instrumentation or lubrication used.

Systematic examination

The examination should follow a structured approach, but focusing on areas as indicated from the history. The presence (or absence) of any abnormalities in the following anatomical sites should be recorded:

- Thighs
- Buttocks and perineum
- Pubic area
- Pubic hair
- Labia majora
- Labia minora
- Clitoris
- Posterior fourchette
- Fossa navicularis
- Vestibule
- Hymen (recording of position of abnormalities is done using a clock-face technique—anterior being 12 o'clock and posterior being 6 o'clock)
- Urethral opening
- Vagina (note ease and comfort of passage of speculum)
- Cervix.

Terminology

Care should be taken to use standard anatomical terms to describe female genital parts. Diagrams may be useful in recording the exact site and extent of injuries (see Fig. 11.2).

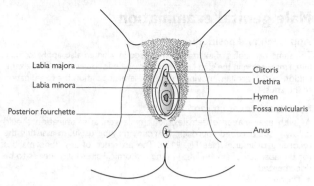

Labia majora

Labia minora

Posterior fourchette

Clitoris

Urethra

Hymen

Fossa navicularis

Anus

Fig. 11.2 Diagram of female genital anatomy.

Male genital examination

Approach and positioning

The same principles of examination as used in women also apply to men. Initial inspection in the standing position may be followed by supine examination of the genitals, moving to the left lateral position for examination of the anus.

Systematic examination

As with examination of females, adult male genital examination should follow a standardized approach. Diagrams may be useful in assisting the recording of injuries (see Fig. 11.3). The presence of any abnormalities (or the absence of any findings) in the anatomical sites listed needs to be documented:

- Thighs
- Buttocks and perineum
- Pubic area
- Pubic hair
- Scrotum
- Testes (note if both present)
- Penile shaft
- Penile glans
- Penile coronal sulcus
- Foreskin.

Particular focus

Irrespective of finding any injury or apparent abnormality, the examining doctor needs to record the following information:

- The presence (or absence) of normal adult male penile anatomy (recording whether or not the individual has been circumcised).
- The presence, size, and position of the testes.
- The presence of normal adult male secondary sexual characteristics (e.g. presence and pattern of pubic hair).
- The presence of any piercings and/or tattoos in the genital area.

Terminology

It is important to use standard terminology to describe adult male genital parts (see Fig. 11.3).

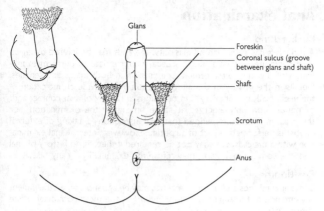

Fig. 11.3 Diagram of adult male genital anatomy.

Anal examination

Background

Although it has some natural elasticity, the anus may be injured by digital or other penetrative assault. It is usually appropriate to perform examination of the anus after genital examination in both males and females. Details in the history of the alleged assault will provide an indication of the likelihood of anal injury. On occasions, a history of anal contact and/or penetration only emerges at some time after the examination. For this reason, it is recommended that anal inspection (± taking of external swabs) is performed as part of a routine. However, internal anal examination with a proctoscope may not be required if there is no history of anal assault—some complainants may refuse this examination in any case.

Positioning

Some anal injuries and/or abnormalities may be apparent when the patient is examined in the supine position. However, the most comfortable and appropriate position for examining the anus is the left lateral position with hips and knees flexed.

Procedure

Examination should include inspection of:
- Buttocks
- Natal cleft
- Perianal area
- Anus.

Spreading the buttocks apart may reveal bruising, lacerations, and other injuries (e.g. fissures). Injuries and other abnormalities (e.g. warts, haemorrhoids) at the anal margin should be recorded in terms of their position on a clock face, with anterior being 12 o'clock and posterior being 6 o'clock.

Proctoscopy

The anal canal and rectum may be examined using a proctoscope. The size of the proctoscope and nature of lubricant used should be documented.

Examination of suspects

Objectives

Medical examination of those suspected of having been responsible for adult sexual assault aims to search for physical and trace evidence which may assist the investigation. The presence of physical injuries may help to confirm or refute an allegation or alternative explanation (or have no influence either way). The same principles apply to the presence or absence of trace evidence (especially DNA).

Avoidance of cross-contamination

Due to the potential for cross-contamination of evidence, complainants and suspects should never be examined by the same doctor or at the same location. If there is more than one suspect in a particular case, different examiners and different locations are employed in order to avoid the risk of unintentional (and unrecognized) transfer of important trace evidence.

Consent

From a medical standpoint, issues of consent are similar for both complainants and suspects, despite the latter being in police custody. A medical practitioner cannot undertake examinations or take samples without the consent of the individual. However, a doctor/nurse can, of course, record those injuries which are apparent from external inspection without examination (e.g. an obvious facial laceration or swollen hand).

The suspect needs to appreciate the potential implications of both allowing and refusing to allow an examination and/or the taking of samples. Usually, the suspect's legal representative is involved in providing this advice.

Prior to the medical examination, the examining doctor should discuss the medical aspects of the assessment, including the nature, purpose, and process. The doctor should explain that he/she will observe the duty of confidentiality with regard to irrelevant medical issues, but that in most jurisdictions (including England and Wales) the court has the power to order disclosure of confidential information. Confidential information for which consent for disclosure has not been given must not be disclosed to the police, unless the doctor reasonably believes that withholding that information will place another person at risk of harm. Different jurisdictions have different rules regarding the obtaining of samples, but doctors will not usually take samples if consent is refused.

Procedure

Examination of a suspect involves the same basic process as that described earlier for complainants, except for the way that the history of the incident is handled. It is usually not appropriate for the examining medical practitioner to ask any direct questions relating to the incident. Instead, the basic information regarding the allegation is provided by the investigating police officers. This information will enable the examination to be focused and for findings to be put in context.

During the examination, the suspect may need to be reminded that information and accounts which he/she provides about the origin of injuries, marks, or other abnormalities may be recorded and potentially used in court. Explanations which the suspect does provide for injuries, marks, and other abnormalities should be recorded verbatim. On occasions, the suspect's legal representative may be present during medical examination and sample taking.

Collecting forensic samples

Purpose of taking samples

The purpose of taking forensic samples in sexual assault cases is to assist in determining one or more of the following:

- To confirm contact between two parties.
- To confirm nature of sexual contact and/or locus.
- To ascertain gender and possible identity of the assailant.

In order to fulfil these functions it is necessary to identify appropriate sites for sampling, take samples appropriately, and ensure that the sample becomes part of a chain of custody whereby its origins and passage through the medical, police, science, and legal system is identifiable throughout. This means that identifiable and traceable labelling of samples (together with records of who has handled the samples) are clear, transparent, and reviewable at any stage from sampling to analysis.

Potential cross-contamination

In addition to the requirements of having separate locations to examine complainants and suspects, separate doctors (and police officers) need to be arranged to avoid other potential routes of transfer of trace evidence.

Sample sites

The samples that are required in any case will be guided by the particular details of the case. Sites that may need to be sampled include:

- Blood (for both DNA analysis and alcohol/drug levels).
- Urine.
- Hair (scalp and pubic).
- Nails.
- Body orifices and other sites including mouth, ears, nose, skin.
- Genitalia: vulva, vagina, cervix, penis, anus, anal canal, rectum.

Less obvious sites that have allowed recovery of identifiable DNA include contact lens (from ejaculation into the eye). For all specimens, sealed sampling kits need to be quality assured and supplied by commercial companies with agreed quality standards. Sampling should follow locally agreed protocols. Specialist agencies will advise on the most appropriate sampling methods (these need regular review).

Types of sample

Table 11.1 summarizes what may be achieved from analysis of various samples. In all cases, if there is any uncertainty, confirm with forensic science laboratories the type of specimen required and how it should be stored to ensure optimum preservation. Samples should be taken in light of the known history and accounts of events. If there is any doubt whether a particular sample may be relevant, it is better to take it and retain it for later analysis. In the case of a suspect, legal requirements need to be observed in order to appropriately request samples. Control swabs are likely to be required, depending on local protocols and operating procedures.

Table 11.1 Examples of analysis from various samples

Sample site or type	What may be found
Blood	Alcohol; drugs (prescribed; licit and illicit); volatile solvents; DNA
Urine	Alcohol; drugs (prescribed; licit and illicit)
Hair (head)—cut and combed	Body fluids (wet and dry); foreign material (e.g. vegetation, glass, fibres); comparison with other hairs found on body; past history of drug use (prescribed; licit and illicit)
Hair (pubic)—cut and combed	Body fluids (wet and dry); foreign material (e.g. vegetation, glass, fibres); comparison with other hairs found on body; past history of drug use (prescribed; licit and illicit)
Buccal scrape	DNA profiling
Skin swabs (at sites of contact)	Body fluids (e.g. semen, saliva—wet and dry); cellular material; lubricant
Mouth swabs	Semen
Mouth rinse	Semen
Vulval swab	Body fluids (e.g. semen, saliva); foreign material (e.g. hairs, vegetation, glass, fibres)
Low vaginal swab	Body fluids (e.g. semen, saliva); foreign material (e.g. hairs, vegetation, glass, fibres)
High vaginal swab	Body fluids (e.g. semen, saliva); foreign material (e.g. hairs, vegetation, glass, fibres)
Endocervical swab	Body fluids (e.g. semen, saliva)
Penile swabs (shaft, glans, coronal sulcus)	Body fluids (e.g. semen, saliva)
Perianal swabs	Body fluids (e.g. semen, saliva)
Anal swabs	Body fluids (e.g. semen, saliva)
Rectal swabs	Body fluids (e.g. semen, saliva)
Fingernail swabs, cuttings or scraping	Foreign material (e.g. skin cells), matching of broken nails

Persistence of forensic material

How long does forensic evidence last on the body?

Police officers tasked with the investigation of allegations of sexual assault often seek advice from the examining doctor as to whether or not there may be a chance of important forensic material still being preserved despite a significant time delay since the alleged incident occurred. The question is not always easy to answer with certainty! The persistence of evidentially relevant materials varies according to the exact type and site of sample and the evidential material being sought. Table 11.2 provides some indication of the approximate times after contact for which evidentially relevant material has been identified.

It should be noted that data on the persistence of foreign material is limited in certain sites (e.g. on the skin). As mentioned earlier with the type of material being sought, if there is any doubt or uncertainty about the time that has lapsed since an offence is alleged to have occurred, it is better to take a sample and retain it for later analysis. Again, in the case of a suspect, the doctor should advise the police investigators regarding which sample(s) are needed, as legal requirements have to be observed in order to appropriately request samples.

Table 11.2 Approximate times after contact for which evidentially relevant material has been identified

Sample site or type	What may be found
Blood Urine	The persistence of alcohol and drugs is dependent on the quantities and type consumed. In general, if an incident occurred within 72h, blood and urine samples should be taken and if between 72h and up to 96h, urine alone
Hair (head)—cut and combed Hair (pubic)—cut and combed	Dried foreign material may persist for many days and if there is visual evidence of such material, it should always be sampled. Hair sampling for drug history cannot be utilized until at least 4 weeks after ingestion
Skin swabs (at sites of contact)	Foreign trace material is considered to be identifiable up to 48h after contact, however experimental data suggests persistence in certain sites up to 1 week. Thus, if a site of contact can be identified and no washing or showering has taken place, consideration should be given to sampling after longer periods than 48h
Mouth swabs Mouth rinse	Semen has been detected up to 48h after oral penetration
Vulval swab	As for skin
Low vaginal swab High vaginal swab Endocervical swab	Body fluids have been detected for up to 7 days after vaginal intercourse and up to 12h after digital penetration.
Penile swabs (shaft, glans, coronal sulcus)	Body fluids if intercourse within 48h
Perianal swabs Anal swabs Rectal swabs	Body fluids if anal intercourse within 3 days or digital penetration within 12h
Fingernail swabs, cuttings, or scraping	No specific time limit—variety of materials may be recovered

Sexual assault examination kit

Most forensic practitioners become accustomed to using a locally agreed, standardized forensic sexual assault examination kit (often referred to as a 'rape kit'). This contains most of the equipment required for the examination and collection of forensic samples from complainants and suspects of adult sexual abuse.

Typical contents

- List of contents of kit and instructions for use.
- Pro forma for doctor to complete (includes body diagrams, tick-list of samples taken, with space to write time taken).
- Black ball point pen.
- Sterile gloves.
- Paper bags (to collect clothes etc.).
- Measuring tape.
- Large brown paper sheet (for complainant to stand on whilst undressing—potentially catching trace material).
- Numerous 'general purpose' cotton-tipped swabs within individual sealed plastic containers.
- Plastic sealable sample bags (various sizes).
- Sterile water (for control swabs).
- Plastic nail 'stick' for nail scrapings.
- Nail clipper.
- Plastic container for nail clippings.
- Comb (to try to collect particulate matter within scalp and pubic hair).
- Scissors (to cut hair).
- Blood sampling kit.
- Blood tubes (for full blood count, alcohol and drug levels, baseline serology for storage and later testing as necessary).

Completing the examination

At the end of the examination, the complainant is usually offered a shower or bath and the opportunity to clean teeth and put on some fresh clothes, prior to having a hot drink and completing any treatment considerations (pregnancy, infection, etc.—see 📖 p.374).

The medical practitioner and police officer need to ensure that all samples ('exhibits') are appropriately labelled, signed, and sealed. Any unopened and unused contents are retained within a large, sealed, labelled sample bag as an exhibit to be available for inspection if required. All exhibits are handed over to the police officer who takes responsibility for transporting them to a forensic laboratory (possibly via a refrigerator if there is likely to be a delay).

Documentation of findings

Documentation of findings should be in written form (ideally using a black ball point pen and standardized pro forma). Descriptions of injury and abnormalities should be recorded in enough detail that they may be clearly and unambiguously interpreted by third parties. Body diagrams should accompany all written notes. Wherever possible, photographic images should be taken of all abnormalities, under the direction of the doctor, with colour bars and rules in all images. If colposcopy has been used for genito-anal assessment, photographic or DVD images may be used (but need to be carefully and securely stored).

Interpretation of genital findings

Interpretation and the doctor

On occasions, a relatively inexperienced doctor may be called on to examine, assess, and document injuries after sexual assault. It is essential that interpretation of findings from such an examination is only undertaken by a doctor experienced in such assessments and who is fully aware of current research about physical findings after sexual assault.

Myths about sexual assault

Injuries can be divided into genito-anal injuries and those which are present elsewhere on the body. It is generally (and wrongly) believed that a sexual assault will inevitably result in injury to the victim, whether adult or child. This is not correct—any sexual assault (including rape and penetration) may occur without any visible physical injury to the genitalia or to the rest of the body. Indeed, studies suggest that evidence of naked eye injury to the genitalia is only seen in a minority of rape victims.

Conversely, consensual sexual activity (sexual activity between consenting adults) can result in injury to the body and genitalia. Thus, the presence or absence of injuries in association with allegations of sexual assault do not indicate by themselves one way or another whether the particular activity was consensual or non-consensual, and it is essential that these facts are understood when reporting and interpreting findings.

Research into injuries after sexual assault

A number of studies in adults have explored the type of injury seen and the frequency with which injuries have been noted following clinical examination of complainants of sexual assault:

- The method of assessment/examination (e.g. a colposcope) may increase the number of 'positive' findings because of better imaging.
- The incidence of non-genital injury is generally higher than genital injury, and the significance of extra-genital injuries may be much greater in the context of allegations of sexual assault.
- The presence of genito-anal injury is of the order of 20–30% in some series, whilst extra-genital injury may be present in >50%.
- The type of and aggressiveness of any sexual assault can increase the likelihood of visible injury.
- Studies suggest that most females do not have visible genito-anal injuries, but the likelihood of sustaining genito-anal injury during a sexual assault is higher among females without prior sexual intercourse experience, females subject to anal penetration, and postmenopausal females.
- Consensual sexual activity has been shown to result in a range of blunt trauma injuries and consequently, bruises, abrasions, and lacerations to genital and non-genital sites may be present.
- The severity and site of injury varies according to many factors: type of sexual activity, relative sizes, positions and intoxication of participants, menopausal state, previous sexual activity.

Factors influencing injury

The accounts between two participants may differ substantially in the description of the degree of force used and the medical findings may add more weight to one account over the other. The same factors that may influence the degree and severity of injury and the anatomical site of the injury are the same as for non-consensual activity and thus may include some or all the following—each of which may have differing influences at different times:

- Age of the complainant.
- Type of sexual activity.
- Relative positions of the participants.
- Previous sexual activity and degree of intoxication of either or both of the participants.
- Consensual insertion or attempts at insertion of a finger or fingers, penis, or any other object into the vagina may result in bruises, abrasions, and lacerations of the labia majora, labia minora, hymen, and posterior fourchette.
- Consensual digital vaginal penetration may result in unintentional fingernail damage or injury to parts of the female genital tract which may not be noticed by either party.

Serious injury and death

Death has been reported in a female who sustained an injury during consensual sexual activity. Vaginal injuries may result in bleeding. If penile–vaginal penetration follows digital–vaginal penetration, then it seems likely that any injury or bleeding may be exacerbated. Cases have been reported where consensual vaginal sexual activity resulted in injury causing bleeding, which necessitated internal iliac artery ligation.

Sexual assault with no visible injury

A study of adolescents with and without a history of prior penetrative sex concluded that 'genital and or body injuries are not routinely found in adolescents after an allegation of rape or sexual assault even when there has not been previous sexual experience. The absence of injury does not exclude the possibility of intercourse, whether with or without consent'.

Interpretation of anal findings

Consensual anal sexual activity

Anal intercourse is part of the normal sexual repertoire of many hetero-sexual and homosexual couples. Consensual anal intercourse may (in the same way as vaginal sex) be pain- and discomfort-free and would not nor-mally leave any residual injury. Repeated anal intercourse results in easier penetration over a period of time. Lubrication such as saliva or K-Y® Jelly can be used to ease penetration.

Non-consensual anal sexual activity

Non-consensual anal intercourse, if done without force, with or without lubrication, and without physical resistance on the part of the person being penetrated may leave no residual injury and may be pain-free. The effects of drugs and alcohol may make penetration easier. In an individual who is otherwise used to anal intercourse, no pain or discomfort may be experienced.

Injury following non-consensual anal intercourse

The likelihood of pain or injury in non-consensual anal intercourse may be increased by:
• Someone who has not previously experienced anal intercourse.
• The absence of lubrication.
• The use of force.
• Great disparity between the size of the anus (which varies little in the adult) and the penis (which may vary a lot).

Forced anal intercourse can result in stretch injuries that damage the lining of the anal canal or the skin surrounding the anus (the perianal region). Such stretching can cause damage to the blood vessels supplying the local tissues and such damage to blood vessels can cause blood to leak out into the tissues resulting in bruises, or can tear the surface of the anal canal and the perianal region, causing fissures, tears, or lacerations. Because of the nerve supply, such fissures, tears, or lacerations (the terms are used interchangeably), even if minor, can be exquisitely painful.

The incidence of fissures in non-consensual anal intercourse is uncertain, as there are only a few studies that have explored these issues, and there is some blurring of definition of terms such as fissure, tear, or laceration (see 📖 p.401).

Anal fissure

The term anal fissure refers to breaks or a tear in the skin around the anus. Fissures may be acute or chronic. Acute fissures (i.e. developing and healing within a couple of weeks) are caused by some form of trauma. Chronic fissures (i.e. persistent and not healing) may be initiated by trauma and be prolonged by certain diseases or illnesses. Chronic constipation, requiring straining to defecate, associated with the passage of hard stool, is one cause of acute fissure development.

Other possible causes of acute and chronic fissure include sexually transmitted disease, diarrhoea, inflammatory bowel disease (e.g. Crohn's disease), skin diseases. Another cause of the development of anal fissures is the passage of objects into the anal passage for sexual purposes. This may include items such as dildos or a penis. In the absence of repeated trauma, any fissures, tears, or lacerations would be expected to heal within 2 weeks or so and leave no residual marks.

Treatment, counselling, and follow-up

Police may understandably primarily focus on investigations and gathering evidence, but the complainant may have different priorities, including:
• Treatment of physical injuries.
• Fear and prevention of pregnancy.
• Fear of sexually transmitted disease.
• Changing clothes, brushing teeth, having a shower and a hot drink.
• Long-term psychological effects.

Doctors need to empathize with the complainant and consider priorities.

Treatment of physical injuries

There can be a tension between whether to initially focus on treating injuries or gather forensic evidence. One factor underlying this is that the quality of the forensic evidence deteriorates with time. The forensic physician must weigh up the priorities regarding medical care and forensic sampling and determine which, from the examinee's viewpoint, is in their best interests. In general terms, serious injuries take priority and need to be treated at hospital first, although steps can be taken to try to preserve forensic evidence (e.g. not having a drink/shower first). Sometimes, it may be reasonable (with the complainant's agreement) to gather forensic samples first and then attend to relatively minor injuries.

Emergency contraception

The risk of pregnancy following unprotected sexual intercourse is an understandable concern. The risk is greatest during the 5 days around ovulation, but is present at other times also. The principal choices are oral levonorgestrel (usually the preferred option if the complainant presents within 72h of intercourse) or insertion of intrauterine contraceptive device (up to 5 days after intercourse).

Levonorgestrel

Previously known as the 'morning after pill' (a term now discouraged), levonorgestrel can be bought over the counter and is available for complainants from SARCs. Contraindications are: acute porphyria, pregnancy, and focal migraine. Properly taken, it has a low failure rate (~1–2%). Give 1.5mg of levonorgestrel (increase dose if on enzyme-inducing drugs—see BNF) as soon as possible and advise GP follow-up in 3 weeks to ensure that menstruation has occurred. If the complainant vomits within 3h of taking the medication, she needs to take a replacement dose. Advise use of condoms (see 'Sexually transmitted disease' later in this section) and explain about theoretical risk of ectopic pregnancy. Levonorgestrel can be used when patients present at 72–120h of unprotected intercourse. As this is an unlicensed indication for the drug, the advice of an expert in family planning should be sought in such circumstances.

Intrauterine contraceptive device

This may be appropriate for complainants who present 3–5 days after unprotected intercourse. It usually requires specialist referral.

Sexually transmitted disease

There is a huge potential range of sexually transmitted diseases, including *Chlamydia trachomatis*, gonorrhoea, trichomoniasis, syphilis, hepatitis, and HIV. It is standard practice to discuss antibacterial prophylaxis (follow local protocols and see following paragraph) and to screen for bacterial infections at genitourinary clinic at 10–14 days (although many complainants ask for an earlier appointment). Complainants are usually given a brief letter from the examining doctor to take to the clinic, where an appointment can be arranged at a convenient time. They should also be advised to use condoms and avoid unprotected sexual contact with their usual partner until they have been screened at genitourinary clinic and/or completed a course of prophylactic antibiotics.

Prophylactic antibiotic regimens

When a complainant may default, is unable to tolerate the distress of a repeat examination, or requires an intrauterine contraceptive device, the following prophylactic antibiotic combination may be offered:
- Azithromycin 1g orally stat + cefixime 400mg orally stat.
- Or if penicillin allergic: azithromycin 1g stat + ciprofloxacin 500mg stat.

Hepatitis and HIV

It is important to consider potential risks of hepatitis B/C, and HIV (± specialist advice and/or protocols) and treat accordingly (this may require involvement of hospital and/or GP):
- Take a baseline sample for storage for serology.
- Hepatitis B is a significant risk following male rape and that risk increases with additional factors such as multiple assailants, intravenous drug use, or rape in a high prevalence area. Hepatitis B cover for those at risk who have not previously been immunized includes giving hepatitis B immunoglobulin and starting an accelerated active immunization course (give first dose with arrangements for subsequent doses).
- The risk of HIV seroconversion may be reduced by postexposure prophylaxis. This prophylaxis is more effective the sooner that it is given, but it is not without side effects—expert advice may need to be obtained before starting it.

See ℘ http://www.careandevidence.org/Assets/HIV%20PEP.pdf

Liaison with general practitioner

The initial emphasis after a reported sexual assault centres around the investigation and collection of forensic evidence, but complainants may have medium- and long-term needs which need to be addressed. The police victim liaison officer is able to arrange contact with appropriate counsellors and victim support. It may also be helpful for the complainant's GP to be informed about the assault. This is a decision for the complainant to make and some complainants do not wish their GP to know. One way of allowing the complainant to 'take control' of this process is for the examining doctor to write a brief letter summarizing the type of assault, investigations, and treatment provided and then to give this letter to the complainant to take to their GP.

Appearance in court

Background

The wider aspects of professional and expert court appearances are considered in detail on 📖 pp.22–25. There are specific considerations relating to appearing in court to give evidence in sexual offence cases. Some forensic practitioners are apprehensive about attending court in these cases. Sometimes this reflects a misunderstanding about their role (professional witness or expert).

Professional witnesses

Medical witnesses giving evidence in court in sexual offence cases within England and Wales may do so either as professional witnesses or as expert witnesses. Professional witnesses may be asked to give evidence as to their findings of fact at examination of a complainant or suspect. They are not expected to give detailed opinions and indeed, are usually best advised to acknowledge the limits of their expertise and not to try to provide expert opinion.

Expert witnesses

Expert witnesses may not necessarily have seen the complainant, nor the suspect, but they will have reviewed all the evidence in the case. They will give opinion evidence on the findings and the ways, in the context of the case, that the medical evidence can be interpreted. Often, medical evidence is 'neutral' as far as the outcome of the case is concerned. For example, where penetrative sexual intercourse is agreed and confirmed by forensic science and either no injury or only minor injury is present, then the medical findings alone are not able to assist in the determination of consent, which may be the key issue at trial. It is important that the doctor does not get coerced into giving likelihoods of events having happened when it is not possible to make such a determination. The examiner should remember to apply basic medical principles and ensure that the information provided to the court assists in appropriate justice being dispensed.

Child abuse and neglect

Background and historical perspective

Recognition

In 1962, Henry Kempe identified 'the battered child syndrome' but the awareness of the prevalence of child sexual abuse was only truly highlighted towards the end of the 1970s. The term 'non-accidental injury' achieved common currency in describing injury which was considered to be inflicted—by inference in an assaultative manner. In 2005 in the USA, 1460 children were considered to have died from maltreatment, of which approximately two-thirds were neglect or physical abuse, with the remainder a mixture of all types of abuse.

Definitions

Article 1 of the United Nations Convention on the Rights of the Child defined children as persons under 18 years of age. Different cultures and jurisdictions vary in how that age limit is applied. The UN Convention places a duty on the state to promote the well-being of all children in its jurisdiction. Article 3 states that any decision or action affecting children (either as individuals or as a group) should be focused on their best interests.

Child abuse is not a new problem, but reflects a greater awareness of the degree of abuse of all kinds in societies and also in part reflects the evolution of a culture or society's understanding of what is acceptable or not. Whereas child sexual abuse may be universally condemned, there remain areas, such as exploitation of children for cheap labour, which may not necessarily always be viewed as abuse.

Child abuse can be defined in a number of ways and many governments have systems in place to ensure that health professionals recognize that they have an overriding duty to report concerns if they believe that the child may be at risk of harm. The World Health Organization defines the physical abuse of a child as 'that which results in actual or potential physical harm from an interaction or lack of interaction which is reasonable within the control of a parent or person in a position of responsibility, power or trust'. Recognition of such incidences is essential for the welfare of children. In the USA, each state has a mandatory child abuse reporting law and the trend is for other countries to develop some form of duty to report.

Risk factors for abuse

The risk factors for abuse can be classified according to the child themselves, the parents, environmental and social factors:

- *Child risk factors:* behavioural issues, disability, being adopted.
- *Parental risk factors:* drug, alcohol, or mental health issues, domestic violence, history of abuse as a child.
- *Environmental and social factors:* poverty, unemployment, single parent.

Obviously for many children, multiple predisposing factors for increased risks of abuse are present.

Effects of abuse

The effects of child abuse can be dramatic and extensive. There are obvious and immediate physical outcomes of injury and death. Psychiatric, psychological, and behavioural disorders (persisting into adulthood) may ensue, together with developmental delay, growth retardation, and failure to thrive. Drug and alcohol misuse and self-injurious behaviour may be observed. There is also a clear increased risk of children who have been abused, becoming abusers themselves as adults.

Types of child abuse

Current definitions of child abuse and neglect within the UK include the following terms:

Physical abuse

Physical abuse may involve hitting, shaking, throwing, poisoning, burning, scalding, drowning, suffocating, or otherwise causing physical harm to a child. Physical harm may also be caused when a parent or carer feigns the symptoms of illness, or deliberately causes ill-health to a child they are responsible for looking after. This situation may be described by a variety of terms, including factitious illness by proxy, fictitious illness by proxy, fabricated and induced illness, or Münchausen syndrome by proxy (see 📖 p.408).

Emotional abuse

This is the persistent emotional ill-treatment or neglect of a child such as to cause severe persistent adverse effects on the child's emotional development. It may involve conveying the impression to children that they are worthless or unloved, inadequate, or valued only insofar as they meet the needs of another person. Emotional abuse may feature developmentally inappropriate expectations being imposed on children. These may include interactions that are beyond the child's developmental capacity, as well as overprotection and limitation of exploration and learning, or preventing the child participating in normal social interaction. It may also involve seeing or hearing the ill-treatment of another. It may involve serious bullying, causing children frequently to feel frightened or in danger or the exploitation or corruption of children. Some level of emotional abuse is involved in all types of ill-treatment of a child, although it may occur on its own.

Sexual abuse

This is involving, forcing, or enticing a child or young person to take part in sexual activities, including prostitution, whether or not the child is aware of what is happening. The activities may involve physical contact, including penetrative or non-penetrative acts. They may include non-contact activities, such as involving children in viewing or producing pornographic material. Other non-contact activities include involving children in watching sexual activities or encouraging children to behave in sexually inappropriate ways.

Neglect

This is the persistent failure to meet a child's basic physical or psychological needs, likely to result in the serious impairment of the child's health or development. It may involve a parent or carer failing to provide adequate food, shelter, and clothing, failing to protect a child from physical harm or danger, or the failure to ensure access to appropriate medical care or treatment. It may also include neglect of, or unresponsiveness to, a child's basic emotional needs.

Medical approach to child abuse

Every episode of child abuse that is missed has the potential for a fatal outcome. In the UK the British Medical Association (2009) published *Child protection—a toolkit for doctors* in part in response to a number of high profile cases where serious cases of child abuse were unrecognized. The toolkit aims to provide an accessible guide to best practice in child protection cases, where it is believed a child may be at risk for neglect or abuse. It is emphasized that the best interests of the child must guide the decision-making process. Due recognition must be given about the child's own capacity to make decisions on their own behalf. The toolkit highlights basic principles, definitions of abuse and neglect, methods of responding to initial concerns, and participation in statutory child protection procedures.

Basic principles for doctors

- Responsibility is to the child—if at risk of serious harm, the interests of the child over-ride those of parents.
- All doctors and others in contact with children should be able to recognize and know how to act upon signs that a child may be at risk of abuse and neglect.
- If a contact with a child raises concerns, follow-on care and a full examination prior to discharge must be ensured.
- Efforts should be made to include children in decisions made about them.
- Wherever possible and appropriate, involvement and support of those with parental responsibility, or those who care for the child should be encouraged.
- If concerns about deliberate harm have been raised, clear, accurate, and comprehensive notes must be kept, which also identify a care plan and a professional with lead responsibility.
- All doctors must be familiar with relevant local child protection procedures.
- All doctors should ensure that safeguarding and promoting the child's welfare form an integral part of care.
- If a doctor sees a child who may be at risk they must ensure systems are in place to ensure follow-up.
- If a child presents to a hospital, enquiries should be made about previous admissions.
- If a child is admitted to hospital, a named consultant must be given overall responsibility for any child protection aspects of the case.
- Any child admitted to hospital for suspected deliberate harm must receive a thorough examination within 24h.
- When an 'at-risk' child is discharged from hospital, a plan for future care must be drawn-up and documented.
- An 'at-risk' child must not be discharged from a hospital without being registered with a GP.
- All professionals must be clear about their own responsibilities and who has specific responsibility for child protection.

Children Act 1989 and 2004 (England and Wales)

Most jurisdictions now have laws, statutes, or codes in place aimed at protecting children and identifying those children at risk. It is crucial that all healthcare professionals who have any contact with children are aware of their own duties and responsibilities towards children, whether identifying those at risk or initiating further assessment by those with specialist skills.

In England and Wales, the Children Act 1989 (implemented in 1991) identified a number of principles:

- The child's welfare is the court's paramount consideration ('the paramountcy principle').
- The parents have prime responsibility for bringing up children.
- Local authorities should provide supportive services to help parents in bringing up children.
- Local authorities should take reasonable steps to identify children and families in need.
- Every local authority should have a register of children in need.
- There should be sensitivity to ethnic considerations in assessing a child's needs and providing services.
- Local authorities should work in partnership with parents.

Protection Orders

In addition, the Act created protection orders for children 'at-risk':

- *Emergency Protection Order*—for which any person may apply to court and then has parental responsibility for the child. The order lasts 8 days and may be appealed after 3 days.
- *Police Protection Provision*—a police officer can take a child into police protection without assuming parental responsibility. This lasts for 3 days.
- *Child Assessment Order*—allows proper assessment of a child up to 7 days.
- *Care and Supervision Orders*—allow the child to placed in the care of, or under supervision of, the local authority—up to 8 weeks.

Significant harm

The 1989 Act utilized the term 'harm' to describe the effects of ill-treatment and poor care leading to injury impairment of health or development of a child. The term 'significant harm' was utilized to determine the severity of the ill-treatment. This differential becomes an important concept when determining both legal and medical issues. 'Significant harm' is the threshold for compulsory intervention in child protection cases. Decisions as to the risk of significant harm must take into consideration the effect of any ill-treatment on the child's overall physical and psychological health and development.

Local authority enquiries

Under Section 47 of the 1989 Act, a duty is placed on every local authority to make enquiries when it has 'reasonable cause to suspect that a child who lives, or is found, in their area is suffering, or likely to suffer, significant harm'. Social services lead these enquiries in conjunction with other bodies such as the police, health bodies, and schools.

All police services within the UK should now have specialist Child Abuse Investigation Units tasked with investigating suspected cases of child abuse.

2004 Act

The 2004 Act imposed a duty on local authorities to establish Local Safeguarding Children Boards. These have overall responsibility for deciding how relevant organizations work together to safeguard and promote the welfare of children in their area. Where statutory child protection proceedings have been initiated, a local authority social care worker is tasked with taking the lead in supporting and safeguarding the child.

Human Rights Act 1998

In the UK, the Human Rights Act 1998 also has a bearing on the rights of children and their parents. These rights may conflict with each other and need to be taken into account. The particular relevant Articles are:
• Article 2—the right to life.
• Article 3—prohibition of torture, inhuman or degrading treatment, or punishment.
• Article 6—right to a fair trial.
• Article 8—respect for private and family life.

Physical abuse: medical perspective

Physical abuse takes many forms—different societies may take very different views on its exact nature. Opinions have evolved (and continue to evolve) considerably over time. Distinguishing 'reasonable chastisement' from abuse when children are disciplined by parents, other carers, or teachers is difficult—medical practitioners may be asked to assist with this process.

The nature of child abuse is such that it is very difficult to determine the overall incidence of it in any of its forms. An apparent increase in incidence may well simply reflect much better understanding of what constitutes abuse and the clearer mechanisms to identify and report it.

Medical history

The medical history is a crucial aspect of the assessment. It is essential that the following elements are clearly explored.

History of presenting symptoms or injuries

Relevant features that may support the suspicion of abuse include various discrepancies in the history:
- The account may change when repeated or when given to another.
- The history may be vague and lack detail.
- There may have been delay in seeking help (reasons given for any delay should be clearly documented).
- There may be a denial of pain or minimization of symptoms (from both child and carer).

Past medical history

This should also include the mother's pregnancy history, the birth history, and the child's illnesses, growth patterns, immunizations, medications, and allergies. Specific enquiry should be made regarding conditions such as haemophilia, von Willebrand disease, idiopathic thrombocytopenic purpura, factor IX deficiency; osteogenesis imperfecta, rickets, scurvy.

Emotional, behavioural, and developmental history

Should include the child's development, including school performance and achievement; the presence of any behavioural issues.

Nutritional history

Note regular intake, type of feed, dietary anomalies, food intolerances.

Family history

Includes genetic or inherited disorders and specific questions regarding brittle bones, easy fracture or bruising, and mental health issues.

Social history

Includes family status, family unit, drug and alcohol use, mental health issues, and interpersonal violence.

Environmental history

Covers housing conditions and adequacy, enquiry about the child's room in relation to others in the home.

Non-abusive injury

Children are prone to injury as a result of accident, play, and sports. The type and site of injury relates to the activity as well as the child's mobility (e.g. immobile neonate compared with the active but unsteady toddler, compared with the teenager).

The prevalence, number, and location of bruising relates to motor development. Young children often have ('normal' or non-abusive) bruises over the shins and superficial abrasions over the knees. Non-abusive bruises tend to be small, sustained over bony prominences and found on the front of the body. Non-abusive bruising to the head, face, neck, abdomen, and genitalia is unusual (but can occur).

Further reading

National Institute for Health and Clinical Excellence (2009). *When to suspect child maltreatment*. Available at ℰ http://www.nice.org.uk

Presentation of physical abuse

Patterns of physical abuse

In children alleged to have been subject to abuse, bruising is common. Any part of the body is vulnerable. Bruises which are the result of abuse may be located away from bony prominences: the commonest site is head and neck (particularly face), followed by the buttocks, trunk, and arms. Bruises following abuse are often large, multiple, and occur in clusters. However, it is most important that bruising—as with other examination findings in suspected child abuse—must be assessed in the context of medical, social, and developmental history, the explanation given, and the patterns of non-abusive bruising.

The presentation of different types of abuse is variable and may overlap, thus indicators of physical abuse, should also raise awareness of the possibility of emotional abuse, sexual abuse, or neglect. Thus, children may present to a healthcare professional with a wide range of signs or symptoms of possible injuries that should raise the possibility of physical abuse.

Injuries which should arouse concern

Examples of patterns of injury that should raise the possibility of physical abuse are listed here:
- Multiple facial bruises
- Multiple discrete round or ovoid bruises
- Bruising to the ear
- Bruises to the neck
- Bruises to the abdomen
- Multiple bruises to the back
- Bruises on the inner aspect of legs
- Linear bruising
- Petechiae in any location
- Multiple old scars
- Mouth bleeding
- Isolated or discrete burns
- Cigarette burns
- Bite marks
- Torn tongue frenulum
- Possible ligature marks (abrasions or bruises) to limbs or neck.

In addition, there are certain patterns of injury which in the absence of any credible explanation, must raise suspicions of non-accidental causation. Thus, bruises in non-mobile infants, bruises over areas of soft tissues, patterned bruises, and multiple similar-shaped bruises should raise concerns.

Scalds

Research shows that intentional scalds are often immersion injuries caused by hot water affecting the extremities (glove and sock distribution), buttocks, or perineum. They tend to be symmetrical with well-defined clear upper margins. Unintentional scald injuries are more commonly due to spill injuries of other hot liquids, affecting the upper body with irregular margins and variable depth of burn.

Fractures

When considering infants and very young children (aged <18 months), physical abuse must be considered in the differential diagnosis when they present with a fracture in the absence of clear history of trauma or a known diagnosis causing bone fragility.

Other research indicates that the following factors may be used to inform decisions about the likelihood of abuse when bone fracture is present, although it must be emphasized that these are not 'diagnostic', but indicative that abuse should at least be considered:

- Multiple fractures are more common after physical abuse than after accidental injury.
- A child with rib fractures has a 7 in 10 chance of having been abused.
- A child with a femoral fracture has a 1 in 3–4 chance of having been abused.
- Femoral fractures resulting from abuse are more commonly seen in children who are not yet walking.
- A child aged <3 years with a humeral fracture has a 1 in 2 chance of being abused.
- Mid-shaft fractures of the humerus are more common in abuse than in non-abuse, although supracondylar fractures are more likely to have non-abusive causes.
- Infants or toddlers with a skull fracture have a 1 in 3 chance of having been abused.
- There is no clear difference in patterns of skull fracture between abused and non-abused children.

Further reading

National Institute for Health and Clinical Excellence (2009). *When to suspect child maltreatment.* Available at ♪ http://www.nice.org.uk

Physical abuse: examination

Approach to examination

A child who is suspected of having sustained physical abuse needs to undergo a comprehensive head-to-toe examination with appropriate consent. Particular features that must be recorded in addition to assessment of cardiovascular, respiratory, abdominal, and neurological signs where relevant are:

- Height (with reference to relevant centile chart).
- Weight (and calculation of body mass index), with reference to centile chart.
- Head circumference.
- Scars.
- Healing/old injuries.
- New injuries (all features to be noted).

Each injury, scar, or mark must be examined and documented in appropriate detail (preferably in written form, on body diagrams and photo-documented), so that they are capable of subsequent proper external review and interpretation. If injury is noted, consideration should be given to repeat examination and serial photography to record the evolution of injury or scars.

Examination routine

Specific examinations that must always be undertaken to ensure occult injury is not missed include:

- Examination of scalp through hair (looking for areas of hair loss, petechiae, bruises, abrasions, reddening, scars).
- Examination behind ears (bruising from direct impact, pinching).
- Examination in ears (blood or effusion behind tympanic membrane).
- Examination of eyes—sclera, evert eyelids, retina. Subconjunctival haemorrhages can be caused by direct trauma or persistent coughing and vomiting. Retinal haemorrhages may be seen after childbirth and may be seen after accidental trauma. Their presence may reflect a child who has been shaken or struck, but interpretation should always be sought from an ophthalmologist.
- Mouth examination for ulcers, petechiae, torn frenulum, teeth injury, tongue injury—may all reflect accidental or deliberate injury.

In each case, it is important that such findings are sought so that they can be included in an overall assessment to make a determination as to whether the findings are consistent or not with physical abuse.

Skeletal survey

If physical abuse is suspected, then consideration must be given to a full radiographic skeletal survey, which must subsequently be reviewed by a paediatric radiologist. The American Academy of Pediatrics Section on Radiology (2000) advised the following required images and technique for a skeletal survey:

- Views of the appendicular skeleton:
  - Humeri (AP)
  - Forearms (AP)
  - Hands (oblique PA)
  - Femurs (AP)
  - Lower legs (AP)
  - Feet (AP)
- Views of the axial skeleton:
  - Thorax (AP and lateral)
  - Pelvis (AP: including mid and lower lumbar spine)
  - Lumbar spine (lateral)
  - Cervical spine (lateral)
  - Skull (frontal and lateral)
- Technique:
  - High resolution film
  - Screen/film speed not to exceed 200
  - Low kVp
  - Single emulsion or special film-screen combination.

Laboratory tests

In addition, laboratory based investigations may also be required and include:

- Full blood count (screening for anaemia).
- Liver function tests (screening for hepatic trauma).
- Amylase (may indicate pancreatic trauma).
- Calcium, phosphorus, and vitamin D (screening for metabolic bone disease).
- Coagulation studies (screening for coagulation problems).
- Urinalysis (screening for renal trauma and infection).

Physical abuse: interpreting findings

Interpretation of physical findings in physical abuse cases requires a full understanding of mechanisms of injury and how those mechanisms apply with respect to accounts of causation (of which there may be several) given. It is generally appropriate to be cautious in giving definite opinions as to causation of injury with regard to legal (as opposed to therapeutic) needs when first assessing a child, as such opinions may subsequently be challenged in non-medical settings, such as courts. It is entirely appropriate to indicate clearly in the medical records that the findings seen are consistent with the account given.

The interpretation of injuries and the determination that those injuries are representative of child abuse is often a complex and difficult process. The consequences of such a determination may have huge significance for the child and their carers. Such determination must be undertaken by those with appropriate expertise.

Injuries resulting from physical abuse

Head injury

Includes the full range of severity, from external bruising alone to cranial fracture with significant brain injury and/or associated haemorrhage. Different mechanisms of injury (direct or indirect impact, rotation, or shaking injury) may give very different patterns of injury. Repeated pulling of scalp hair may result in traumatic alopecia. The 'shaken-baby' syndrome is an extremely complex area, requiring multiprofessional input and assessment in order to determine the relevance of clinical and radiological findings.

Skin injury

Cuts, grazes, lacerations, bruises, burns may all occur. The presence of patterns and clustering of injuries is often crucial in determining whether a particular event was abusive. In particular, it is important to recognize possible slap marks, punch marks, grip marks, pinching and poking marks. In addition to injuries caused by hands and fingers, any implement with a shape has the potential to leave an imprint of the pattern on the skin. If a patterned bruise of unknown origin is identified, it is important to inform those tasked with investigating the case, so that they can attempt to identify the causative implement, perhaps at a home address. Seizure of such an implement may allow forensic sampling linking the implement with the child. Additionally, those with darker skins are more likely to have visible evidence of previous injury to the skin, because of a tendency of healed tissue to develop hyper- or hypopigmentation compared with uninjured skin. Such marks may persist for many years, providing long-term evidence of abuse or assault. Certain injuries (e.g. cigarette burns: localized <1cm diameter circular scars or burns) are readily identifiable but may need to be distinguished from other causes, such as chickenpox or excoriated insect bite scars.

Abdominal injury

Although skin injury is common over the abdomen, physical abuse, often as blunt force injury (kicks or punches), can cause massive and potentially fatal injury. All intra-abdominal organs can be damaged—the two most serious consequences being bleeding (e.g. from ruptured liver or spleen) and infection (e.g. from ruptured bowel or stomach). The outcome of such events is often magnified by delay in presentation.

Chest injury

Unlike the abdomen, the chest contents have a rigid skeleton which offers some degree of protection to the chest contents, but adult assaults on children may still result in substantial injury including rib fractures, lung laceration and contusion, ruptured great vessels, and cardiac contusion. Whilst rib fractures in adults are quite common, the child's thoracic skeleton is much more elastic and so it takes relatively much more energy to cause a rib fracture in a child. Any evidence of blunt force injury to chest or abdomen must take into account that substantial injury may have few symptoms or signs initially.

Skeletal injury

The interpretation of skeletal injury in possible child abuse is a very specialized area. A range of injury may be seen, from obvious fractures, to subtle bony injuries only apparent as a result of subperiosteal new bone formation. In many cases, early imaging may miss pathological changes, so repeat imaging may be required.

Development of sexual characteristics

Background

In order to recognize and place in context those abnormal findings which might imply sexual abuse in children, it is first necessary to understand normal anatomy and sexual development in children.

Prepubertal female genitalia (Fig. 12.1)

The external female genitalia (vulva) comprise the mons pubis, labia majora, labia minora, clitoris, and vestibule. The hymen surrounds the entrance to the vagina. It usually has a single opening, but occasionally there may be two openings, or rarely, no opening at all (imperforate hymen). Along with the changes to the breasts and pubic hair that occur during puberty (see Tanner stages, Table 12.1), the labia minora and vestibule may enlarge and become folded.

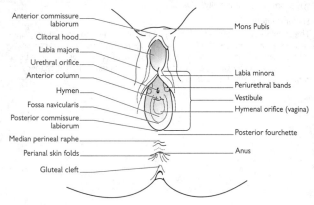

Fig. 12.1 Prepubertal female genitalia.

Puberty in girls

Tanner staging of pubic hair and the breasts are summarized in Table 12.1. In addition:
- 8–13 years: onset of puberty.
- ~12 years: axillary hair appears.
- ~13 years: menstruation commences.

Table 12.1 Tanner staging of female secondary characteristics

Stage	Pubic hair	Breasts
1	Prepubertal: no pubic hair	Elevation of breast papilla only
2	Sparse growth of downy hair along labia	Breast bud becomes elevated with a small mound
3	Starting to curl, becoming darker and spreading over the mons	Continuing enlargement of the breasts and areola
4	Adult type, coarse, curly hair, but limited to the mons pubis	Areola and papilla form a secondary mound
5	Adult type, coarse, curly hair, but limited to the mons pubis	Mature: adult type breast contour which includes areola with projection of papilla only

Puberty in boys
- 9–14 years: onset of puberty with enlargement of the testicles.
- 12–13 years: pubic hair and axillary hair starts to grow.
- 13–14 years: change in voice.
- 15–20 years: growth of facial hair.

Sexual abuse: presentation

Background

Sexual abuse may be chronic and long term or it may be an acute or single episode. The UK Department of Health showed 2600 child protection registrations for sexual abuse in 2006. This figure is considered a substantial underestimate, with figures for those convicted of sexual offences against children nearer to 20 000. In 2002, over 88 000 children were confirmed victims of sexual abuse in the USA. Research suggests that many individuals experience sexual abuse, but never disclose it. Disclosure may be delayed for days or many years, but this may result in loss of forensically supportive evidence. Research confirms that girls are more likely to have significant genital signs if examined within 7 days of the last episode of abuse. Anal signs in particular are more likely to be seen acutely. Delays in proper examination should be avoided when disclosure of recent sexual contact is made.

Managing disclosure

Child sexual abuse may present in many different ways. A child may disclose to an adult (e.g. parent, relation, teacher), friend, or sibling. A healthcare professional may identify a problem as a result of seeing the child for medical problems, injuries, or behavioural issues that may be precipitated by sexual abuse. If a child discloses sexual abuse:

• Listen and accept what is being said without displaying shock or disbelief.
• Reassure the child that they have done the right thing by disclosing.
• Do not make any promises that cannot be kept and do not promise confidentiality as there is a duty to refer.
• React to the situation only as far as necessary for you to establish whether you need to refer. Do not 'interrogate' for details.
• Ask open questions and avoid leading questions.
• Do not comment about or criticise the alleged perpetrator.
• Explain to the child what you have to do next and whom you have to contact.
• Make contemporaneous notes accurately recording the facts. Record verbatim the child's comments. You may need to explain terms used. Record the comments of the parent or carer.
• Record why the examination was requested, who requested it, where the examination took place, and who was present.
• If disclosure occurs during the examination or suspicions arise, note obvious injury or abnormality and record these on body charts (consider photo-documentation).
• If disclosure occurs and there is no medical or forensic urgency, it may be appropriate to defer examination until a forensically trained specialist is available.
• Ensure medical records are accurate, legible, comprehensible, dated, timed, and signed.

Presenting symptoms

Presenting symptoms may be general and non-specific, for example:
- Sleep disturbance
- Abdominal pain
- Enuresis
- Encopresis
- Phobia.

Presenting signs

Certain features are more specific and include:
- Abrasion and bruising of the genitalia.
- Acute or healed tear ins the posterior aspect of the hymen that extends to or nearly to the base of the hymen.
- A markedly decreased or absence of hymenal tissue in the posterior aspect.
- Injury to, or scarring of, the posterior fourchette, fossa navicularis, or hymen.
- Anal bruising or lacerations.

Sexual abuse: approach to examination

Approach

The principles of examination and documentation of the sexually abused child are in many respects similar to those of an adult, but with complexities added by virtue of consent issues and authority for documentation, recording, and storing notes, images, and other evidence such as colposcope recordings.

Guidelines

In 2008, in the UK, the Royal College of Paediatrics and Child Health, in conjunction with the Faculty of Forensic and Legal Medicine, produced guidelines related to child sexual abuse: *Guidelines on Paediatric Forensic Examinations in Relation to Possible Child Sexual Abuse.*

Key points include:
- Paediatric forensic examination will be required whenever a child has made a disclosure of sexual abuse or when a referring agency suspects abuse has occurred.
- Such an examination consists of:
  - Clinical history
  - Clinical examination
  - Detailed documentation (including the use of line drawings) and photo-documentation
  - Relevant forensic sampling.
- Every examiner has a responsibility to ensure that there is a therapeutic and supportive environment for the child and carer during the examination.
- Evaluating significant harm in sexual abuse includes not only the documentation of any genital or anal injury, but also any accompanying physical injury, the possibility of a sexually transmitted infection or pregnancy, and the short/long-term psychological or psychiatric sequelae.
- The assessment should lead the planning of any ongoing investigation or treatment required by the child.

Decision whether or not to examine

The need for examination following disclosure of chronic or historic sexual abuse will need to take into account its relevance. Examination of a female alleging penetrative sexual assault prepubertally, but disclosing in her 30s after vaginal delivery of children will provide no information. Examination of a prepubertal girl alleging vaginal penetration some months earlier may have value. A male alleging historic anal penetration with immediate pain and bleeding at the time may have persistent scarring. The key consideration is to determine whether any other intervening factor between the alleged event and the current time could have accounted for a potential abnormality. Testing for sexually transmitted infections must be done according to local protocols. Pregnancy testing may be appropriate.

Timing of examination

The timing of the examination needs to taken into account:
- The medical care of the examinee.
- The forensic clinical examination.
- The needs of forensic sampling.
- The likelihood of positive culture for sexually transmitted infection.
- Legal requirements.

Sexual abuse: examination procedure

Examining doctors

The assessment may be undertaken by a single doctor if that doctor has the necessary knowledge, skills, and experience for the case. Two doctors with complementary skills (e.g. a paediatrician and a forensic physician) are most appropriate.

Camera and/or colposcope

It is considered essential for a permanent record of the genital or anal findings to be obtained whenever examining a child for possible sexual abuse. A colposcope or camera may be used. The images must be of adequate quality to demonstrate the clinical findings. Further examinations may be required after initial assessments to determine whether abnormalities or features evolve/change.

Examination procedure

Examinations for acute or recent child sexual abuse are similar to those for adult sexual assault. Emphasis must be placed on as much detail of alleged events as possible to ensure proper consideration of body sites to be examined and forensic samples to be taken. Anogenital examination may be particularly stressful for a child and is done at the end of the general assessment and examination. Genital examination can be done in the supine 'frog-leg' position with hips flexed and the soles of the feet touching. If in a female an abnormality is found in the hymen, this should be followed by a prone knee–chest position. The lateral position may be appropriate for some children, whilst others may be comfortable held on a carer's lap. Other positions may be used. The key aim is to ensure clear, full, and unambiguous examination of the genitalia and anal region. In the majority of children, simple labial separation (Fig. 12.2) provides a good view of the hymen, although some children require the labial traction technique in order to obtain the best view (see Fig. 12.3).

Issues of consent will be dependent on the age and capacity of the examinee and advice may need to be sought as to the appropriate person who can (in the absence of the child's consent) consent to an examination and sampling. Examiners must be aware of a potential risk that an examination may further psychologically traumatize an already traumatized child. As with adult sexual assault, therapeutic intervention (e.g. for genital injury) may have priority over forensic examination, but if treatment is required under general anaesthesia, thought should be given to forensic assessment, with appropriate consent at the time of therapeutic intervention.

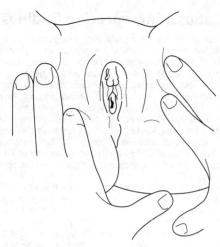

Fig. 12.2 Labial separation.

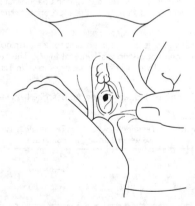

Fig. 12.3 Labial traction technique.

Sexual abuse: interpreting findings

The interpretation of physical signs found after genito-anal assessment is a minefield for the unwary. It is also important to understand that as the term 'child' includes those above the age of consent, issues of consensuality vs non-consensuality, as with the adult patient may also have great relevance. Thus, the presence of abnormality or injury may be associated with consensual as well as non-consensual contact. As with adult sexual assault, most complainants of child sexual abuse have no genito-anal abnormalities when examined after alleged sexual abuse. Kellogg and the Committee on Child Abuse in the USA reviewed the evaluation of child sexual abuse in 2005, and more recently (2008) in the UK the Royal College of Paediatrics and Child Health and the Faculty of Forensic and Legal Medicine published an evidence-based review on the physical signs of child sexual abuse.[1]

It is important to understand that the evidence-base is growing continually and this must be taken into consideration when interpreting findings from such reviews. In addition, when referring to publications such as these, it is essential that the primary sources of research are familiar so that appropriate interpretation is made. The 2008 publication uses precise terminology to describe the normal anatomy of the female, so that ambiguity in description is avoided (see 📖 Recommended terminology, p.401). Additionally, the publication draws attention to the need for precise terminology in the description of abnormality and injury, and gives clear recommendations as to the appropriate terms.

Hymenal disruptions

One of the areas where it is most important to use terminology which is generally agreed and understood is hymenal injury. The recommended terms used to describe hymenal disruptions are shown in Table 12.2.

Table 12.2 Recommended terminology to describe hymenal disruptions

Depth of hymenal disruption	Terminology to use when acute	Terminology to use when non-acute
Partial	Laceration	Notch (may be superficial or deep)
Complete to base of hymen	Laceration	Transection

Reference

1 Royal College of Paediatrics and Child Health in collaboration with the Royal College of Physicians of London and its Faculty of Forensic and Legal Medicine (2008). *The Physical Signs of Child Sexual Abuse*. London: RCPCH.

Recommended terminology

The following terms are those recommended in the 2008 publication: *The Physical Signs of Child Sexual Abuse* (by RCPCH and FFLM):

- *Abrasion*—superficial injury not extending through the full epidermis.
- *Anal fissure*—break or split in perianal skin radiating from anus (may be superficial or deep).
- *Anal gaping*—separation of the buttocks results in an open anus in a fixed way (of greater degree than anal laxity).
- *Anal laxity*—decreased muscle tone of anal sphincters.
- *Anal skin tag*—a protrusion of anal verge tissue interrupting the symmetry of the perianal skin folds (a projection of perianal skin).
- *Annular hymen*—the hymenal membrane extends completely around the circumference of the vaginal orifice.
- *Crescentic hymen*—hymen with attachments anteriorly with no hymenal tissue visible between the two anterior attachments.
- *Cribriform hymen*—a hymen with multiple openings.
- *Fimbriated hymen*—a hymen with highly folded edges, resulting in a flower-like appearance.
- *Fossa navicularis*—concavity of the lower part of the vestibule situated posterior to the vaginal orifice and extending to the posterior fourchette.
- *Hymenal bump*—a solid, localized, rounded, and thickened area of tissue on the edge of the hymen.
- *Hymenal laceration*—a fresh wound/tear (may be partial or complete).
- *Hymenal notch*—an indentation in the hymen not extending to its base.
- *Hymenal orifice*—opening to the vagina through the hymenal membrane.
- *Hymenal remnants*—small elevations or rounded mounds around the vaginal orifice.
- *Hymenal tag*—an elongated projection of tissue arising from any location on the hymenal rim. Commonly found in the midline.
- *Hymenal transection*—a (healed) discontinuity in the hymenal membrane that extends through the width of the hymen so there appears to be no hymenal tissue remaining at this location.
- *Hymenal width*—the visible amount of the membrane from its free margin to its base attachment to the vagina (measurement not recommended as it is difficult to obtain accurate measurements).
- *Imperforate hymen*—a hymenal membrane with no opening.
- *Median (perineal) raphe*—a ridge or furrow that marks the line of union of the two halves of the perineum.
- *Perianal fissure*—a split (break) in the perianal skin and/or mucosa that radiates out from the anal orifice, is confined to the anal margin and is usually <1cm in length.
- *Perianal lacerations*—acute tears in the anus and tissues around it:
  - First degree—superficial and <1cm long and/or not perpendicular to the anal margin.
  - Second degree—a laceration of the perianal skin and/or mucosa which involves the underlying musculature.
  - Third degree—extends through the underlying musculature and opens the anal canal or rectum.
- *Vulva*—the external genitalia (or pudendum) of the female.

Female child genital findings

The following summarizes key points for clinical practice taken from the RCPCH/FFLM 2008 publication *The Physical Signs of Child Sexual Abuse*, and should be interpreted having read this publication, and in the entire context of background, history, and all clinical findings of the individual case and any more recently published data by those with special expertise.

Genital erythema/redness/inflammation

- Genital erythema, redness, or inflammation has been reported in sexually abused prepubertal girls and 1% of girls selected for non-abuse. In pubertal girls, erythema is seen in a proportion of girls who allege penile penetration and are examined within 72h.
- Early examination is more likely to detect erythema. If the sign is of concern then re-examination should be undertaken. Other possible causes of erythema should be considered (e.g. acute trauma, infection, skin conditions, allergies, poor hygiene).

Oedema (swelling)

- There is insufficient evidence to determine the significance of oedema in prepubertal girls. In pubertal girls, oedema is seen in a proportion of girls who allege penile vaginal penetration and are examined within 72h after the abuse.
- Early examination is more likely to detect oedema. If this sign is of clinical concern, then the child should be re-examined. Other causes of oedema are inflammation, infection, and trauma.

Genital bruising

- Genital bruising has been reported in prepubertal girls alleging vaginal penetration examined soon after the abusive episode. It has not been reported in the only study of prepubertal girls selected for non-abuse that looked for it. There is some evidence that genital bruising is associated with sexual abuse in pubertal girls.
- Early examination is more likely to detect genital bruising. If this sign is of clinical concern then the child should be re-examined. There are many other causes of bruising or apparent bruising: haematological disorder, lichen sclerosis, and haemangioma. Sexual abuse should always be considered if bruising is present.

Genital abrasions (grazes)

- Genital abrasions have been reported in prepubertal girls with a history of vaginal penetration. In one study of prepubertal girls selected for non-abuse, abrasions were not been reported. In pubertal girls, genital abrasions are seen in a proportion of girls who allege penile penetration and are examined within 72h.
- Early examination is more likely to detect abrasions. If this sign is of concern then the child should be re-examined to assist. Other causes of abrasions which should be considered are infection, inflammation, and excoriation due to itchy skin. Sexual abuse should always be considered if abrasions are present.

Hymenal/posterior fourchette and fossa navicularis lacerations/tears

- Hymenal lacerations/tears have been described in prepubertal girls with a history of vaginal penetration/fondling. These were not seen in girls selected for non-abuse. In pubertal girls, hymenal lacerations/tears are seen in a small proportion of girls, 90% of whom alleged penile penetration.
- Posterior fourchette/fossa tears have been reported in prepubertal girls with history of vaginal penetration, but not in girls selected for non-abuse. In pubertal girls, tears are seen in a large proportion who allege penile penetration and are examined within 72h.
- All girls with acute genital bleeding need assessment within 24h to determine the cause of bleeding. If lacerations are found on the genitalia, sexual abuse should be strongly suspected in the absence of a clear history of accidental injury.

Hymenal transections

- Are seen in a small proportion of prepubertal girls with history of penetrative abuse. They are not seen in girls selected for non-abuse. They are seen in a small proportion of pubertal girls with alleged vaginal penile penetration.
- Hymenal injuries heal rapidly and unless large, can leave no residue.
- Scars to the hymen or posterior fourchette have been reported at the site of acute injuries in a small proportion of prepubertal and pubertal sexually abused girls. Scars appear to be associated with sexual abuse.
- A hymnenal transection is strongly suggestive of penetrative injury.
- It is not possible to time injury from the presence of a scar.

Hymenal clefts and notches

- Clefts and notches in the anterior hymen have been described in newborns and in prepubertal sexually abused and non-abused girls. Superficial notches have been reported in prepubertal girls with a history of vaginal penetration and those selected for non-abuse.
- Deep clefts or notches in the posterior half of a non-fimbriated hymen have only been reported in prepubertal girls with a history of vaginal penetration. In pubertal girls, such findings have been reported more often in girls with a history of vaginal penetration/consensual sexual intercourse than in girls denying this.

Hymenal diameters

- Hymenal diameters are difficult to measure. Hymenal diameter is non-discriminatory in prepubertal girls for abuse or non-abuse.
- There is insufficient evidence to determine the significance of hymenal diameter in pubertal girls.

Labial fusion

- Extensive and partial labial fusion is seen in both prepubertal girls reporting vaginal penetration and girls selected for non-abuse.
- There is insufficient evidence to determine the significance of labial fusion in prepubertal girls.
- Re-examination should be undertaken (after treatment if necessary) if labial fusion is seen.

Anal findings in suspected child abuse

The evidence is summarized as follows.

Anal/perianal erythema

- Is seen in a small proportion of children who allege sexual abuse (including anal penetration) and in children selected for non-abuse.
- It is more likely to be seen in an abused child if examined early.
- Other causes for these findings must be considered including: injury, infection, threadworm, poor hygiene, faecal soiling, and skin conditions.

Perianal venous congestion

- Appears to be present in both abused and non-abused children.

Anal/perianal bruising

- Has been reported in a small proportion of children alleging sexual abuse (including anal penetration). Not been reported in children selected for non-abuse. Early examination is important and re-examination to note resolution/evolution of abnormalities.
- Other causes for these findings must be considered including: trauma, haematological disorder, lichen sclerosus, haemangioma.

Anal fissures, lacerations, scars, and tags

- One study indicates that acute and chronic anal fissures are a frequent finding in anally abused children. Anal fissure has been reported in a study of children selected for non-abuses.
- Tears and lacerations are associated with sexual assault and have not been reported in non-abused children.
- Anal scars appear to be associated with anal abuse. Anal scars have not been seen in those selected for non-abuse.
- Skin tags are found in and away from the midline in children who have been anally abused. Midline skin tags have been observed in children selected for non-abuse.
- Other causes for anal fissure (e.g. current constipation or passage of a large hard stool) must be considered.
- It is sometimes difficult to distinguish between fissures and lacerations.

Reflex anal dilatation

- Refers to the dynamic action of the opening of the anus due to relaxation of the external and internal sphincters with minimal buttock traction. Usually examined in left lateral position and observation maintained for 30s after parting the buttocks.
- Has been described in children who allege anal abuse and sexual abuse. Very little data on the prevalence in children selected for non-abuse, although it has been noted in this group.
- Should raise the possibility of sexual abuse.

Sexual abuse and infections

Vaginal discharge in prepubertal girls

- Is seen more often in sexually abused prepubertal girls than in prepubertal girls selected for non-abuse. It is seen more frequently in girls who have experienced penile vaginal penetrative abuse than other types of abuse.
- Although common it may often be culture negative. If persistent, screening for sexually transmitted infection should be undertaken.

Infections

The presence of certain infections may have relevance in sexual abuse enquiries:

- Sexual abuse is the most likely mode of transmission in pubertal and prepubertal children with gonorrhoea. Evidence does not help to establish the age at which the possibility of vertical transmission can be excluded.
- Penetrative sexual contact is the most likely mode of transmission in prepubertal children with genital infection caused by *Chlamydia trachomatis*. Evidence does not help to establish the age at which the possibility of vertical transmission can be excluded.
- Sexual abuse is a likely source of *Trichomonas vaginalis* infection in girls. Evidence does not help to establish the age at which the possibility of vertical transmission can be excluded.
- There are insufficient data in children to determine the significance of bacterial vaginosis in relation to child sexual abuse.
- There are insufficient data in children to determine whether genital mycoplasmas are sexually transmitted in children.
- There are insufficient data to determine whether sexual contact is a likely route of transmission in children with syphilis.
- A significant proportion of children with anogenital warts have been sexually abused. Evidence does not help to establish the age at which the possibility of vertical transmission can be excluded.
- Very limited data exist on whether sexual abuse is likely to be the mode of transmission in children with genital herpes, although a small number of cases have been described.
- There are insufficient data to determine the significance of hepatitis B and C in child sexual abuse.
- Sexual abuse is a likely source of infection in children with HIV in whom the possibility of mother–child transmission or blood contamination has been excluded.

Neglect and emotional abuse

Neglect is the persistent failure to meet a child's basic physical or psychological needs, which is likely to result in the serious impairment of the child's health or development. It must be diagnosed at an early stage as any prolongation of neglect may have severe long-term physical, emotional, and social consequences.

Features

Noticeable behaviour characteristics include:
- Age inappropriate social skills (e.g. inability to use knife and fork)
- Bedwetting and soiling
- Inability to use toilet or potty
- Inability to self-dress
- Smoking
- Drug and/or alcohol misuse
- Sexual precocity
- Failure to attend school.

Assessment

It is important to remember that an assessment should necessarily entail observation prior to a physical examination. Certain features should be considered and may be associated with neglect on such assessment and physical examination and include:
- Dirty habitus/unkempt child
- Ill-fitting, dirty, or absent items of clothes
- Matted hair, nits
- Dirty or uncut nails
- Local skin infections/excoriations
- Poor dental hygiene
- Low centiles for weight and height.

Failure to thrive

Occurs when a child fails to grow at the expected rate due to inadequate nutrition. In the UK this may apply to up to 5% of those under 5 years. Most have no physical illness, but may be neglected or emotionally abused.

Emotional abuse

Emotional abuse often occurs with neglect and may involve conveying to children that they are worthless or unloved, inadequate, or valued only insofar as they meet the needs of another person. It may feature age or developmentally inappropriate expectations being imposed on children. These may include interactions that are beyond the child's developmental capacity, as well as overprotection and limitation of exploration/learning or preventing the child participating in normal social interaction. It may involve seeing or hearing ill-treatment of another. It may involve serious bullying, causing children frequently to feel frightened or in danger or the exploitation or corruption of children. Some level of emotional abuse is involved in all types of child ill-treatment, but may occur alone.

Children at particular risk of emotional abuse are:
- Unplanned or unwanted children
- Children of the 'wrong' gender
- Disabled children
- Children who are ill
- Children with behavioural issues
- Children in unstable or chaotic family settings.

It is estimated in the UK that of children on the child protection register, 16–18% are on it under the category 'emotional abuse'. Emotional abuse is most prevalent in the 5–15-years age group, although overall 'neglect' is the most common reason for children to be on the register. These proportions vary from country to country and one of the reasons for this may be the variable definition and reporting techniques. Types and definitions of emotional abuse vary. The term ***psychological maltreatment*** is used by the American Professional Society on the Abuse of Children and describes six forms of such abuse which enable the concept of emotional abuse to be grasped:
- Spurning (verbal and non-verbal hostile rejection or degradation).
- Terrorizing (behaviour that threatens or is likely to harm physically the child or place the child or the child's loved objects in danger).
- Exploiting/corrupting (encouraging the child to develop inappropriate behaviours).
- Denying emotional responsiveness (ignoring the child's need to interact, failing to express positive affect to the child, showing no emotions in interactions with the child).
- Isolating (denying the child opportunities for interacting and/or communicating with peers or adults).
- Mental, health, medical, or educational neglect (ignoring or failing to ensure provision of the child's needs).

Approach when addressing these issues
The following approach may help:
- Confirm the presence of harmful or potentially harmful carer or parent behaviours.
- Define the nature of the interaction between carer and child and the adequacy of the level of physical and psychological care in the context of the potentially harmful behaviours.
- Consider the presence or absence of intent to harm and if such intent appears to be present notify statutory authority—if not present, consider mental-health based management (although local jurisdiction may compel reporting).
- Mental management needs to establish the carer's comprehension and acceptance of their harmful behaviour and to review the child's need for protection and the psychological adequacy of the care environment. Based on this an intervention programme can be established.

Fictitious illness by proxy

Fictitious illness by proxy (also known as factitious illness by proxy, fabricated illness by proxy, Münchausen syndrome by proxy, or induced illness) is a term used to describe a setting in which a parent or carer presents a false history or appearance of illness for their child to healthcare professionals. There are many ways in which illness can be claimed, fabricated or induced and include:

- Manipulation of required drug therapy (e.g. in epilepsy).
- Suffocation.
- Apnoeic attacks.
- Administration of noxious substances.
- Injury (e.g. to mimic bleeding from the urinary tract).

Presentation

The child may present or be presented to healthcare professionals with a range of symptoms, including one or more of: vomiting (e.g. after administration of salt), diarrhoea (e.g. administration of laxatives), bleeding (e.g. scratching of inside of mouth), fever, convulsions, rashes, failure to thrive, drowsiness/altered consciousness.

Motivation

The motives behind such behaviour are very complex and often not determined. Examples of reasons for parents or carers creating fictitious illnesses have been said to include:

- Emotional relationship with child.
- Behavioural disorder.
- Personality disorder.
- Attention-seeking.
- Financial (award of disability or carer grants).
- Wanting to establish relationships with healthcare professionals.
- Seeking acclaim or support from families or friends.

Behaviour underlying fabricated and induced illness is variable in nature—some situations involving active interventions (commission) and others involving omission (e.g. failure to administer medication).

Features

Features which may be part of fictitious illness are:

- Frequent visits to primary care physician.
- Referrals to different hospital specialists and many Emergency Department attendances.
- Illness course is not typical of the illness described.
- Illness fails to respond to prescribed therapies.
- Parent or carer is very familiar with medical terminology.
- Resentment at suggestion that there is no illness.

Investigation of suspected fictitious illness is complex and sensitive. All agencies/professionals need to agree to the best course of action, which may include the involvement of GP, health services, social care services, and police. Covert surveillance is controversial, but may be the only way of confirming the suspected pattern of behaviour.

Management of child abuse

The management of child abuse depends on the type of abuse or abuses experienced and many other factors such as their health and where they are living. Every jurisdiction has its own legal requirements, policies, protocols and procedures. Relevant UK procedures in child abuse management have been referred to earlier in this chapter. It is the responsibility of every healthcare professional working with children, parents, or carers to acquaint themselves with this information so that they carry out their duties, requirements, and responsibilities to the benefit of the potentially abused child. Doing nothing is not an option.

Further reading

British Medical Association (2009). *Child protection – a toolkit for doctors*. Available at ℗ http://www.bma.org.uk/ethics/consent_and_capacity/childprotectiontoolkit.jsp

Children Act 1989. Available at ℗ http://www.opsi.gov.uk/acts/acts1989/Ukpga_19890041_en_1.htm

Donald T. (2005). Children: emotional abuse. In: Payne-James JJ, Byard RW, Corey TS, Henderson C (eds) *Encyclopedia of Forensic & Legal Medicine*. Oxford: Elsevier Academic Press.

Jenny C (2005). Children: physical abuse. In: Payne-James JJ, Byard RW, Corey TS, Henderson C (eds) *Encyclopedia of Forensic & Legal Medicine*. Oxford: Elsevier Academic Press.

Kellogg N and the Committee on Child Abuse and Neglect (2005). The evaluation of sexual abuse in children. *Pediatrics* **116**:506–12.

Kemp AM, Dunstan F, Harrison S, *et al.* (2008). Patterns of skeletal fractures in child abuse: systematic review: *BMJ* **337**:859–62.

Maguire S, Mann MK, Sibert J, Kemp A (2005). Are there patterns of bruising in childhood which are diagnostic or suggestive of abuse? A systematic review. *Arch Dis Child* **90**:182–6.

Royal College of Paediatrics and Child Health in collaboration with the Royal College of Physicians of London and its Faculty of Forensic and Legal Medicine (2008). *The Physical Signs of Child Sexual Abuse: an evidence-based review and guidance for best practice*. London: RCPCH.

Royal College of Paediatrics and Child Health/Faculty of Forensic and Legal Medicine (2007). *Guidelines on Paediatric Forensic Examinations in Relation to Possible Child Sexual Abuse*. Available at ℗ http://www.rcpch.ac.uk/doc.aspx?id_Resource=3379

Watkeys, JM, Price LD, Upton PM, Maddocks A (2008). The timing of medical examination following an allegation of sexual abuse: is this an emergency? *Arch Dis Child* **93**:851–6.

Psychiatric aspects

Introduction

Background

Forensic physicians and healthcare professionals working in a custody environment will inevitably be called upon to consider many problems relating to the mental health of detainees. Often the request to attend will be the result of positive answers from detainees about a past history of mental health problems or self-harm. These matters form part of the routine risk assessment made by custody staff in order to assess the medical risk or need for medical attention of those brought into police custody.

Although there is an increased incidence of psychiatric illness and self-harm amongst people in police custody, the psychiatric conditions of individuals who are in custody are no different from those found in the general population. The clinical assessment should be conducted as it would be elsewhere in a more normal setting. However, the range of options and recommendations available to the forensic practitioner following a mental health assessment in police custody are different and need to be clearly understood.

Psychiatric roles of the forensic practitioner

In a custody context, the forensic practitioner needs to be able to do the following:

- Conduct an assessment under the relevant mental health legislation.
- Consider diversion from the criminal justice system.
- Assess the impact of a detainee's mental illness on fitness for interview.
- Advise on the need for an appropriate adult (see 📖 p.186).
- Assess the risk of suicide or self-harm.

Definitions of some common terms

- *Comorbidity*—the simultaneous presence of two or more disorders, often referring to combinations of severe mental illness, substance misuse, learning disability, and personality disorder.
- *Delirium*—an organic mental state in which altered consciousness is combined with psychomotor over-activity, hallucinosis, and disorientation.
- *Depersonalization*—a subjective feeling of altered reality of the self (e.g. 'I feel unreal, I'm not myself anymore').
- *Derealization*—a subjective feeling of altered reality of the environment (e.g. 'Things aren't the same anymore, everything seems like in a dream').
- *Delusion*—a false belief out of keeping with the patient's cultural and intellectual background.
- *Dual diagnosis*—dual diagnosis is a term used to describe people with a combination of substance misuse (including alcohol) and mental illness. This is a particularly common problem amongst those with a history of offending and involvement in the criminal justice system—forensic practitioners should be diligent in enquiring about a history of substance misuse in all those detainees with a mental disorder and vice versa.
- *Flight of ideas*—accelerated thinking in which associations between ideas are casual, but where links are detectable and the flight can be followed. Typical of hypomanic and manic illnesses.
- *Hallucinations*—a perception occurring in the absence of an outside stimulus.
- *Ideas of reference*—a perception that events and objects have a special significance to the individual.
- *Mental disorder*—defined in the Mental Health Act 2007 as 'any disorder or disability of the mind'.
- *Passivity*—a feeling of bodily influence or control by outside agents.
- *Personality disorder*—this term covers a variety of clinically significant conditions and behaviour patterns, which tend to be persistent and arise in childhood or adolescence. They are not secondary to other mental disorders, but may coexist with them.
- *Psychopathic disorder*—a persistent disorder or disability of mind (whether or not including significant impairment of intelligence) which results in abnormally aggressive or seriously irresponsible conduct on the part of the person concerned.
- *Thought disorder*—a disturbance of the process of conceptual thinking that in its mild forms may manifest itself as a subjective inability to think clearly whereas, in its severe form, patients' speech may be reduced to fragmented nonsense or 'word salad'.

Anxiety disorders

Generalized anxiety disorder (GAD)

This is a long-term condition that fluctuates in severity and nature, often beginning in adolescence. The essential feature of GAD is excessive anxiety and worry occurring for a period of at least 6 months. It may be associated with:

- Restlessness or feeling 'keyed up' or 'on edge'.
- Easy fatiguability.
- Difficulty concentrating (important when considering fitness to interview).
- Irritability.
- Muscle tension.
- Disturbed sleep.

Phobias

These have similar symptoms to GAD, but limited to certain situations. The five main features are:

- Marked and persistent fear, cued by the presence or anticipation of a specific object or situation (e.g. needles, enclosed spaces).
- Exposure to the phobic stimulus almost invariably provokes an immediate anxiety response.
- The person recognizes that the fear is excessive or unreasonable.
- Avoidance of the phobic situation.
- Anticipatory anxiety when there is the prospect of encountering the phobic situation.

Panic disorder

Panic attacks are very common, but panic disorder is uncommon. The term refers to a chronic disorder whose essential feature is the presence of recurrent, unexpected panic attacks followed by persistent concern about having further panic attacks.

Panic attacks

Discrete periods of intense fear or discomfort which have a sudden onset and build to a peak rapidly (usually within 10min) and are associated with four or more of the following symptoms:

- Palpitations
- Sweating
- Trembling or shaking
- Shortness of breath
- Feeling of choking
- Chest pain or discomfort
- Nausea
- Dizziness or light-headedness
- Derealization or depersonalization
- Fear of losing control
- Fear of dying
- Numbness or tingling
- Chills or hot flushes.

Substance-induced anxiety disorder

This is characterized by prominent symptoms of anxiety which are judged to be the direct physiological consequence of a drug of abuse, a medication, or toxin exposure.

Post-traumatic stress disorder (PTSD)

Caused by experiencing or witnessing a traumatic event and characterized by:
- Intrusive recollection—thoughts, flashbacks, nightmares.
- Avoidance behaviour.
- Increased arousal—anxiety, irritability, insomnia, poor concentration.

Obsessive–compulsive disorder

This tends to present in young adults and is characterized by obsessions (which cause marked anxiety or distress) and/or by compulsions (which serve to neutralize anxiety). Often patients are aware that what they are thinking or doing is irrational and are too embarrassed to tell anyone.

Mixed anxiety and depression

Combinations of anxiety and depression are relatively common, particularly amongst women. When anxiety and depression occur together, symptoms tend to be more severe and there is an increased functional impairment.

Mood disorders

Mood disorders are relatively common amongst the general population.

Major depression

Essential features of a major depressive episode are illness of ≥2 weeks with either depressed mood or loss of interest or pleasure in doing things in association with five or more minor symptoms of depression:

- Change in appetite
- Insomnia or hypersomnia
- Fatigue or loss of energy
- Poor concentration
- Lethargy
- Low self-esteem
- Psychomotor agitation or retardation
- Sense of worthlessness or guilt
- Recurrent thoughts of death or suicidal ideation
- Feeling of hopelessness.

Psychotic symptoms (hallucinations or delusions) can occur.

Mild depression

Some of the listed symptoms of major depression (but not enough to make a diagnosis of major depression) associated with some functional impairment.

Dysthymia

Chronic minor depression characterized by at least 2 years of depressed mood for more days than not, accompanied by additional depressive symptoms that do not meet the criteria for a major depressive illness.

Mania and hypomania

Mania refers to a period of abnormally and persistently elevated, expansive, or irritable mood lasting at least 1 week associated with:

- Inflated self-esteem or grandiosity
- Decreased need for sleep
- Increased pressure of speech
- Flight of ideas
- Distractibility and poor concentration
- Increased sexual desire
- Decreased insight
- Spending sprees
- Over-assertiveness and disinhibition
- Hallucinations.

Hypomania

This is a less severe form of mania.

Bipolar disorder or manic depression

In this condition, individuals have episodes of mania (bipolar I) or hypomania (bipolar II) against a background of depression.

Psychotic illness

A class of illnesses characterized by three key features:
- Hallucinations
- Delusions
- Thought disorder.

Psychotic illnesses can be subdivided into:
- Affective psychoses—psychotic depression, mania, and hypomania.
- Delusional psychoses—schizophrenia and paranoid psychoses.
- Organic psychoses—the dementias, acute confusional states.

Schizophrenia

This is a frightening and disabling condition in which the patient is unable to distinguish between fact and fantasy.

First rank symptoms

These are generally reliable markers of schizophrenia, the presence of one or more being suggestive of the condition.
- Auditory hallucinations in the form of commentary.
- Hearing thoughts spoken out loud.
- Hearing thoughts referring to the patient, made in the third person.
- Somatic hallucinations.
- Thought broadcasting.
- Thought withdrawal, insertion, and interruption.
- Delusional perception.
- Feelings of passivity.

Paranoid psychosis

This is a form of schizophrenia in which delusions or auditory hallucinations are prominent, in the context of a relative preservation of cognitive functioning and affect. Delusions are typically persecutory.

Acute confusional states (delirium)

Most common in the elderly (particularly with a background of dementia) in whom there is sudden deterioration in cognitive functioning. Acute confusional states in police detainees are most likely to be drug-related.

Causes

- Infection.
- Drugs—opiates, cocaine, amphetamines, major tranquillisers, L-dopa.
- Metabolic—hypoglycaemia, uraemia, liver failure, hypercalcaemia.
- Alcohol or drug withdrawal.
- Hypoxia.
- Stroke and transient ischaemic attack.
- Head injury, space-occupying lesions (tumours, intracranial haematomas).
- Thyroid disease.
- Carcinomatosis.
- Nutritional deficiency—B12, thiamine or nicotinic acid deficiency.
- Epilepsy.

Learning disability

Individuals with learning disability are over-represented amongst those detained in police custody (incidence 5–8%). Individuals with learning disabilities are very likely to have deficits in communication, memory, and problem solving that can affect the outcome of their cases—hence the importance of identifying them and putting in place safeguards to protect their interests (such as an appropriate adult, see 📖 p.186).

Definition of learning disability

Learning disability is defined as a state of arrested or incomplete development of mind which includes significant impairment of intelligence and social functioning. Learning disability is to be preferred to the older terms mental handicap and mental retardation.

Learning disability should not be confused with specific 'learning difficulties'. The latter does not imply any disorder and usually refers to a person who finds one particular thing hard, but manages well in everything else. For example, a child can have a specific learning difficulty in reading, writing, or understanding what is said to them (e.g. dyslexia), but have no problem with learning in other areas of life.

Categories of learning disability

Causes of learning disability include: genetic factors, infection before birth, brain injury at birth, brain infections, or damage after birth (e.g. Down's syndrome, Fragile X syndrome, and cerebral palsy). However, in nearly one-half of children affected, the cause of the disability remains unknown.

The degree of disability can vary greatly. Some children never learn to speak and even when they grow up need help to look after themselves—feeding, dressing, or going to the toilet. On the other hand, the disability may be mild, allowing the child to grow up to become independent.

Learning disability should not be diagnosed or categorized solely on the basis of an intelligence test or intelligence quotient (IQ) because it is a condition not only of reduced intellectual functioning, but also a diminished ability to adapt to the daily demands of normal life.

Nonetheless, as a rough guide the condition is divided into four groups:
• Borderline: IQ of 70–79.
• Mild: IQ of 50–69.
• Moderate: IQ of 35–49.
• Severe: IQ of 20–34.

People with severe learning disability almost invariably need to be cared for by others. Although they may exhibit violent behaviour, their ability to gain insight into the criminality of their actions is likely to be seriously restricted and they are usually diverted away from the criminal justice system. Therefore, individuals with a mild–moderate or borderline learning disability will form the majority of those seen as a forensic practitioner.

Recognizing detainees with learning disability

There is no easy way to know if a detainee has a learning disability, so the forensic practitioner needs to be alert to the possibility whenever assessing detainees in custody. Many individuals with mild or borderline learning disability appear very 'street wise' and are adept at hiding their disability.

Problems exhibited by detainees with learning difficulty

Individuals with learning disability *may* have difficulty:

- Speaking.
- Moving.
- Understanding.
- Reading and writing.
- Telling the time.
- Remembering their date of birth, age, address, telephone number.
- Knowing the day of the week, where they are, and who you are.

In addition, they *may*:

- Also have physical disabilities, visual or hearing impairments (but most people with physical disabilities do not have learning disabilities).
- Appear very eager to please and/or repeat what is said to them.

Questions to identify learning disability

There are a number of questions that the forensic practitioner can ask in order to help identify a detainee with learning disability. These include asking:

- Where they live (do they live in a group home, hostel, hospital, or, as an adult, still live with their parents?).
- Where they work (do they attend a special work scheme?).
- Where they went to school (was it a special school?—if it was, their IQ is almost certainly <70).
- If they carry special identification.
- If they have a social worker or key worker.
- If they go to a Day Centre.
- If they get a disability living allowance.
- If people say that they have learning disabilities or are mentally handicapped.

If the pattern of answers suggests that a person might have a possible learning disability, the forensic practitioner should consider conducting a Mini-Mental State Examination (see 📖 p.425). A score of 20 or less would support the diagnosis of a learning disability.

Psychiatric illness, alcohol, and drugs

Dual diagnosis (the coexistence of substance misuse and mental illness) is common amongst those who come into contact with the criminal justice system. It should be noted, however, that dependence on alcohol or drugs alone is not considered to be a disorder or disability of the mind for the purposes of the Mental Health Act 2007 (MHA 2007). This means there are no grounds under the Act for detaining a person in hospital (or using other compulsory measures) purely on the basis of alcohol or drug dependence. By contrast, when alcohol or drug dependence is accompanied by, or associated with, a mental disorder which does fall within the Act's definition, it is possible to detain people who are suffering from mental disorder, even though they are also dependent on alcohol or drugs, as long as the relevant criteria for compulsory admission are met. This is true even if the mental disorder in question results from the person's alcohol or drug dependence.

The MHA 2007 does not exclude other disorders or disabilities of the mind related to the use of alcohol or drugs. These disorders (for example, withdrawal state with delirium or associated psychotic disorder, acute intoxication, and organic mental disorders associated with prolonged abuse of drugs or alcohol) remain mental disorders for the purposes of the Act.

Excited (agitated) delirium

This is one of the most dangerous drug-induced states the forensic practitioner is likely to encounter amongst those detained in police custody, as detainees with this condition are at risk of sudden collapse and death. Although there is controversy about the precise definition of the condition, the clinical features are generally accepted to be:

- Bizarre and/or violent behaviour.
- Agitation.
- Impaired thinking.
- Hallucinations.
- Hyperpyrexia, sweating, and excessive thirst.
- Unexpected physical strength.
- Insensitivity to pain and apparent ineffectiveness of restraint sprays.

Excited delirium can be caused by drug intoxication, psychiatric illness, or a combination of both. Cocaine (see ⌑ p.472) is the best known cause of drug-induced excited delirium, although many other drugs have been implicated, including prescribed neuroleptics.

One particular concern about excited delirium is that it is often necessary to restrain individuals exhibiting signs and symptoms previously listed for their own protection and the protection of others. However, there appears to be a correlation between physical restraint (in particular, certain types of physical restraint such as 'hog-tying') and sudden death in these patients (see ⌑ p.272). Thus, the police need to be aware of the symptoms of excited delirium and to appreciate that attempts at physical restraint should be avoided unless absolutely necessary.

Drug-induced psychosis

The essential features of a drug-induced psychosis are prominent hallucinations or delusions that are judged to be due to the direct physiological effects of a drug of abuse, a medication, or exposure to a toxin. The diagnosis should only be made when the psychotic symptoms (e.g. hallucinations) are in excess of those usually associated with intoxication or withdrawal from the particular drug.

Psychosis in association with intoxication can occur with:
- Alcohol
- Amphetamine and related substances
- Cannabis
- Cocaine
- Hallucinogens
- Hypnotics
- Opioids
- Phencyclidine and related substances
- Sedatives
- Solvents.

The time taken for the psychosis to develop varies considerably depending on the substance involved. For example, cocaine-induced psychosis may develop within minutes of ingesting high doses of the drug, whereas days or weeks of high-dose intake of alcohol or sedatives are usually required before the onset of psychosis with these drugs.

The clinical features of the psychoses induced by intoxication with cocaine and amphetamines are similar, with persecutory delusions usually developing rapidly after drug use. Although the psychotic features typically settle promptly after cessation of drug use, this is not always the case—there are reports of psychotic states persisting for several weeks despite stopping the drugs and treatment with neuroleptics.

Psychosis in association with withdrawal can occur with:
- Alcohol
- Anxiolytics
- Hypnotics
- Sedatives.

The commonest withdrawal-associated psychosis is that which occurs after heavy alcohol misuse in those with alcohol dependency. Vivid, persistent, and frightening hallucinations (typically auditory, but there may also be tactile or visual hallucinations) develop within 48–72h of stopping or reducing alcohol intake.

Assessing the mental state of those who are intoxicated

Where a detainee is subject to the effects of sedative medication, or the short-term effects of drugs or alcohol, the forensic practitioner should wait until, or arrange to return when, the effects have abated before conducting an assessment of the patient (unless this is not possible because of the patient's disturbed behaviour and the urgency of the case).

Violent/disturbed behaviour

Persons detained by the police not infrequently exhibit violent and/or disturbed behaviour. Such acute behavioural disturbance usually occurs in relation to misuse of alcohol and drugs (both intoxication and withdrawal), but may also be associated with physical illnesses (e.g. head injury, hypoglycaemia) and psychiatric conditions.

Predicting violent/disturbed behaviour

Disturbed/violent behaviour cannot be predicted with 100% accuracy. However, this does not mean that a risk assessment should not be carried out.

Risk factors

There are a number of factors that increase the risk of violent behaviour, including:

- Misuse of substances and/or alcohol.
- Drug effects (disinhibition, akathisia).
- Active symptoms of schizophrenia or mania.
- History of disturbed/violent behaviour.
- Previous expression of intent to harm others.
- Previous use of weapons.
- Previous dangerous impulsive acts.
- Verbal threat of violence.

Warning signs

Certain features can serve as warning signs to indicate that a detainee may be escalating towards physically violent behaviour, including:

- Facial expressions—tense and angry.
- Increased or prolonged restlessness, body tension, pacing.
- General over-arousal of body systems (increased breathing and heart rate, muscle twitching, dilating pupils).
- Increased volume of speech, erratic movements.
- Prolonged eye contact.
- Discontentment, refusal to communicate, withdrawal, fear, irritation.
- Thought processes unclear, poor concentration.
- Delusions or hallucinations with violent content.
- Verbal threats or gestures.
- Reporting anger or violent feelings.

Managing disturbed/violent behaviour

It is important to establish, as soon as possible, the likely cause for a detainee's disturbed behaviour and arrange immediate hospitalization if there is an underlying illness that poses a serious threat to health.

De-escalation

Once the decision has been taken to manage the detainee in custody, it is appropriate to consider recommending a period of de-escalation ('time-out') where the detainee may calm down (away from arresting officers).

Rapid tranquillization

If a period of de-escalation fails to curb disturbed behaviour, rapid tranquillization (also called urgent sedation) may need to be considered. Rapid tranquillization involves use of medication to lightly sedate the patient, inducing a state of rest in which verbal contact is maintained. The aims of rapid tranquillization are threefold:

• To reduce further suffering for the patient—psychological and physical (through self-harm or accidents).
• To reduce the risk of harm to others.
• To do no harm (by safe prescribing and monitoring physical health).

The decision to employ rapid tranquillization must be reasonable and proportionate to the risk it seeks to address. Use of medication for rapid tranquillization in a police station is a serious step because of risks of:

• Loss of consciousness instead of tranquillization.
• Sedation with loss of alertness.
• Compromised airway and breathing.
• Cardiovascular and respiratory collapse.
• Interaction with medicines already prescribed or illicit substances taken (can cause side effects such as akathisia, disinhibition).
• Possible damage to patient–doctor relationship.
• Underlying coincidental physical disorders.

Choice of medication[1,2]

Evidence suggests oral drugs can be as effective as intramuscular medication. Due to greater risks associated with parenteral treatment, rapid tranquillisation in custody should be restricted to oral therapy.

Lorazepam is recommended as the first-line drug of choice for use in police custody. The drug should be offered orally in a dose of 1–2mg—an appropriately trained healthcare professional should be in attendance to monitor the effect of the drug.

Specific risks associated with lorazepam use in these circumstances are:

• Loss of consciousness.
• Respiratory depression or arrest.
• Cardiovascular collapse (particularly detainees who may be receiving both clozapine and benzodiazepines).

If there is insufficient effect, the drug can be repeated up to 2 times at 45-min intervals up to a maximum dose of 4mg.

References

1 NICE (2005). *Violence: the short term management of disturbed/violent behaviour in in-patient settings and emergency departments.* Available at ℅ http://www.nice.org.uk
2 FFLM (2008). *Acute Behavioural Disturbance, Guidelines on Management in Police Custody.* Available at ℅ http://www.fflm.ac.uk

Assessment of the mental state

Clinical assessment of a detainee with a suspected mental disorder should begin by obtaining as much background information as is readily available from arresting officers, custody staff, relatives, friends, or healthcare workers already involved in the care of the detainee.

A police station is not an ideal environment to conduct a mental state examination, but efforts should be made to put the patient at ease as much as possible. Examinations should usually be performed in a medical room or an interview room, rather than a police cell. Both the forensic practitioner and the patient should be seated. Careful thought should be given to whether a police officer should be present in the room during the interview—the detainee's right to medical confidentiality should not outweigh considerations of personal safety.

When examining the detainee's mental state, it is important to avoid asking leading questions and/or antagonizing the patient if he/she appears to be evasive or uncooperative. The interview begins by introductions and explaining what the purpose of the examination is. Adopting a consistent style and approach to the mental state examination is far more likely to detect variations from the norm. A useful scheme for a mental state examination involves considering:

- Appearance—clothing (e.g. dishevelled, dirty), facial expressions, and whether they are appropriate (e.g. anxious, irritable, etc.).
- Behaviour—observing how the patient behaves during the interview, noting points such as disinhibited, withdrawn, preoccupied, distracted, aggressive behaviour.
- Motor—retardation, over-activity, Parkinsonism, tardive dyskinesia.
- Talk—noting both form and content (the simplest way of doing the latter is by recording a verbatim sample). Rate and quantity (fast, pressured, slow, monosyllabic, long pauses); volume and tone; flow (e.g. interruptions due to thought block or distraction, flight of ideas, loosening of associations) can also be noted.
- Mood—depression, anxiety, elation, irritability, lability.
- Delusions—often only elicited by careful questioning (e.g. thought interference, delusions of control, paranoid, grandiose, guilt, religious, hypochondriacal, amorous).
- Hallucinations—auditory, visual, tactile, olfactory, gustatory.
- Obsessive–compulsive phenomena.
- Cognition—orientation, attention and concentration, short-term memory, remote memory.
- Insight into what is happening.
- Suicidal or homicidal thoughts.

The examination of a detainee with a suspected mental disorder does not stop short at the mental state examination. The forensic practitioner should also take a general medical history, noting in particular any history of substance misuse and conduct a physical examination as appropriate. It is important to remember that many individuals with mental illness have co-existent physical disease and indeed, may have physical disease contributing to or causing their mental disorder.

Mini-Mental State Examination (MMSE)

When assessing the cognitive function of a detainee a modified Folstein MMSE may be useful. The MMSE is not suitable for making a diagnosis, but can be used to indicate the presence of cognitive impairment, such as in a person with suspected dementia or following a head injury. It is far more sensitive in detecting cognitive impairment than the use of informal questioning or overall impression of a patient's orientation. The test takes only about 10min and provides measures of orientation, registration (immediate memory), short-term memory (but not long-term memory), as well as language functioning, providing an overall total score. The MMSE has been validated in a number of populations. Scores of 25–30 out of 30 are considered normal; 18–24 indicate mild to moderate impairment; scores of 17 or less indicate severe impairment.

Table 13.1 The Mini-Mental State Evaluation

Score	Section	Task
	Orientation	
5	e.g.	What is the date?
	Registration	
3	e.g.	Listen carefully. I am going to say three words. You say them back after I stop. Ready? Here they are ... APPLE (pause), PENNY (pause), TABLE (pause), Now repeat those words back to me. (Repeat up to 5 times, but only score the first time)
	Language	
2	e.g.	What is this? (Point to a pencil or pen)
3	e.g.	Please read this and do what it say. (Show examinee the words on the stimulus form.) CLOSE YOUR EYES.
30	Total score	
Score results		
30-29	Normal	
28-26	Borderline cognitive dysfunction	
25-18	Marked cognitive dysfunction—may be diagnosed as demented	
<17	Severe dysfunction—severe dementia	

Assessment of suicide risk

The incidence of successful suicides in police custody has decreased in recent years. This is a result of many factors, including greater police awareness, routine suicide risk assessment by custody officers, and improved cell design to ensure absence of ligature points. Nonetheless, suicide remains a significant cause of deaths in police custody and assessment of suicide risk is an essential part of the forensic practitioner's role. The computerized 'Detained Person's Medical Form' that should be completed after each encounter with a detainee in police custody contains an obligatory field in which the forensic practitioner is required to indicate whether assessment of the risk of self-harm is considered to be standard, medium, or high. Although it will never be possible to predict every potential suicide in police custody, a careful risk assessment should identify most of those who are likely to harm themselves, thus allowing special precautions to be put in place.

General principles of risk assessment

There are a number of general principles of risk assessment that the forensic practitioner should be aware of:
• Risk can be assessed and managed.
• Risk varies over time.
• Risk varies according to circumstances.
• Some risks are general, others more specific.
• Interventions can decrease or increase risk.
• Demographic factors are poor predictors of risk.
• Assessment requires information from many sources.
• Assessment of risk should involve colleagues whenever possible.
• The outcome of the assessment process should be shared with others and recorded adequately.

Suicide risk factors

There are a number of factors that should alert to the increased risk of suicide. Some are general to all patients with mental illness:
• Demographic factors (male sex; younger age; single status; and living alone).
• History (previous suicidal behaviour; short duration of mental illness; several hospital admissions and/or admission within the last year; recent change in chronic illness; substance misuse).
• Mental state examination (depressed mood; feelings of hopelessness; psychosis; suicidal thoughts; communication of suicidal intent; suicidal content to psychotic phenomena).

Other factors are specific to the police custodial environment:
• Nature of offence (e.g. offences of sex, violence, and child abuse).
• Feelings of guilt associated with the offence.
• First time in custody.
• Early hours of detention.
• Alcohol and drug intoxication or withdrawal.

Assessing an episode of self-harm in custody

Acts of deliberate self-harm (DSH) are relatively common amongst those detained in police custody. Many of these acts may constitute attention seeking behaviour or an attempt to try and evade police custody. The challenge for the forensic practitioner is to assess whether there was serious suicidal intent behind an act of DSH. When assessing an act of DSH it is important to:

- Attempt to establish an adequate rapport with the detainee.
- Try to gain an understanding of recent events.
- Enquire about personal and social circumstances.
- Take a history of any substance misuse (including alcohol).
- Take a psychiatric history and conduct a mental state examination.

*Factors associated with an act of DSH that indicate a
high risk for suicide are:*

- A medically serious act of DSH.
- The writing of a suicide note.
- Precautions having been taken against being found.
- Stated wish to die.
- Belief that the act would have proved fatal.
- Expressed regret that the act failed.
- Previous episode of DSH.
- Depression and psychoses.
- Substance misuse.
- Comorbidity.
- Impulsive and aggressive personality traits.
- Loneliness and lack of a social network.

Advice to the police after an act of DSH

Having assessed a detainee following an act of DSH, the forensic practitioner should communicate the outcome of the suicide risk assessment to the custody staff both verbally and in writing (in the custody record). When the risk is considered to be high, custody staff should be instructed to keep the detainee under constant supervision and a request be made for an urgent psychiatric assessment.

Where you consider the risk of further self-harm to be moderate, the forensic practitioner should consider advising the police to:

- Move the detainee to a cell that can be closely monitored (e.g. by CCTV if available).
- Remove any objects from the cell and detainee that could be used to self-harm.
- Make frequent checks of the detainee at irregular intervals so that the detainee cannot anticipate when the next check will be made.
- Arrange for a further psychiatric assessment where appropriate.

Management of poisoning in police custody

Whenever a detainee is seen, or believed, to have swallowed drugs either in an attempt to conceal those drugs from the police or to self-harm they should be considered to have taken an overdose and be transferred to hospital for assessment and monitoring.

Fitness to interview

False confessions

The custodial interrogation of suspects is an important means of solving crime. The confessions and other inculpatory statements made during such interrogations are often relied on to provide evidence of guilt in criminal trials. Studies suggest that such evidence is crucial in about 30% of cases that proceed to Crown Court in England and Wales. However, it has long been recognized that, in certain circumstances, vulnerable individuals can make false and misleading admissions against their own interest. For example, the emotional shock experience by the victims of the Salem witch trials distorted their memory and led many to make what were frequently absurd confessions. More recently, a number of well-publicized miscarriages of justice in which the convictions depended heavily on admissions and confessions to the police that were subsequently shown to be untrue, have served to highlight the problem of false confessions. The challenge for the courts and the police since these judgments has been to preserve the value of the police interview as a means of solving crime whilst, at the same time, introducing safeguards to minimize the risk of involuntary and false confessions. The forensic practitioner's assessment of a detainee's fitness to be interviewed is one of these important safeguards.

Categories of false confessions

There are three principal categories of false confession:

Voluntary false confessions

These occur when individuals confess to a crime without any external pressure from the police. Such confessions may be motivated by a morbid desire for notoriety; an unconscious need to expiate guilt feelings through receiving punishment; a desire to protect someone else; or an inability to distinguish between fact and fantasy (e.g. in schizophrenia).

Coerced-compliant false confessions

These are typically elicited during persuasive interrogation where the person perceives that there is some immediate instrumental gain from confessing. Suspects do not confess voluntarily, but come to give in to the demands and pressures of the interrogators. They are fully aware of not having committed the crime and the confession is usually retracted.

Coerced-internalized false confessions

By contrast, coerced-internalized false confessions are made as a result of suspects coming to believe that they really have done the act in question. Either suspects have no memory at all of the alleged offence (e.g. due to alcohol-induced memory loss) or, as a result of subtle manipulative techniques employed by the interrogator, they begin to distrust their own memory and beliefs. These false confessions will only be retracted if and when the individuals realize that they are, in fact, innocent.

Factors that increase the likelihood of a false confession

Individuals may be vulnerable to making false confessions by virtue of their **P**ersonality, **H**ealth, the **I**nterview characteristics or the **T**otality of circumstances (PHIT).

Personality

False confessions are more common with increased suggestibility, compliance, and acquiescence:

- *Suggestibility*—the way leading questions produce distorted responses because they are phrased in such a way as to suggest the expected response (associated with anxiety, lack of assertiveness, poor self-esteem, and low IQ).
- *Compliance*—the tendency to obey the instructions of others when you don't really want to (associated with eagerness to please, wish to avoid conflict, feelings of guilt).
- *Acquiescence*—answering questions in the affirmative irrespective of the content (associated with low IQ, poor education).

Health

The risk of providing a false confession may be increased by physical or mental illness (including substance misuse).

- *Physical illness*—can increase a person's vulnerability due to factors associated with physical illness in general (e.g. physical illness is often associated with anxiety and depression which can both result in increased vulnerability) or disturbances in cognitive functioning specific to the disease in question.
- *Mental illness*—can affect the reliability of testimony in a number of ways (e.g. the distorted thought processes of schizophrenia cause inability to distinguish between fact and fantasy; lack of judgement and delusional ideas associated with hypomania; increased suggestibility and compliance associated with anxiety and depression; and the impact of learning disability).
- *Substance misuse*—intoxication by alcohol or drugs can adversely affect cognitive functioning, whereas withdrawal from alcohol and drugs can increase anxiety and induce depression. Individuals may consider that the risks entailed in providing a false confession are worthwhile in order to achieve early release and access to their supply of drugs or further alcohol.

Interview characteristics

The manner in which a police interview is conducted will have a major bearing on the ultimate reliability of any confession made by a suspect. Generally speaking, the more serious the offence is perceived to be, the more coercive the police interview is likely to be and the greater the risk of a false confession.

Totality of the circumstances

The final consideration is the overall totality of circumstances pertaining to the individual's arrest and custody (e.g. access to legal advice, adequacy of rest periods, and presence of significant social distractions).

Definition of fitness to interview

Annex G of PACE Codes of Practice, Code C, contains general guidance to help police officers, forensic physicians and other healthcare professionals assess whether a detainee might be at risk in an interview:

> A detainee may be at risk in an interview if it is considered that:
> (a) conducting the interview could significantly harm the detainee's physical or mental state;
> (b) anything the detainee says in the interview about their involvement or suspected involvement in the offence about which they are being interviewed might be considered unreliable in subsequent court proceedings because of their physical or mental state.

The role of the healthcare professional

The forensic practitioner should assess detainees' fitness for interview and advise the custody officer of the outcome of that consideration whenever asked by custody staff. Before starting an examination, forensic practitioners should routinely ask custody staff if a detainee will be interviewed and if so, whether an assessment of fitness for interview is required. If a detainee is deemed at risk in an interview, the forensic practitioner should try to quantify the risk and inform the custody officer:
• Whether the person's condition is likely to improve.
• Whether the condition requires or is amenable to treatment.
• How long it may take for any improvement to take effect.

Illnesses that might be significantly worsened by interview

The forensic practitioner should advise that a detainee will be unfit for interview if he/she has a physical or mental illness that is likely to deteriorate significantly because of the delay in obtaining treatment that the interview will engender and/or the stress of the interview.
  Examples of conditions that might fall into this category are:
• Detainee with chest pain and known ischaemic heart disease.
• Asthmatic with bronchospasm.
• Diabetic with either hypoglycaemia or hyperglycaemia.
• Detainee with migraine, severe anxiety, or panic attacks.

Assessing the likely reliability of a detainee's confession

In making this assessment the forensic practitioner should consider:
• How the detainee's physical or mental state might affect the ability to understand the nature/purpose of interview, to comprehend what is being asked, and to appreciate the significance of any answers and make rational decisions about whether to say anything.
• The extent to which the detainee's replies may be affected by their physical or mental condition rather than representing a rational and accurate explanation of their involvement in the offence.
• How the nature of the interview, which could include particularly probing questions, might affect the detainee.

Thus, it is important to consider various vulnerability factors that render an individual more likely to provide an unreliable confession (see 📖 p.429).

Scheme of examination

The history

Before interviewing the suspect the forensic practitioner should obtain as much background information as is practicable, including:

- Reason for the arrest.
- Any unusual factors surrounding the circumstances of the arrest.
- Any unusual behaviour since arrest.
- Any warnings on the PNC or concerns raised by the risk assessment.
- The proposed time and likely length of the interview.
- Any relevant property (medication, drug paraphernalia, etc.).

The following information should then be obtained from the detainee:

- A general medical history.
- Psychiatric history (including any previous suicide attempts).
- Medication (prescribed or over-the-counter).
- Use of illicit drugs and/or alcohol.
- Last meal.
- Sleep pattern, last period, and length of sleep.
- Social history.
- Forensic history (previous arrests, imprisonment).
- Occupation.
- Educational background (questions such as 'Do you have difficulty in reading and writing?' 'While at school did you receive some extra help because of learning difficulty?', and 'Did you attend a special needs school?' can all be useful.)

The examination

The nature and extent of the examination will depend on the circumstances of the case. It should include an appropriate general physical examination, looking in particular for signs of drug dependency, intoxication, and withdrawal. A brief mental state examination should be performed in all cases (is the detainee oriented, rational, and coherent?). Where there are concerns about mental health, a more detailed examination will be required. Finally, it is necessary to make a functional assessment of the detainee by considering factors such as:

- Is he/she aware of why he/she is at the police station?
- Does he/she know and understand his/her rights?
- Does he/she understand the police caution? (It may be necessary to explain it carefully first before assessing comprehension).

Fitness to be charged/plead

Fitness to be charged

PACE requires that suspects are dealt with expeditiously once arrested and that they are not detained for longer than necessary. Thus, the custody officer has a duty to determine, as soon as practicable, whether there is sufficient evidence with which to charge a detainee with the offence for which he/she was arrested. Once the custody officer determines that there is sufficient evidence to charge the detainee then the detainee must:

• Be charged; or
• Be released without charge, either on bail or without bail.

However, the custody officer can keep detainees in detention until such time as they are in a fit state to be dealt with under these provisions (i.e. fit to be charged).

Definition of fit to be charged

Detainees will be fit to be charged if they are capable of:

• Understanding the meaning of the written notice detailing the particulars of the offence (which should be stated in simple terms as well as following the precise wording of the offence in law); and
• Understanding the meaning of the statutory warning that precedes the details of the charge.

The statutory warning is:

'You are charged with the offence(s) shown below. You do not have to say anything. But it may harm your defence if you do not mention now something which you later rely on in court. Anything you do say may be given in evidence.'

Assessing fitness to be charged

This role is usually performed by the custody officer but, on occasions, the forensic practitioner may be asked to assess a detainee's fitness to be charged. Crucial to this is a functional assessment of the detainee's ability to understand the particulars of the offence and the statutory warning—it may be necessary to explain the meaning of these to the detainee before assessing whether he/she can understand it.

It should be noted that fitness to be charged is not the same as fitness to be interviewed, as those vulnerabilities that render an individual more likely to give a false confession to the police are not relevant when considering fitness for charge. However, if someone is deemed fit to be interviewed they will also be fit to be charged, unless there is any material change in their condition.

Fitness to plead

Under Article 6 of the European Convention of Human Rights, everyone is entitled to a fair trial. In order for trials to be fair, it is essential that defendants should be able to understand their situation and instruct their lawyers. This general capacity is known colloquially as 'fitness to plead'.

Definition of fitness to plead

A defendant will be deemed unfit to plead if he/she suffers from a disability (mental or physical illness) that renders him/her unable to:
- Understand the charge.
- Distinguish between a plea of guilty and not guilty.
- Instruct a lawyer.
- Challenge a juror to whom he/she might object.
- Understand the evidence.

Assessing fitness to plead

A finding of 'unfitness to plead' can only be returned by a jury and it is thus a matter for the court rather than doctors or nurses. However, in reaching its determination, the court will usually be assisted by psychiatric reports that may be commissioned by the defence, the Crown or the Court. When advising on a person's fitness to plead, psychiatrists are obliged to consider the mental condition of the defendant at the time of the trial, their mental condition at the time of the offence being of no relevance.

Generally speaking, only the most serious of psychiatric disorders are likely to affect fitness to plead (e.g. psychoses, organic brain disease, or severe learning disability). It is extremely unusual for a defendant to be found unfit to plead as a result of physical disability, although the forensic practitioner may be asked to make recommendations to facilitate a fair trial for those with physical illness (e.g. regular rest periods, access to medication).

Mental capacity and the 2005 Act

The Mental Capacity Act 2005 (MCA) provides a comprehensive framework for decision-making on behalf of adults aged 16 and over who lack capacity to make decisions on their own behalf. The Act applies to England and Wales only (see 🕮 p.16).

Defining capacity

For the purpose of the Act a person lacks capacity if, at the time a decision needs to be made, he or she is unable to make or communicate the decision because of an 'impairment of, or a disturbance in the functioning of, the mind or brain'. The Act contains a two-stage test of capacity:

• Is there an impairment of, or disturbance in the functioning of, the person's mind or brain? If so,
• Is the impairment or disturbance sufficient that the person lacks the capacity to make that particular decision?

Basic principles

The MCA sets out five statutory principles—the values that underpin the legal requirements in the Act (see also 🕮 p.16):

• A person must be assumed to have capacity unless it is established that they lack capacity.
• A person is not to be treated as unable to make a decision unless all practicable steps to help him to do so have been taken without success.
• A person is not to be treated as unable to make a decision merely because he makes an unwise decision.
• An act done, or decision made, for or on behalf of a person who lacks capacity must be done, or made, in his best interests.
• Before the act is done, or the decision is made, regard must be had to whether the purpose for which it is needed can be as effectively achieved in a way that is less restrictive of the person's rights and freedom of action.

Assessing capacity

Assessment of capacity is 'task-specific', that is to say it focuses on the specific decision that needs to be made at the specific time the decision is required. Under the Act, a person is regarded as being unable to make a decision if, at the time the decision needs to be made, he or she fails:

• To understand the information relevant to the decision;
• To retain the information relevant to the decision;
• To use or weigh the information; or
• To communicate the decision (by any means).

Admission to hospital of patients who lack capacity

Prior to the MCA, if at the time of admission a patient was mentally incapable of consent but did not object to entering hospital and receiving care or treatment, admission was often arranged on an informal basis. The patient was effectively deprived of his or her liberty without recourse to review by the likes of a Mental Health Tribunal (the so-called 'Bournewood gap'). Now, under the provisions of the MCA, treatment may be provided in the best interests of mentally disordered patients who are aged 16 or over and who lack capacity to consent to treatment.

This may be possible, even if the provision of treatment unavoidably involves depriving patients of their liberty. Deprivation of liberty for the purposes of care or treatment in a hospital or care home can be authorized in a person's best interests under the deprivation of liberty safeguards in the MCA. The MCA deprivation of liberty safeguards can be used only if the six qualifying requirements listed are met:

- The person is at least 18 years old.
- The person has a mental disorder.
- The person lacks capacity to decide whether to be in a hospital or care home for the proposed treatment or care.
- The proposed deprivation of liberty is in the person's best interests and it is a necessary and proportionate response to the risk of them suffering harm.
- The person is not subject, or potentially subject, to specified provisions of the Mental Health Act in a way that makes them ineligible.
- There is no advance decision, or decision of an attorney or deputy which makes the proposed deprivation of liberty impossible.

In all other circumstances, the admission of mentally disordered patients who lack capacity to consent to admission must be made under the provisions of the Mental Health Act 1983 as amended.

Mental health legislation

Mental Health Act 1983 (England and Wales)
In England and Wales, the legal framework that managers, doctors, nurses, social workers and the police must follow is set by the Mental Health Act 1983 (MHA 1983). An accompanying Code of Practice gives guidance on how the Act should be applied and should be used by everyone who works with people with mental health problems, whether or not they are patients formally detained under the Act.

The MHA 1983 is a comprehensive act that amended and consolidated previous legislation. The Act is divided into 10 parts and, when enacted, its most important features were to:
- Pass control of mental hospitals and mental nursing homes to the National Health Service.
- Encourage informal admission to hospital.
- Make the procedure for compulsory admission to hospital more clinical and less formal and intimidating.
- Define the role of the local authority in mental health services.
- Establish a Mental Health Act Commission that can inspect hospitals, and hear patients' complaints.

Mental Health Act 2007 (England and Wales)
Since its enactment, the MHA 1983 has become increasingly out of date. Through the MHA 2007, the Government has updated the 1983 Act to ensure it keeps pace with the changes in the way that mental health services are (and need to be) delivered. A comprehensive revision of the Codes of Practice has also been undertaken. The new Codes of Practice came into effect in November 2008.

The main changes to the 1983 Act made by the 2007 Act are summarized as:

Definition of mental disorder
Mental disorder is defined as 'any disorder or disability of the mind'. In somewhat tautologous guidance, the Code of Practice states that you should determine whether a patient has a disorder or disability of the mind in accordance with good clinical practice and accepted standards of what constitutes such a disorder or disability.

The Code lists a number of clinical conditions that are intended to fall within the definition of mental disorder (the list is not intended to be exhaustive):
- Affective disorders, such as depression and bipolar disorder.
- Schizophrenia and delusional disorders.
- Neurotic, stress-related, and somatoform disorders, such as anxiety, phobic disorders, obsessive–compulsive disorders, PTSD, and hypochondriacal disorders.
- Organic mental disorders such as dementia and delirium (however caused).
- Personality and behavioural changes caused by brain injury or damage (however acquired).
- Personality disorders.

- Mental and behavioural disorders caused by psychoactive substance use.
- Eating disorders, non-organic sleep disorders, and non-organic sexual disorders.
- Learning disabilities.
- Autistic spectrum disorders (including Asperger's syndrome).
- Behavioural and emotional disorders of children and adolescents.

Approved mental health professionals (AMHPs)
AMHPs replace approved social workers (ASWs) for the purposes of the Act. Local social service authorities may appoint persons from a number of different backgrounds to become AMHPs (e.g. social workers, nurses, occupational therapists), but registered medical practitioners are expressly excluded from taking on this role.

Criteria for prolonged detention
The MHS 2007 introduces a new 'appropriate medical treatment' test which will apply to all the longer-term powers of detention (such as detention under Section 3) and which replaces the old 'treatability test'. Long-term compulsory detention will only be possible if medical treatment which is appropriate to the patient's mental disorder and all other circumstances of the case is available to that patient. 'Appropriate medical treatment' means treatment that is intended to alleviate, or prevent a worsening of a mental disorder, its symptoms, or manifestations and also includes nursing, psychological intervention, and specialist mental health habilitation, rehabilitation, and care. Some commentators see this as a means of allowing the prolonged compulsory detention of persons with dangerous personality disorder who, in the past, could not be detained because their condition was not considered treatable.

Supervised community treatment (SCT)
The Act introduces SCT for patients following a period of detention in hospital. SCTs are designed to address the previous problem whereby some patients left hospital and did not continue with their treatment, their health deteriorated, and they required detention again—the so-called 'revolving door'.

Mental Health (Care and Treatment) (Scotland) Act 2003
The MHA(S) 2003 came into force in October 2005 and replaced the previous 1984 Act. The new Act introduced the Mental Health Tribunal for Scotland and clarified and enhanced the role of the Mental Welfare Commission for Scotland, which is responsible for ensuring that patients receive appropriate care.

Compulsory hospitalization

Compulsory admission to hospital under the MHA 1983 (as amended) may be used if:
- Voluntary admission is not possible or appropriate; and
- The patient has a mental disorder.
- And admission is necessary for one or more of the following reasons:
  - In the interests of his or her health; or
  - In the interests of his or her own safety; or
  - For the protection of other people.

Informal or compulsory admission?

Where admission to hospital is considered necessary and the patient is willing to be admitted informally, this should, in general, be arranged. However, even when a patient consents to admission, compulsory admission powers can still be exercised if:
- Detention is necessary because of the danger the patient presents to him/herself or others.
- The patient's current mental state, together with reliable evidence of past experience, indicates a strong likelihood that he or she will have a change of mind about informal admission prior to actually being admitted to hospital.

Section 2: Admission for assessment

(The most commonly used section in the community)

Purpose:	Admission for observation and assessment (or for assessment followed by treatment).
Duration:	28 days.
Applicant:	AMHP or nearest relative.
Nearest relative:	Must be informed (when possible) but cannot block application.
Medical signatories:	Two doctors, one of whom must be s.12 approved.
Exam^n requirements:	Must be no more than 5 clear days between the examinations by the two doctors, who should always discuss the patient with each other. At least one of the doctors must discuss the case with the applicant (AMHP or nearest relative).
Psychiatric condition:	Mental disorder.

Section 3: Admission for treatment

Purpose:	Admission for treatment ('appropriate medical treatment' must be available).
Duration:	Up to 6 months.
Applicant:	AMHP or nearest relative.
Nearest relative:	Must be consulted before the Order is made (where reasonably practical) and has the right to object to the Order being made.
Medical signatories:	Two doctors, one of whom must be s.12 approved.
Exam^n requirements:	As for section 2.
Psychiatric condition:	Mental disorder.

Section 2 or 3?

Section 2 should be used if:
- The full extent of the nature and degree of a patient's condition is unclear;
- There is a need to carry out an initial in-patient assessment in order to formulate a treatment plan, or to reach a judgement about whether the patient will accept treatment on a voluntary basis following admission; or
- There is a need to carry out a new in-patient assessment in order to re-formulate a treatment plan, or to reach a judgement about whether the patient will accept treatment on a voluntary basis.

Section 3 should be used if:
- The patient is already detained under section 2 (detention under section 2 cannot be renewed by a new section 2 application); or
- The nature and current degree of the patient's mental disorder, the essential elements of the treatment plan to be followed and the likelihood of the patient accepting treatment on a voluntary basis are already established.

Section 4: Emergency admission for assessment

Purpose:	Emergency admission to hospital in circumstances where admission is urgent and compliance with Section 2 would cause undesirable delay. Must never be used for administrative convenience.
Emergency criteria:	To be satisfied that an emergency exists there must be evidence of:
	• An immediate and significant risk of mental or physical harm to the patient or to others; and/or
	• The danger of serious harm to property; and/or
	• The need for physical restraint of the patient.
Duration:	72h
Applicant:	AMHP or nearest relative
Nearest relative:	Must be informed (when possible) but cannot block application.
Medical signatories:	Any doctor, does not have to be s.12 approved.
Psychiatric condition:	Mental disorder.

Scotland

The Mental Health (Care and Treatment) (Scotland) Act 2003 provides for compulsory admission under Part 5 for 72h. The application is made by a fully registered medical practitioner in consultation with a mental health officer, unless this is impracticable. In hospital Part 6 (lasting 28 days) can be applied and then, if necessary, Part 7 (Compulsory Treatment Order) for 6 months.

Further reading

Departent of Health (2008) Code of Practice *Mental Health Act 1983*. London: DH.

Sections 136 and 135 (Mental Health Act 1983)

Section 136: Police power to remove to a place of safety

The extent to which this section is used varies considerably around the country. Forensic practitioners are only likely to be involved in assessments under the provisions of this section if the local place of safety in the area they work is the police station (something that is being actively discouraged).

Purpose:	To remove a person in a public place to a place of safety, in order to facilitate a formal assessment under the MHA 1983 by a doctor and AMHP. The doctor should wherever possible be approved under s.12 of the Act.
Implemented by:	A police officer in respect of a person in a public place who is causing risk to themselves or others, and the police officer believes that the person is suffering from mental disorder.
Duration:	Up to 72h.
Place of safety:	The identification of preferred places of safety is a matter for local agreement. It is preferable for a person thought to be suffering from a mental disorder to be detained in a hospital or other healthcare setting where mental health services are provided (subject, of course, to any urgent physical healthcare needs they may have). A police station should be used as a place of safety only on an exceptional basis. It may be necessary to do so because the person's behaviour would pose an unmanageably high risk to other patients, staff or users of a healthcare setting. Under the MHA 2007 it is now possible to transfer a person from one place of safety to another.
Nearest relative:	There is no obligation or requirement to contact the nearest relative. This should not be done without the permission of the patient.
Authority to treat:	The section confers no powers to treat any illness.
Patient rights:	A person removed under s136 is deemed to be 'arrested' for the purposes of PACE 1984 and is subject to the rights and provision of that Act
Manner of discharge:	Ordinarily the patient should not be discharged until after an assessment by both a doctor and an AMHP. However, where the doctor, having examined the individual, concludes that he or she is not mentally disordered within the meaning of the Act then the individual can no longer be detained and should be immediately discharged from detention. This applies whether or not the doctor is s.12 approved.

Section 135: Power to search for and remove patients

This gives a police constable authority to enter and search premises under the terms of a warrant issued by a Justice of the Peace in order to remove a patient to a place of safety for assessment. In issuing the warrant, the Justice of Peace must be satisfied, subsequent to information laid on oath by an AMHP, that the person believed to be suffering from a mental disorder:

- Has been, or is being, ill treated, neglected, or kept otherwise than under proper control; or
- Being unable to care for him/herself, is living alone

When exercising these powers, the police constable must be accompanied by a registered medical practitioner and AMHP, and the forensic practitioner may occasionally be asked to assist in this respect.

A person can be detained in a place of safety pursuant to this section for a maximum period of 72h.

Diversion from the criminal justice system

There is a growing recognition that mentally disordered offenders are best dealt with by treating their mental disorder outside the criminal justice system where possible and appropriate. Such diversion can occur at a number of stages.

Court diversion schemes

These schemes have been developed to divert mentally disordered offenders away from the criminal justice system at an early stage as possible. The objectives of such schemes are:

- To divert mentally disordered offenders from prosecution by assessing them in police custody, on remand in prison, or bail.
- To provide information to the CPS on the nature and severity of the mental disorder to enable the CPS to exercise its right not to prosecute or to discontinue proceedings on the grounds of public interest.
- To reduce the number of mentally disordered offenders remanded to prison for psychiatric reports.
- To reduce the number of mentally disordered offenders serving a custodial sentence.
- To re-establish links between mentally disordered offenders and community psychiatric services when contact has been lost.
- On release from prison seek to prevent further offending by liaising with appropriate services for provision of a suitable package of care.

Forensic practitioners should be aware of any court diversion schemes operating in their area and should play an active role in supporting the objectives outlined in the list. Although their primary concern should be for the health (both physical and mental) of the detainee, they should remember that the ultimate decision regarding the diversion of a mentally disordered offender from police custody rests with the custody officer, whose decision must take into account wider public safety issues.

Remand of accused persons to hospital under MHA 1983

Section 35

Purpose:	Remand to hospital for psychiatric report.
Duration:	28 days (renewable for further periods of 28 days up to 12 weeks).
Authority required:	Magistrates' or Crown court.
Medical signatories:	Written/oral evidence of one s.12 approved doctor.
Psychiatric condition:	Reason to suspect mental illness, psychopathic disorder, severe mental impairment, or mental impairment.
Additional:	Bed must be available within 7 days.

Section 36

Purpose:	Remand to hospital for treatment.

Duration:	28 days (renewable for further periods of 28 days up to 12 weeks).
Authority required:	Crown Court only.
Medical signatories:	Written/oral evidence of two doctors (one must be s.12 approved doctor).
Psychiatric condition:	Mental illness or severe mental impairment.
Additional:	Bed must be available within 7 days.

Hospital orders for convicted prisoners

The most frequent route to treatment for a mentally disordered offender is provided after conviction. There are a number of psychiatric disposals available to the Court after conviction but the commonest is a hospital order (Section 37(2) MHA 1983).

Section 37(2)

Purpose:	Detention to hospital for treatment.
Duration:	6 months (renewable).
Authority required:	Magistrate's or Crown Court. The offence must be one punishable by imprisonment and not one for which the sentence is fixed (e.g. murder).
Medical signatories:	Written/oral evidence of two doctors (one must be s.12 approved doctor).
Psychiatric condition:	Mental disorder.
Additional:	The court must be satisfied that arrangements have been made for the prisoner's admission to hospital within 28 days

Transfer of prisoners to hospital under the MHA 1983

The MHA 1983 has provision for transferring prisoners from prison to hospital.

Section 47

Purpose:	Transfer of sentenced prisoner to hospital for treatment.
Duration:	6 months (renewable).
Authority required:	Secretary of State, Home Office.
Medical signatories:	Written evidence of two doctors.
Psychiatric condition:	(a) Mental illness or severe mental impairment;
	(b) psychopathic disorder or mental impairment if treatment will alleviate or prevent deterioration.
Additional:	Bed must be available within 14 days.

Section 48

Purpose:	Transfer of remand prisoner to hospital for treatment.
Duration:	May be terminated by trial or report from RMO that treatment is no longer required or effective.
Authority required:	Secretary of State, Home Office.
Medical signatories:	Written evidence of two doctors.
Psychiatric condition:	Mental illness or severe mental impairment.

Forensic psychiatry

Background

Forensic psychiatry is a subspecialty of psychiatry. Although it has no official definition, the term refers to the overlap, interface, and interaction between psychiatry and the law in all its aspects. In practice, forensic psychiatrists are primarily involved in the clinical assessment and treatment of mentally disordered offenders in a variety of settings and under a range of circumstances. However, people with mental disorders who have never been involved with the criminal justice system might also be treated in forensic psychiatric services if they cannot be safely managed elsewhere.

Forensic psychiatric services

Mentally disordered offenders may be treated in various settings:
- Special hospitals
- Regional forensic psychiatric services
- General adult psychiatric services
- Independent sector.

Special hospitals

The NHS provides inpatient services under conditions of maximum security for mentally disordered offenders who are considered too dangerous to be treated elsewhere at three special hospitals in England and Wales (Broadmoor hospital, London; Ashworth hospital, Liverpool; Rampton hospital, Nottinghamshire) and one in Scotland (The State Hospital, Carstairs). Most patients are admitted from prisons and courts, with only a small minority of inpatients being non-offenders who have shown serious violence. When appropriate, transfer to a unit with lesser security is more common than discharge to the community.

Regional forensic psychiatric services

Regional forensic psychiatric services and regional secure units (RSUs) were developed after the Butler report in 1975. RSUs provide medium-security inpatient facilities, as well as acting as the administrative, teaching, research, and clinical base for the regional forensic psychiatric service.

General psychiatric services

These provide services for mentally disordered offenders who can be managed in conditions of low security.

The independent sector

Private forensic healthcare mainly provides long-stay inpatient services for offender patients. There are now a number of independent or private hospitals providing these services, particularly in areas that have inadequate NHS resources.

The forensic psychiatrist as an expert witness

It has been estimated that about 2% of persons appearing before Magistrates' Courts are remanded for psychiatric reports. Ideally, a forensic psychiatric opinion should be sought in all cases where an offender appears to be suffering from a mental disorder at the time the offence was committed or at the time of the trial. In practical terms, psychiatric assessments of mentally disordered offenders are usually requested only in the relation to the following:

- Fitness to plead.
- Automatism.
- Pleas of diminished responsibility or insanity.
- Consideration of psychiatric disposal (e.g. psychiatric probation order, hospital order, restriction order, transfer form prison, or guardianship order).

Forensic psychology

Definition

Forensic psychology is the application of psychology (the science of human behaviour and experience) to crime and the criminal justice process. Forensic psychologists should have Charter status conferred by the Division of Forensic Psychology of the British Psychological Society.

The role of the forensic psychologist

Forensic psychologists are able to advise on a range of issues:
- Vulnerabilities:
  - Suggestibility
  - Compliance
  - Acquiescence
  - Low self-esteem.
- Psychological disorders:
  - Psychotic and neurotic states
  - Personality disorders
  - Stress disorders including PTSD.
- Learning disabilities and difficulties.
- Likelihood of false confessions.
- Distortion/contamination of witness testimony following exposure to post-event information (including recovered memory—see later in this section).
- Forensic autopsy and psychological autopsy (see later in this section).

Recovered memory

There are probably few areas so controversial in the forensic world than that of the role of recovered memory. Proponents of the technique explain that 'forgotten' memories of experiences in early childhood may be 'recovered' by experts and so reveal evidence of (usually) sexual abuse. Sceptics argue that it is difficult, if not impossible, to distinguish imagined events from reality.

Psychological autopsy

In recent times, the concept of a 'psychological autopsy' has emerged. It has been applied to situations where there is uncertainty as to whether deaths were the result of an accident or were due to suicide. By examining in detail the actions, behaviour, and actions of an individual in the time prior to death (in the context of their lifestyle), it is believed that additional insight (adding to the physical autopsy) may be gained into how and why death occurred.

Forensic toxicology

Introduction to forensic toxicology

History and perspective

Self-inflicted poisoning accounts for significant numbers of hospital admissions. The majority of these do not have fatal results, but the resource implications for health services are considerable. Deaths due to poisoning have been recorded throughout history: notable cases being Socrates (hemlock, 399 BC) and Cleopatra (traditionally attributed to the bite of an asp, although the actual poison remains unknown, 30 BC). Napoleon's death has been attributed to arsenic poisoning, but the official cause of death (stomach cancer) is more prosaic. More recently, important examples include accidental poisonings such as the Bhopal (methyl isocyanate, 1984) and the (non-fatal) Seveso (dioxin, 1976) disasters and deliberate poisonings such as the assassinations of Markov (ricin, 1978) and Litvinenko (polonium, 2006). The use of chemical and biological toxins and agents in warfare is a continuing threat, despite international conventions attempting to control and limit their use. The activities of Harold Shipman between 1993 and 1998 should remain as an important reminder to all practitioners of the danger of underestimating the need for postmortem toxicological analysis. One of the first recorded uses of postmortem toxicological analysis for court purposes was that of Orfila, whose work secured the conviction of Marie LaFarge in France in 1840.

Clinical toxicology

Within hospital practice, clinical toxicologists mostly focus upon the clinical management of patients who are suffering from the effects of poisoning. Such poisoning may be unintentional ('accidental') or intentional, with the latter mostly being deliberate self-poisoning rather than deliberate poisoning of one person by another. There are several poison centres in the UK where specialists are available to advise on the management of poisoned individuals. The telephone number for the UK National Poisons Information Service is 0844 892 0111. There is a large database on clinical toxicology (called 'TOXBASE') available to health professionals on the internet via ॐ http://www.toxbase.org.

Environmental toxicology

Human activity is increasingly associated with complex chemical and biochemical processes. Environmental toxicology is concerned with the toxic characteristics of all substances of anthropological origin. These include numerous industrial, agricultural, and biochemical substances. Although reported cases of mortality are unusual and rare, the toxicologist is particularly concerned when an individual's exposure risk (whether environmental, relating to employment, or as the result of a single event) is significantly increased during life.

Arsenic poisoning

In historical terms, arsenic has a prominent (if not pre-eminent) place amongst poisons. Arsenic was much feared as a poison and for good reason. Colourless and tasteless, relatively small amounts can kill within hours of ingestion, causing symptoms prior to death which resemble natural gastrointestinal disease. Perhaps most importantly, from early times right through until the 19th century, there was no test which could reliably detect it. This situation changed when James Marsh (who worked at the Woolwich Arsenal) developed a laboratory test and published his findings in *The Edinburgh Philosophical Journal* in 1836. The use of arsenic as a poison subsequently declined.

The history of arsenic poisoning over thousands of years makes interesting reading. Some examples of serial killers who employed it are outlined here.

Agrippina

This ancient Roman is believed to have used arsenic to kill a variety of individuals, including her husband, thereby freeing her to marry the emperor Claudius, who she poisoned in 54 AD, enabling her son Nero to become emperor.

Cesare Borgia

At the end of the 15th century, the powerful Borgias family living in Rome are said to have killed large numbers of people by using arsenic. It is postulated that they got a recipe to make arsenic trioxide from the Spanish Moors and certainly, the family had Spanish connections, as Cesare's father was a Spanish cardinal who became Pope Alexander VI, but died mysteriously after a banquet …

Mary Ann Cotton

This daughter of a coal miner was born in Durham in 1833, married young, and moved to Cornwall, where three of her four children died suddenly of a 'gastric' illness. The fourth died shortly after she moved back to County Durham, along with numerous other members of her family. She was arrested after it was found that her stepson had died with high levels of arsenic in his body. The bodies of other victims were exhumed and also found to contain high levels of arsenic. She was convicted with the murder of her stepson and was executed by hanging at Durham jail in 1873.

Common drugs and poisons

A range of drugs/poisons are encountered in forensic practice:

Suicide

Prescribed medication

- Antidepressants (tricyclic, SSRI, etc.)
- Benzodiazepines
- Barbiturates
- Analgesics:
  - Dihydrocodeine
  - Dextropropoxyphene
  - Morphine.

'Over-the-counter' preparations

- Paracetamol
- Products containing paracetamol.

Other

- Bleach and household chemicals

'Accidental drug-related' death

Prescribed medication

- Methadone
- Dihydrocodeine
- Benzodiazepines.

Illicit drugs

- Heroin
- Methadone (diverted)
- Dihydrocodeine
- Benzodiazepines
- Cocaine*
- Cannabis*
- Amphetamine*
- LSD*
- Ecstasy.*

Other

- Solvents, glues, etc.

* It is arguable as to whether these are commonly encountered drugs in the practice of forensic **pathology**. In terms of clinical forensic practice, law enforcement, and drug use they are, however, common drugs. The use of poison as a method of committing homicide is relatively rare, primarily because of the controlled nature of most toxic substances and their limited availability (the Shipman case, see 📖 p.486, being an obvious exception). Note, however, the use of household substances such as common salt in poisonings associated with fabricated and induced illness.

It is noted that the lists make no reference to the common drugs and poisons of the past: arsenic, opium, paraquat, strychnine, strong acids and alkalis. These are rarely encountered in modern forensic practice. Note also that all the drugs listed under one heading could also have been included in the other—this is especially true when considering comorbid ('dual diagnosis') patients who have access to a wide range of prescribed and non-prescribed drugs.

Barbiturates were once the most common drug of dependence. With increased control and reduced prescribing, they are now relatively rarely implicated in poisoning. However, drugs such as phenobarbitone, do continue to have a useful role in managing certain patients with epilepsy and barbiturates are still widely used in veterinary practice.

Toxicology and sudden death

When is toxicology required?

Although there are no fixed guidelines, toxicology should be considered in all sudden deaths. Toxicology should be considered **necessary** in any apparent or suspected suicide, drug-related death, homicide, death of a child, death of an apparently healthy individual, or as part of a defined protocol (e.g. research into drug use in road traffic fatalities). The presence of disease or pathology sufficient to cause death does not mean that drugs or poisons were not involved—to dismiss toxicology as being unnecessary following an apparently natural death is to ignore the lessons of Shipman (see 📖 p.486).

Manner of death

Manner of death is difficult to determine from toxicology alone. The fact of a deliberate overdose in a drug user does not indicate suicidal intent (indeed, a drug user effectively needs to 'overdose' in order to overcome the effect of tolerance). It is vital to take account of all additional information in order to establish whether a death was a suicide or an accident (or indeed, homicide). This emphasizes the importance of a comprehensive police enquiry into sudden death and, crucially, a team approach to the investigation.

Toxicology and public health

Although the primary remit of the forensic investigation into a sudden death is to provide a cause of death in that individual case, poisoning and drug-related deaths have significant implications from a public health perspective. Information from postmortem toxicological analysis is vital to psychiatric and drug services as it provides insight into compliance with prescribed medication, illicit drug use, and comorbidity. It is important, therefore, that the forensic services participate in or at least facilitate, the communication of information to primary care providers and specialist drug treatment services—whether through formal local/national Confidential Enquiries or via informal channels.

Further information

The following resources may prove to be useful:
- Drug Misuse and Dependence—Guidelines on Clinical Management, Department of Health (see 🖰 http://www.dh.gov.uk).
- European Monitoring Centre for Drugs and Drug Addiction (see 🖰 http://www.emcdda.europa.eu).
- DrugScope (see 🖰 http://www.drugscope.org.uk).

Signs of poisoning at autopsy

Physical evidence

At autopsy, it is important to look for signs of toxic substances or drug use. These include:

- The classic 'cherry-pink' skin colouration of **carboxyhaemoglobin** resulting from carbon monoxide inhalation.
- The 'almond' smell associated with cyanide.
- Aromas associated with alcohol and/or volatile solvents.
- Skin marks of recent or old drug injection sites.
- Remnants in the stomach.

Although such signs may be characteristic of the substance, they are almost invariably not diagnostic of the cause of death. In conjunction with the circumstances of the death (for instance, a domestic fire with evidence of smoke inhalation), such evidence **may** sometimes be considered sufficiently persuasive to certify the cause of death. However, most poisons, drugs, and toxic substances do not reliably produce macroscopic characteristic changes in tissues and the presence of these substances can only be demonstrated by toxicological analysis. If there is any possibility of legal proceedings, toxicology should be deemed necessary.

Indirect evidence

Indirect evidence of drug use and/or poisoning may also be found at the scene. This evidence includes drug paraphernalia (syringes, needles, wraps, etc.), suicide notes, empty medication containers, empty alcohol bottles, evidence of faulty gas appliances, or deliberate diversion of gases.

The forensic team

The pathologist works as a team with the forensic toxicologist. The laboratory needs to be informed what was found at autopsy and what substances are indicated by the scene, circumstances of death, and medical history of the deceased (particularly any period in hospital and associated treatment and intervention). This enables the toxicologist to focus the initial analysis and is likely to lead to quicker results.

Postmortem toxicology

Interpretation of postmortem toxicology (see 📖 p.456) requires an understanding of sensitivity (resistance), tolerance, and idiosyncrasy. The investigator should always be prepared to suspect more than the circumstantial evidence of the case might initially indicate. Observing significant pathology at autopsy does not rule out accidental or deliberate poisoning. A full and comprehensive toxicological screen in every case is neither feasible nor practical. Careful sampling, collection, and storage will enable additional tests to be performed if required.

Postmortem sample collection

Collection of samples for analysis is a routine part of the autopsy. It is clearly much easier to dispose of unused samples than attempt to retrieve samples from a body at a later date. Containers should be clean and appropriately labelled (case reference, date, pathologist's name) and processed to ensure continuity of evidence and minimize any possibility of cross-contamination.

Blood

If possible, blood is taken from the exposed iliac or femoral vein. The vessel should not be 'milked', as this is likely to increase the quantity of extraneous fluid. Pooled blood should never be taken, as it is likely to be contaminated with other fluids (especially stomach contents). Similarly, blood should not be taken from the heart or great vessels of the chest, as postmortem diffusion will lead to unreliable results. Coagulated blood can be submitted for analysis if no other blood sample is available—this may be a problem if, for example, the body is incinerated.

Consideration should be given to taking three samples:

- 10–20mL plain labelled container.
- 10mL labelled container with anticoagulant (e.g. EDTA or heparin).
- 5mL labelled container with sodium fluoride (for alcohol analysis).

Urine

Urine is collected from the bladder. Even a small quantity of urine may be sufficient for a range of immunoassays for common drugs.

Vitreous humour

Fluid from the eye has the advantage of being anatomically isolated. The fluid is replaced with saline for cosmetic reasons—doing so during the autopsy will also encourage better relations with undertakers. However, the results obtained from analysis are difficult to interpret, as there is a lack of comprehensive data on *in vivo* normal/therapeutic concentrations.

Other

Modern analytical techniques are able to detect drugs in almost any body tissue. Unfortunately, however, many give only a qualitative analysis as to whether the drug was or was not present. Although this is not sufficient to determine an exact cause of death, in some cases it can be important and useful information. If the sample gives a quantitative result, this will require very careful interpretation as reliable reference data are rare.

Liver samples will often enable the presence of drugs (or their metabolites) to be demonstrated after blood levels have fallen to unquantifiable or undetectable limits.

Lung samples can be useful to detect inhaled solvents—note that the sample should be stored in a nylon impervious bag.

Hair samples can be used to generate a time-line of drug use. Since hair is easily taken and stored, it is worth considering whether this should be a routine sample, even if no subsequent analysis is required.

Analysis of skeletal remains

When dealing with skeletal remains, concealed or exhumed bodies, samples should be taken from the remaining tissues and also from the local environment (soil, fluids, maggots, etc.), as with time-consuming and expert investigation poisons and evidence of poisoning may be recovered. This evidence is usually of qualitative value only.

Interpretation of postmortem toxicology

The concept of a minimum fatal dose has no relevance to forensic practice and the concept of a minimum fatal blood concentration (or any other measurable postmortem value) even less so! Postmortem toxicology is subject to a wide range of variables which make simplistic statements about numerical values meaningless. Postmortem blood is not the same as blood obtained from a living person and comparisons between ante- and postmortem concentrations are also of limited value.

Sensitivity

Different individuals have different sensitivities (or resistance) to whatever substances they are exposed to. There is no measure of sensitivity and indeed, an individual's sensitivity varies with time. Sensitivity has a genetic basis, and is also related to characteristics such as weight (body mass index), physical health, and environmental factors.

Tolerance

Individuals have a genetically determined tolerance to various drugs. This is based on enzyme profiles and receptor sites. In this context, 'tolerance' usually refers to the acquired tolerance as a result of chronic or previous use. Tolerance to a substance occurs when an individual's response to a given dose diminishes over a period of time and with repeated administration. Therapeutically, this causes problems when administering analgesia (especially opioids) and is highly significant for drugs of misuse (especially opioids and amphetamines). A high concentration (an order of magnitude higher than a fatal level in a non-tolerant user) of a drug in a known drug user is not conclusive of a fatal level. There is no simple postmortem measure of tolerance and the importance of a comprehensive police investigation into the death cannot be overestimated. An important corollary to tolerance is the opposite phenomenon—loss of tolerance once exposure to the drug ceases. This is observed in drug users who after a period of voluntary (e.g. drug-free or 'clean' rehabilitation) or involuntary (e.g. imprisonment) abstinence revert to their original dose, with often fatal consequences. Avoid relying solely on a postmortem toxicology result unless there is a good proxy indicator of tolerance (e.g. evidence of drug use over an appropriate period). One effect of tolerance is that drug users constantly have to 'overdose' in order to achieve the desired effect—thus increasing the risk of death. The term 'overdose' should be avoided when certifying death unless it is intended to convey a deliberately *fatal* overdose.

Idiosyncrasy

An idiosyncratic reaction may be the result of anaphylaxis or an abnormal response to exposure to a tiny quantity of a substance. Although this can occur with any substance, cocaine and volatile solvents are particularly hazardous. It is important to record idiosyncratic deaths (particularly those associated with substances such as ecstasy) as they may attract extensive publicity which needs to be accompanied by a balanced statement of the risks.

Postmortem changes and redistribution

The shorter the postmortem interval, the more accurately toxicological findings reflect the antemortem situation. Drugs which are bound to tissues in life are released into the blood postmortem, thus rendering concentrations to be artificially elevated. Postmortem biochemical changes (enzymatic and microbial), as well as physical processes such as osmosis and diffusion, may also affect concentrations and produce site-specific results. The effects of postmortem changes and redistribution mean that reference tables and databases have limited value. It is important to adhere to standardized practices and procedures when collecting blood and other samples to reduce variability between cases.

Interpretation of toxicology

This requires an understanding of the relationship between the postmortem concentration and the drug dose *in vivo*. There are a number of potential factors which determine how accurately the postmortem analysis of a toxic substance reflects levels when the individual was alive. These include:

- The way that drug concentrations decrease as a result of metabolism.
- The way that concentrations of metabolites will increase with metabolism.
- The time interval between consumption and death.
- Hospital admission and appropriate intervention will, in some cases, remove all traces of the original toxic substance.
- Some drugs are more sample-site specific than others.
- Postmortem redistribution.
- Postmortem metabolism: some drugs (e.g. heroin, nitrazepam) continue to be metabolized after death.
- The way that the sample was collected, stored, and analysed.

Lawyers may ask a doctor in court to use a known postmortem value to calculate the amount of drug consumed or the probable blood concentration at some time in the past. The wise doctor will answer such questions with care—often a simple 'I do not know'.

Modern scientific techniques have the ability to provide quantitative and/or qualitative evidence about a huge range of substances found in a body or at a scene. However, this information does not necessarily state how/why/when the substance got there. Nor does it necessarily mean that these substances caused death. The objective, numerical result of the toxicologist's science must be carefully interpreted using all relevant information—over-reliance on the 'number' is likely to mislead.

Controlled drugs legislation

Legislation relating to the possession, supply, and use of 'drugs' is complex and outside the scope of this book. However, the concept of controlling drugs and medicines is one applicable to most legal jurisdictions. In the UK, the main statutes regulating the availability of controlled drugs are the Misuse of Drugs Act 1971 (as amended, e.g. Misuse of Drugs Regulations, 2001) and the Medicines Act 1968. The Controlled Drugs (Supervision of Management and Use) Regulations 2006 governs prescribing, record keeping and destruction of controlled drugs. The Crime and Disorder Act 1998, Drugs Act 2005, and the various Road Traffic Acts are also important.

Medicines Act 1968

The Medicines Act governs the manufacture and supply of medicines. It rarely has implications for the public.

Misuse of Drugs Act 1971 (MDA)

The MDA differs from the Medicines Act in that it includes drugs with no current medical use and it also prohibits unlawful *possession* (with associated police powers to stop and search). Drugs under this Act are known as 'controlled drugs' and it divides drugs into three 'classes':

Class A

Legally, the Class A substances are considered to be the most 'dangerous' and include cocaine (and 'crack cocaine'), MDMA (ecstasy), heroin, LSD, methadone, methamphetamine (crystal meth), and any injected Class B drug. Magic mushrooms (fungus which contains psilocin or psilocybin) were added to the list of Class A substances by the Drugs Act 2005, prior to which only prepared or dried mushrooms were included.

Class B

The most important Class B drugs are amphetamine and codeine. Cannabis was reclassified as a Class B drug in 2008.

Class C

Class C drugs include amphetamines, anabolic steroids, and minor tranquillizers. Cannabis was controversially reclassified from Class B to Class C in 2004, but reclassified back to Class B in 2008. Ketamine was added as a Class C drug in 2006. Note that it is illegal to possess temazepam and flunitrazepam (Rohypnol®) (the so-called 'date-rape' drugs) without a prescription.

  The classifications outlined here take no account of the type or context of use and the debate as to whether Class A drugs do, in fact, cause the greatest (medical and/or social) harm will continue. The MDA lists offences and penalties relating to the manufacture, supply, and possession of the controlled drugs. The maximum penalties for the possession and supply of a Class A drug are 7 years (plus a fine) and life imprisonment (plus a fine) respectively. There is some evidence that police policy and court sentencing practices vary significantly between regions within the UK.

Alcohol

The laws relating to alcohol are particularly complex. It is not illegal for anyone aged over 5 years to consume alcohol away from licensed premises, although it is illegal to sell alcohol to anyone aged under 18 years. The laws relating to the consumption of alcohol with a meal differ from those relating to consumption without food and further, in some areas, the consumption of alcohol in a public place is, irrespective of age, an offence.

Other drugs

Some other drugs which are not included within the remit of the MDA include:

- *Khat leaves*, when chewed have a stimulant effect. Possession and supply is not an offence. Khat is sold in markets primarily to an immigrant African community and is not widely used.
- *Poppers* (liquid gold, amyl or butyl nitrate) are sold primarily in sex shops. They are not illegal to use or buy. Whether they are covered by the Medicines Act 1968 has never been tested in court.
- *Solvents* (including aerosols, glues, gases) are not illegal to buy, possess, or use. It is, however, an offence to sell 'glue sniffing kits' to anyone under the age of 18 years.
- *Tobacco products* can be used by persons of any age although is it illegal to sell them to anyone who is less than 16 years of age.

Schedules

In addition to the three Classes of controlled drugs, substances are also classified according to one of five schedules (Misuse of Drugs Regulations, 2001) which govern their medical and scientific use.

- Schedule 1 drugs are those having no currently recognized medical use (e.g. LSD, cannabis, MDMA), although licences can be given for research purposes.
- Schedules 2, 3, and 4 are primarily concerned with those drugs which may be prescribed by doctors although only under special circumstances or following certain guidelines (e.g. amphetamines, cocaine, dihydrocodeine, Diconal®, heroin, methadone, morphine, pethidine, Ritalin®, flunitrazepam, and temazepam).
- Schedule 5 includes low-dose, non-injectable, over-the-counter preparations (e.g. cough medicines, mild analgesics) which can be possessed without prescription. Note that such substances cannot legally be supplied to another person.

Alcohol overview

Ethanol (ethyl alcohol or 'alcohol') is widely consumed and causes significant problems for doctors, law enforcement agencies, and society. It is reported that up to 15% of the Emergency Department's workload can be attributed to alcohol. The effects of alcohol are even more significant to the forensic practitioner and the forensic pathologist, given that it is involved in the majority of homicides and assaults. Alcoholics have increased rates of heart disease, malignancy, and stroke, but mortality is often related to injury. Excessive alcohol consumption is a feature of 30% of road traffic fatalities, 25% of fatal work injuries, 30% of drownings, and 50% of domestic fire deaths. Alcohol is involved in ~30% of suicides, ~60% of homicides, and in most assaults.

Methanol may also be encountered in forensic practice. Mixed with ethanol and diluted with water, it is sold relatively cheaply as methylated spirits ('meths') and is associated with social and economic deprivation.

Units

As a standard, easily understood, measure of alcohol consumed, the number of 'units' (approximately 8g of alcohol) is included on packaging.

The number of units equals:

$$\frac{\text{Strength (ABV)} \times \text{volume (mL)}}{1000}$$

One unit is approximately half a pint (300mL) of 'standard' beer (some beers/lagers are much stronger), a 100mL glass of wine, or a 25mL spirit measure. Current advice is a 'safe' limit of 21 units/week (males) and 14 units/week (females). Above these, liver damage may occur.

Alcohol intoxication

Alcohol depresses the nervous system—initial euphoric effects are due to suppression of inhibition by the cerebral cortex. Effects vary between individuals and those listed in Table 14.1 are only a guide. Behaviour, including the propensity to violence, is influenced by environment and social setting. Although death may occur at levels >350mg/100mL, the risk of a harmful or fatal event increases at *any* level: especially road traffic collisions, work and home accidents, and assaults (including sexual assault).

Table 14.1 Effects of alcohol.

Blood alcohol concentration (mg/100mL = mg/dL)	Effects
30–50	Measurable impairment of motor skills
50–100	Reduced inhibitions, 'excitant effect'
100–150	Loss of coordination and control
150–200	'Drunkenness', nausea, ataxia
200–350	Vomiting, stupor, possible coma
350+	Respiratory paralysis, possible death

Alcohol absorption

Alcohol is mostly absorbed from the small intestine and, to a lesser extent, the stomach. Relatively small amounts are also absorbed from the mouth. The rate of absorption depends on a variety of factors, but most particularly the nature of the drink and any associated food consumed (Fig.14.1). Alcohol is absorbed more slowly from dilute drinks (such as beer or wine) as compared with the more concentrated fortified sherry or port. Food in the stomach tends to delay the rate of absorption, partly by delaying the rate at which alcohol reaches the upper small intestine.

Metabolism and elimination

Alcohol is soluble in water and so distributes throughout the body. It is mostly metabolized in the liver by an enzymatic process involving alcohol dehydrogenase, which converts it to acetaldehyde and then to acetic acid (which itself is a form of energy). A relatively small amount of alcohol is excreted unchanged in the urine (and to a lesser extent, also in breath and sweat).

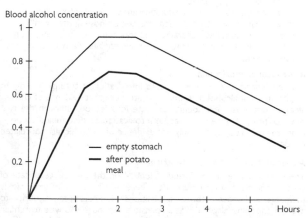

Fig. 14.1 The Widmark curve. Reproduced from Houck MM and Siegel JA (2006). *Fundamentals of Forensic Science*, copyright Academic Press.

Alcohol and sudden death

Autopsy findings

Although not intended as a substitute for toxicology and histology, it is important to recognize the signs of chronic and acute alcohol use at autopsy. The police investigation into any sudden death will almost certainly comment on a history of chronic abuse (particularly if the deceased had received treatment for alcohol dependency) and whether there was reliable evidence of recent excessive consumption. However, such information is not diagnostic and as far as certifying death is concerned, should not be relied upon if not supported by other evidence.

Chronic alcohol misuse

Chronic alcohol misuse typically results in pathologically distinct diseases of the liver:

• *Fatty liver*—a greasy cut surface (histologically, the hepatocytes demonstrate fatty accumulation).

• *Cirrhosis*—on gross examination, the liver exhibits fibrosis and a micronodular appearance.

• *Alcoholic hepatitis*—a jaundiced appearance and oesophageal varices are associated with alcoholic hepatitis and cirrhosis. Histologically, alcoholic hepatitis has a characteristic appearance with degeneration of hepatocytes and inflammation with neutrophils. Mallory bodies may also be seen.

Acute alcohol intoxication

The most noticeable feature of acute intoxication at autopsy is likely to be the smell of alcohol. It is important to note that evidence of chronic alcohol misuse is not evidence of acute intoxication, although the two often coincide. Furthermore, acute intoxication as determined by post-mortem toxicology, is certainly not evidence of a chronic alcohol-related condition.

Alcohol and death certification

The question whether to include 'alcohol' on the medical certificate of cause of death is not an easy one. There may be pressure from family members and indeed, those in positions of medicolegal authority to avoid mentioning 'alcohol' if at all possible. Although it is wise to remain responsive to such opinions, the primary responsibility of the certifying doctor is to provide a cause of death. At a blood alcohol concentration of <300mg/100mL, it is unlikely (although not impossible) that death resulted solely from acute intoxication. At a blood concentration level of >450mg/100mL, it is both justified and reasonable to write 'Acute Alcohol Intoxication' under Part 1(a) of the certificate. The situation is, of course, considerably complicated by the presence of other drugs, but it is important not to be tempted to use the presence of other drugs to underestimate the role of alcohol in causing death.

Less certain, are those cases in which either acute intoxication has played some causal role in the event leading to death (such as a motor vehicle collision, postural asphyxiation, or possibly, suicide), or there is evidence of contributory sequelae of chronic abuse. It is important to remember that the function of the death certificate is to report the medical cause of death—it is not a document on which to record social history.

Toxicological kinetics

The pharmacological kinetics of a toxic substance describes what happens to that substance after it has been administered to the body. This comprises absorption, distribution, metabolism, and elimination. The assumption is that the substance is able to move into the bloodstream and then into the tissues and organs of the body. The blood itself may be the method of transportation or the substance may move from the blood across cellular membranes by diffusion across a concentration gradient or by an active transport mechanism. What happens to the drug *in vivo* has a significant effect on what happens to it postmortem (e.g. relative concentrations at different sites).

Absorption

The absorption pathway of a drug depends on the method of administration. Intravenous administration results in almost immediate and total availability of the drug to the body. Oral administration is slow and often incomplete (the presence of food is also significant). Absorption at the lung–blood interface occurs when vapours are inhaled (e.g. heroin, cocaine—nasal insufflation when inhaled through the nose). Other routes of administration (e.g. intramuscular, ocular, intravaginal, rectal) have specific roles in treatment, but are not common in drug misuse. The bioavailability of a drug is invariably less than the quantity of the drug administered.

Distribution

The distribution of a substance around the body is related to the method of administration (e.g. a drug administered intravenously is immediately available to be circulated around the body within the blood) and how readily the drug distributes into other tissues or cellular fluid. Cannabis has a high affinity for fat, which reduces the bioavailability.

Models of drug distribution are based on the concepts of single or multiple compartments. A single-compartment model assumes that the drug is evenly distributed as if in a single volume. Thus, the concentration in the tissues is the same as that in the plasma. In a two-compartment model it is assumed that initially all the drug is in the plasma (intravascular space) from which it distributes into an extravascular compartment, resulting in a biphasic distribution curve.

Metabolism

Once distributed, drugs are metabolized (broken down or converted into other substances) by two types of biochemical processes known as 'phase 1' and 'phase 2'. The ability of an individual to metabolize a substance has a significant impact on the effect of that substance on the body (including the degree of toxicity). This is particularly important in individuals with defective CYP450 enzymes. The detection of metabolites is an important aspect of postmortem toxicology.

Elimination and clearance

The majority of drugs are eliminated from the body in the urine via the kidneys. Faecal excretion can account for a significant quantity, particularly of an unabsorbed drug taken orally. Metabolites may be excreted in liver bile. Saliva and sweat are of less significance except for volatile solvents.

Although an understanding of the kinetics of a drug is important to forensic investigation, it is important not to rely on antemortem data. Such information is almost invariably obtained from normal healthy individuals with known (and safe) doses. High doses can result in different effects as the bioavailability is significantly increased. The presence of disease (or prescribed medication and/or other drugs) may amend the normal pathway and factors such as obesity, age, and dehydration may also be significant.

Diamorphine (heroin) and morphine

Background

Morphine is very widely used in clinical practice to treat pain. Diamorphine (also known as 'heroin') is also in clinical use, but is perhaps better known for its role as 'heroin' amongst drug users. Both drugs are opioids. Diamorphine and morphine are both highly addictive and have very similar metabolic pathways. The former is initially metabolized to 6-MAM (6-monoacetylmorphine) which is not detected if only morphine was administered. 6-MAM is rapidly broken down into morphine from which point the metabolism is identical. To certify a death as being caused by heroin requires either the presence of 6-MAM at postmortem toxicology and/or other persuasive evidence such as witness statements.

Clinical effects

Heroin is usually either smoked, the fumes inhaled ('chasing the dragon'), or injected. A powerful analgesic and depressant, heroin results in a feeling of euphoria when administered. Clinical signs include pinpoint pupils, slurred speech, and persistent rubbing of the nose and mouth. Tolerance develops rapidly (after which the dose must be increased to achieve the same effect), although physical dependence takes longer. The effects of heroin are short term (typically 2–3h) and withdrawal symptoms appear 8–24h after the last dose. Withdrawal is unpleasant, but is not usually dangerous (some symptoms resemble flu together with diarrhoea lasting 5–10 days). Tolerance is lost after a period of abstinence (e.g. a custodial sentence) and users who return immediately to previous dosage are at increased risk of fatal overdose.

Injecting

Common sites for injecting include the arms, hands, and legs. Repeated injecting damages these vessels, when the groin and neck are then often used. Damage may result in thrombosis, fibrosis, false aneurysms, abscesses, ulceration, and septicaemia. Injecting as the route of administration has a much increased risk of infection (particularly HIV and hepatitis B/C), hence the development of needle exchange programmes to encourage the use of clean equipment. At autopsy, the presence of injection marks may establish that the deceased was an intravenous drug user, although this is not sufficient to prove that the death was drug-related.

Overdose

Deaths from heroin or other opiates may be suicides, but the majority are 'accidental' (unintentional) drug overdoses. Drug-related murder is rare (although see 📖 Shipman, p.486). Overdose causes death principally by causing central respiratory depression (i.e. via the brain)—respiration slows dramatically, causing hypoxia. There may be a reduction in blood pressure and reduced conscious level, often with associated airway obstruction and/or gross pulmonary oedema.

Interpretation of toxicology

A thorough and comprehensive history should be obtained, but note that records of prescribed medication (including 'scripts' issued by specialized drug services) do not necessarily depict the comprehensive history of drug use and must never be assumed to describe the substances taken on a single incident. The risk of death increases if heroin is taken with alcohol, cocaine, or other depressants.

Note: the use of prescribed diamorphine (heroin) to drug-dependent patients remains controversial. Whilst the practice has obvious harm-reduction benefits (lowering the risks associated with injecting—including transmission of HIV and hepatitis—and arguably, the rate of acquisitive crime), some authorities argue that it merely perpetuates drug misuse rather than adopting a zero tolerance policy with the aim of getting patients off drugs.

Methadone (physeptone)

Background

Methadone is widely used in the treatment of opioid-dependent patients ('methadone maintenance treatment'). The main advantage of methadone as an alternative to heroin is that it has a longer duration of action (approximately 36h), enabling a patient to remain relatively stable over a day. It can also be taken orally in liquid form, thereby avoiding the risks associated with injecting. Although methadone has certainly been successful in reducing harm from opioid dependence and misuse[1] it is also true that it has now become one of the main causes of drug-related deaths. Anecdotal reports from users suggest that withdrawal from methadone may be more difficult than from heroin or other opioids.

Supervised consumption strategies have been widely introduced as an attempt to control the quantity of drug diverted onto the street market. As these schemes do not cover all users (often limited to one or all of: high-dose patients, new starts, chaotic users, and randomized samples), some leakage is inevitable. Note too, that many users will supplement a prescription with other drugs obtained on the illicit market—including heroin.

Clinical effects and overdose

Although deemed to be 'safer' than morphine and diamorphine, clinical effects of methadone are similar. Overdose can result in death due to respiratory depression.

Interpretation of toxicology

As with any opioid drug, it is important to obtain a thorough and comprehensive history of drug use. This was highlighted in the Scottish case of Paxton v HMA, (Appeal Court, High Court of Justiciary 1999)[2] in which the Court held that it was reasonable to conclude that methadone caused death, given the evidence relating to the deceased's tolerance and previous drug-taking behaviour. The postmortem blood level in this case was 0.25 mg/L.

References

1 Greenwood J (1990). Creating a new drug service in Edinburgh. *BMJ* **300**:587–9.
2 Paxton v HMA (1999). Scottish Criminal Case Reports, Dec. 869–1108.

Other opioid substitutes

Dihydrocodeine and buprenorphine (Subutex®) are also used to treat opiate-dependent patients.

Dihydrocodeine

Dihydrocodeine (DHC, Diffs, Dfs) is prescribed for moderate to severe pain and tablets are readily available as a diverted ('street') drug. Dihydrocodeine is popular with some users because it is easily transportable in tablet form and the daily dose can be distributed throughout the day to reduce cravings. Some studies have suggested that dihydrocodeine might be just as effective as methadone for the management of opioid dependent patients.[1]

Buprenorphine

Buprenorphine or Temgesic® (licensed for analgesia) is sometimes confused with the benzodiazepine temazepam (both are sometimes known as 'tems'). Suboxone® is a combination of buprenorphine and naloxone—if injected, the naloxone blocks the effect of the buprenorphine and leads to withdrawal symptoms, but this is avoided if taken as directed, sublingually (under the tongue).

Long-term use of opiates can be assessed by hair analysis.

Reference

1 Robertson JR, Raab GM, Bruce M, *et al.* (2006). Addressing the efficacy of dihydrocodeine versus methadone as an alternative maintenance treatment for opiate dependence: a randomized controlled trial. *Addiction* **101**:1752–9.

Stimulants: amphetamines and ecstasy

The term 'stimulants' usually refers to amphetamines and related substances and cocaine. The increased use of 'designer' or 'dance' drugs such as 'ecstasy' is also important. These drugs increase cerebral activity and result in excitement and euphoria. High doses may cause hallucinations and drug-induced psychosis resembling paranoid schizophrenia.

The fatal effects of these drugs are not usually dose-related, so postmortem toxicology tends to be qualitative rather than quantitative. In addition, unlike alcohol, blood levels do not correlate well with levels of impairment.

Amphetamines

Medical uses

These drugs have been prescribed over the years for a variety of conditions. Previously, they were used widely as medical agents for the induction of anorexia, although concerns about dependency and other effects largely stopped this. Amphetamines continue to be used in the treatment of attention deficit hyperactivity disorder.

Effects

Amphetamines have euphoriant effects and cause psychomotor stimulation. They cause a predominately psychological dependence with rapid tolerance, such that it is not uncommon for users to increase their dose by up to 50x to overcome this. The following sympathomimetic effects can be pronounced and last for several hours:

- Dilated pupils
- Tachycardia
- Hypertension
- Tachypnoea.

Deaths due to amphetamine overdose are relatively rare, but can occur, resulting from hyperpyrexia, fits, and heart failure. Long-term consumption of large amounts of amphetamines can cause psychosis, characterized with paranoid ideas and delusions of persecution. Cardiomyopathy has been associated with amphetamine use.

Methamphetamine is chemically similar and is usually smoked (as 'crystal meth' or 'ice').

Withdrawal

Cessation of amphetamine use after chronic consumption may cause a protracted withdrawal syndrome. In the initial period after a 'binge', individuals may experience agitation and craving for the drug. Continuing withdrawal effects can result in fatigue, severe insomnia, and depression.

MDMA (ecstasy, 3,4 methylenedioxymethamphetamine)

A derivative of amphetamine, this stimulant has mild 'psychedelic' effect and at high doses some pseudo-hallucinogenic effect. Often classified as an emphathogen (or enactogen), hence the 'love-drug' association. Chemical variants have similar effects.

Tolerance develops gradually. Long-term use is thought to cause mood disorders (although controlled clinical information is lacking and animal models are not necessarily relevant).

Ecstasy-related deaths

These are rare, but invariably high-profile events, attracting intense media attention. Most ecstasy-related deaths involve at least one other drug. The cause of death is complex and has been attributed to various mechanisms, including exacerbation of undiagnosed heart conditions, hyperthermia, disseminated intravascular coagulation, idiosyncratic reactions, and water retention (renal failure), resulting in cerebral oedema. The extent to which ecstasy deaths can be attributed to 'overdose' or direct intoxication remains unclear.

Toxicologists and those working in forensic units should be aware that following an apparent ecstasy-related death, journalists are likely to request statements and information. It is imperative that a balanced view is maintained.

Cocaine

History

The stimulant effect of the leaves of the coca plant (*Erythroxylum coca*) has been known for thousands of years. Cocaine was extracted from the leaf in Europe during the 1850s. It was the first local anaesthetic to be discovered.

Effects

Psychological and behavioural effects

Its attraction as a drug of abuse relates to its ability to cause a feeling of euphoria, although the short-lived nature of this results in users often attempting to obtain further doses soon after the first. Cocaine is often taken with alcohol and it plays a similar role to alcohol in terms of being implicated in causing road traffic collisions and deaths from trauma (including 'accidents', homicides, and suicides). It causes feelings of increased alertness, irritability, aggressive behaviour, and an increased tendency to take risks. Psychological dependence can develop quite quickly.

Physiological effects

Physiologically, it has a marked stimulant effect on the CNS, causing tachycardia, hypertension, sweating, and tremor. Although regarded by many users as an aphrodisiac, long-term use of cocaine is known to be associated with reproductive problems and sexual dysfunction (erectile difficulties in men and difficulty achieving orgasm in women).

Nasal effects

Snorted intranasally, the effects last for <30min. Vasoconstriction damages the mucous membranes in chronic intranasal users, who can lose the sense of smell and develop perforations of the nasal septum. If cocaine use is suspected, swabs from the nostrils may yield a positive toxicological analysis.

'Crack'

Freebase cocaine ('crack') is produced by mixing cocaine with (usually) sodium bicarbonate (baking soda) and water. Heated, it produces brittle sheets which are 'cracked' into small 'rocks' and smoked. The effects of freebase last for only 5–10min, with dependence reportedly developing rapidly.

Cocaine-related deaths

Cocaine use is associated with a higher mortality rate than amphetamine. It has a direct action on the heart, leading to arrhythmia and fibrillation. It may also cause cardiac artery spasm, resulting in an acute myocardial infarction (which can cause long-term damage to the myocardium, even if not fatal). Convulsions may lead to respiratory arrest and increased blood pressure has been linked to stroke deaths. The risk of death particularly increases if there is pre-existing cardiac disease.

Autopsy findings of the classical signs of heart disease together with a history of cocaine use may be sufficient to certify a death as being cocaine-related, even if toxicology is negative. Cellulose granulomas from adulterants may be found in the lungs of recreational cocaine 'snorters/sniffers'.

Deaths associated with extreme violence

These have also been linked to cocaine use. Acute behavioural disturbance or excited ('agitated') delirium may present as hyperthermia, delirium, respiratory arrest, and death. Law enforcement agencies are often required to detain the individual during the agitated phase, so some of these deaths occur whilst the individual is in custody. Toxicology will not necessarily reveal elevated levels of cocaine. The extraordinary strength a person is able to exercise during the agitated phase requires significant restraint, the evidence of which is often the only finding at autopsy and on occasions, the issue of 'police brutality' may be raised.

The symptoms of excited delirium are similar to other disorders such as neuroleptic malignant syndrome (e.g. patients taking dopamine antagonists). Violence associated with cocaine-induced paranoid psychosis is also reported.

Hallucinogens and related substances

Terminology

The use of the term 'hallucinogen' is a convenient label, but not without controversy. Although these drugs alter how reality is perceived, users can usually distinguish between their vision and the real world. In a true hallucination (e.g. with LSD use), the vision *becomes* reality. The hallucinogens and related substances are not often directly associated with mortality. Indirectly, they may cause death by increasing risk-taking behaviour and causing injuries. There are case reports of cannabis being associated with drowning.

Cannabis (tetra-hydrocannibol, THC)

Cannabis was reclassified as a Class B substance following classification as Class C in 2004 (see 📖 p.458). It is the most widely used and available illegal drug. It may be eaten, infused in water, or smoked. It is available either as a resin ('hash'), in leaf form ('herbal', marijuana, 'grass'), or (rarely in the UK) in the form of a concentrated oil. Plants are easily cultivated at home (using hydroponic techniques under artificial lighting), including the high-yield varieties such as 'skunk'. Seeds can be purchased legally.

Clinical effects (see also 📖 *Effects on driving, p.333*)

Cannabis does not directly cause death. The key clinical effects relate to mood disturbance (euphoria) and altered judgement and perception (important in road users). Possible long-term effects are the subject of much argument, but include delusions and psychotic illness.

Testing

It can be detected more than a month after the last administration in a chronic user (approximately 1 week in a non-chronic user). This has potential significance for randomized testing in, for example, the workplace or prison.

Medical uses

The possession and use of cannabis as self-medication for multiple sclerosis and during chemotherapy remains controversial and is currently still a criminal offence in the UK.

Psilocybin ('magic mushrooms')

Most commonly in the UK, the liberty cap mushroom (*Psilocybe semilanceata*) when eaten or boiled and infused in water produces euphoria and hallucinations which can last for up to 8h. The most significant risk comes from mistakenly eating other varieties of poisonous mushroom and fungi.

The fly agaric (*Amanita muscaria*) is very toxic and can cause cardiac arrest.

LSD (lysergic acid diethylamide)

LSD (along with psilocybin, *infra*) was the drug which launched the psych-edelic age in the 1960s. It is associated with powerful hallucinogenic 'trips' which may be experienced again as 'flashbacks' (including negative experiences or 'bad trips'). It is administered by mouth (often as microdots on squares on paper). There are no physical or psychological withdrawal effects, although flashbacks can be associated with psychological problems (including suicide). It is not addictive.

LSD is often available at clubs and parties where MDMA is used. However, the doses used today are significantly lower than in the 1960s, which may explain why deaths are extremely rare.

In a custody setting, a user who is experiencing a 'bad trip' should be exposed to the minimum of external stimulation. All light and noise levels should be kept as low as possible.

Other related drugs

Ketamine ('special K') produces an effect similar to cocaine and the hallu-cinogenic effects of LSD. It can act rapidly, with the effects lasting up to 3h. Although fatalities are rare, inhalation of vomit is a serious risk if the dose is sufficient to induce anaesthesia. Ketamine may also used in low doses to facilitate sexual assault. Collectively, substances such as ketamine, phen-cyclidine (PCP, 'angel dust') and nitrous oxide ('laughing gas') are known as 'dissociative anaesthetics', as they separate perception from sensation. At the extreme, users experience an 'out-of-body' experience (sometimes known as a 'K-hole') in which they are often unable to move.

Mescaline is found in the Mexican peyote cactus and is the precursor of MDMA and several other psychoactive compounds. Mescaline use is often accompanied by severe vomiting although serious problems have not been reported. As with all psychoactive substances, deaths as a result of drug-induced disorientation and confusion have occurred.

The number of synthetic psychoactive substances will inevitably increase and forensic toxicologists must remain open to new developments and problems. The interpretation of toxicology will remain challenging, particularly as scientific clinical information may be limited.

Benzodiazepines

Readily available (either on prescription or illicitly), the depressant effect of benzodiazepines ('downers') compounds that of opioids, other sedatives/tranquillizers, and/or alcohol. Their use is associated with suicide and unintentional drug-related death. The risk of fatal overdose is low, but increases when used with other drugs, including alcohol. It is also not uncommon to find benzodiazepines used in combination with opioids.

The current widespread use of benzodiazepines has largely replaced the previous use of barbiturates. Drugs such as phenobarbital, which were once common in forensic practice, are now rarely encountered.

Shorter-acting

Temazepam ('tems' not to be confused with Temgesic®, 'jellies'), loprazolam, lormetazepam, lorazepam, oxazepam.

Longer-acting

Nitrazepam (Mogadon®, 'moggies')), diazepam (Valium®, 'vallies'), chlordiazepoxide (Librium®).

The use of a benzodiazepine to 'chill-out' or calm down after the recreational use of MDMA (Ecstasy) or other stimulant is frequently reported. Sudden withdrawal can be dangerous and care must be taken in a custody setting (see 🕮 p.262).

Phenothiazines

This group of antipsychotic (neuroleptics) drugs includes chlorpromazine, fluphenazine, levomepromazine, pericyazine, perphenazine, pipotiazine, prochlorperazine, promazine, trifluoperazine. Drugs having similar clinical characteristics include the butyrophenones (haloperidol), diphenyl-butyl-piperidines (pimozide), thioxanthenes (flupentixol, zuclopenthixol) and the substituted benzamides (sulpiride). The risk of fatal overdose is low, but increases when used in combination with opiates, other sedatives/tranquillizers and/or alcohol.

'Date-rape' drugs

The nature of the problem

Most drug misuse involves self-administration. A smaller number of cases involve the concealed administration to a third party. This may be for a variety of reasons, but one of the most commonly encountered in forensic practice is to facilitate a sexual assault ('drug facilitated sexual assault'). The scale of the problem is unknown, but an increasing number of sexual assault complaints involve an allegation that a substance was administered. On one level, this may be as simple as 'spiking' a drink in the hope of encouraging disinhibited behaviour. At the other extreme, it involves administering an illegal substance to an otherwise unwilling person without their knowledge or consent.

The role of toxicology

Toxicology may be of limited value because of the time delay between the administration of the drug and the reporting of the alleged offence. It is unlikely that traces of substances in a glass will still be available for analysis. However, urine samples are generally taken from the complainant for drug testing.

Drugs involved

Various drugs (often called **'predatory drugs'**) have been implicated, including:

- Gammahydroxybutyrate (GHB, 'easy lay', 'liquid X', 'liquid ecstasy', 'get her to bed') (note that GHB is not related to MDMA despite the name).
- Flunitrazepam (Rohypnol®) (or other benzodiazepine).
- Ketamine ('special K').
- Alcohol (which should be considered to be the most common of all substances used for this purpose).

The common features of these drugs are:

- They render the victim incapable or less likely to resist a sexual advance.
- Victims are unlikely to know that they are ingesting the drug.
- Typically, anterograde memory loss means that victims are less likely to remember the events (often it is only after contact with friends that the person even becomes aware that they are unable to recollect exact events).
- Rapid metabolism means that the drugs are less likely to be detected, thus reducing the physical evidence of assault.

Interpretation of findings

The presence of a typical 'date-rape' drug in the complainant does not prove that a sexual offence has been committed. Whether any sexual encounter was consensual or indeed, whether the drugs were self-administered, are issues to be decided by a jury. The benzodiazepine flunitrazepam (Rohypnol®) has been associated with drug-facilitated sexual assault, although data for this are incomplete.[1,2]

Prevention

As far as the public health and safety message is concerned, it should be emphasized that alcohol remains the most significant contributory factor associated with sexual assault. Many clubs and bars encourage customers not to let their drinks out of their sight, in order to address the opportunistic nature of this problem.

References

1 Beynon CM, McVeigh C, McVeigh J, et al. (2008). The involvement of drugs and alcohol in drug-facilitated sexual assault: a systematic review of the evidence. *Trauma Violence Abuse* **9**:178–88.
2 Scott-Ham M, Burton FC (2005). Toxicological findings in cases of alleged drug-facilitated sexual assault in the United Kingdom over a 3-year period. *J Clin Forensic Med* **12**:175–86 (now the *Journal of Forensic and Legal Medicine*).

Poisonous gases

There are numerous poisonous gases in common use in industrial and laboratory settings. This section covers the three most commonly encountered, as the others are rarely seen in forensic practice.

Carbon monoxide (CO)

Sources

The three main sources of CO are house fires, faulty gas heaters, and vehicle exhaust fumes. The circumstances of death are usually sufficient to deduce the source, although some scenes may be ambiguous as to the manner of death (e.g. an old car left with its engine running in an enclosed space is not necessarily a suicide). Prior to the use of natural ('North Sea') gas in the 1960s, the domestic gas supply ('coal' or 'town' gas) contained up to 20% CO and was responsible for many suicides and accidental deaths.

Risks of CO

CO has an affinity for haemoglobin some 250x greater than that of O_2 and over time even small atmospheric concentrations of CO will disrupt the transport of O_2 to the tissues. Although catalytic converters significantly reduce the amount of CO in exhaust fumes, the cumulative nature of CO toxicity is such that in an enclosed space fatal carboxyhaemoglobin (COHb) concentrations build up relatively quickly. The availability of O_2 in the atmosphere does not prevent death from CO poisoning—this has important safety implication for crime scene and body retrieval teams working in confined, often poorly ventilated spaces.

Autopsy findings

At autopsy, hypostasis and tissues exhibit a cherry-pink colour. A blood CPHb concentration confirms the presumptive diagnosis. A level above 50% saturation can be fatal in healthy adults—lower levels (>25%) may be fatal for the very young, the elderly, and especially those with pre-existing heart disease or compromised respiratory function. Concentrations in excess of 70% are invariably fatal. COHb levels can vary significantly, depending on the source of blood (which can be an issue if the body is also extensively burned). Elevated levels of COHb (>5% in a non-smoker) imply that the person was alive at the time of the fire.

Prevention of smoke inhalation

CO is the major cause of death in house fires and this has resulted in several campaigns to ensure the fitting of effective smoke alarms in domestic properties.

Carbon dioxide (CO_2)

CO_2 is a non-toxic gas which causes death as a result of displacing O_2 in the atmosphere. This occurs in plastic-bag suffocation or when the heavier-than-air CO_2 pools in a confined space as a result of industrial or agricultural processes. 'Dry ice' is a source of CO_2 and fatalities have been reported with its use.

Hydrogen cyanide (HCN)

Cyanide is an extremely toxic substance which inhibits the respiratory enzyme cytochrome oxidase and prevents the utilization of O_2 by cells. Hydrogen cyanide (HCN) is a gas which is released when cyanide salts (sodium or potassium) come into contact with water or acid. Although it is present in most house fires, it is usual that deaths which may be attributed to CO and HCN rarely appear as such on a death certificate. Deaths due to suicide are rare and confined to individuals who have access to laboratory or industrial supplies. Homicides using cyanide have also been reported.

Cyanide poisoning remains an option for the death penalty in five US states. It was also the gas (in the form of the insecticide 'Zyklon B') used by the Nazi regime in the gas chambers during World War II.

Autopsy findings

Hypostasis may appear darker than the cherry-pink associated with CO poisoning and in some cases can appear purple. The most distinguishing feature at autopsy is the 'distinctive' almond smell, although the majority of the population are unable to detect this aroma! The oesophagus and lining of the stomach will often exhibit erosion and haemorrhages.

Elevated blood-cyanide levels may result from postmortem diffusion when exposed to burning.[1] Care must be taken in the autopsy suite to minimize exposure to the team. Breathing hoods should be worn.

Reference

1 Karhunen PJ, Lukkari I, Vuori E (1991). High cyanide level in a homicide victim burned after death: evidence of postmortem diffusion. *Forensic Sci Int* **49**:179–83.

Volatile substances

The misuse of volatile solvents differs from most other forms of drug misuse in that the substances involved are easily available and are not illegal (although their sale may be restricted and controlled). Most households contain at least one substance known to be used in solvent misuse.

Amyl nitrate, butyl nitrate ('poppers')

The alkyl nitrates have been associated with the male gay community, but their use is considerably more widespread. Inhaling the volatile fumes is said to enhance sexual arousal and performance (as a result of virtually instantaneous vasodilation). The rectal sphincter relaxes, facilitating easier anal intercourse.

Adhesives and glues

Approximately one-quarter of all solvent-related deaths involve adhesives and glues. Toluene is the most common solvent used. It is usually inhaled from a paper or plastic bag.

Aerosols

These include deodorants, hairsprays, insect sprays, adhesive sprays, air fresheners, pain-relief sprays, paint sprays, and perfume sprays. Less common than 'sniffing' from a bag, aerosols are usually inhaled directly from the can. Aerosol propellants (e.g. butane) can stress the heart and lead to sudden cardiac failure. General advice is that a person discovered to be inhaling should not be agitated (e.g. chased). Butane itself can be inhaled directly as a gas fuel and is linked to swelling of the larynx causing asphyxiation.

Cleaning agents

Substances containing tetrachloroethane, 1,1,1-trichloroethane, acetone, and related compounds include industrial and domestic cleaning agents, printer corrector fluids, thinners, and nail varnish removers. Usually, they are inhaled directly from the container. Carbon tetrachloride is highly toxic and causes liver and brain damage. All these substances cause irreversible damage if used in the long term. If lung samples are submitted to the laboratory for analysis, they need to be sent in nylon impervious bags.

Antidepressants

Antidepressant drugs are most commonly encountered as suicidal overdoses. Although recent antidepressant drugs are inherently safer than their older counterparts, the availability of any toxic substance to a depressed patient creates an inevitable risk.

Autopsy findings in most cases of suicidal overdose will not reveal macroscopic abnormalities which enable the cause of death to be confidently attributed, but toxicology will usually establish the cause of death. Thorough scene investigation is also required (looking for evidence of missing tablets etc.). This can be particularly important if the deceased is elderly and exhibits sufficient other pathology to explain death—unless the index of suspicion is increased by the examination of the scene, a suicide may go undetected. Note that even if the cause of death is obvious (e.g. hanging or train suicide), toxicology is important as the information is useful to primary care and psychiatric service providers auditing procedure and practice (e.g. was the patient complying with prescribed antidepressants?).

Tricyclics and related antidepressants

Traditional tricyclic antidepressants include amitriptyline, clomipramine, dothiepin, and imipramine. Overdosage carries significant risks to the heart—fatal arrhythmias can occur. In addition, there is often initial excitement (with dilated pupils and tachycardia) and sometimes fits, before unconsciousness ensues. The 'related antidepressants' mianserin and trazodone are generally less cardiotoxic in overdose.

Selective serotonin reuptake inhibitors (SSRIs)

These drugs include citalopram (Cipramil®), fluoxetine (Prozac®), and paroxetine (Seroxat®). They tend to be safer than other antidepressants in overdose.

Monoamine oxidase inhibitors (MAOIs)

Patients prescribed one of the MAOIs (e.g. phenelzine, isocarboxazid) need to avoid certain drugs and foods containing tyramine (red wine, cheese, etc). These drugs result in an increase in the 5-HT (serotonin), noradrenaline, and dopamine levels in the brain. Overdose causes stimulation of the CNS, sometimes causing fits.

A list of commonly encountered antidepressant drugs can be found on 📖 p.492.

Paracetamol poisoning

Background

Paracetamol (called 'acetaminophen' in the USA) is widely available to buy over-the-counter on its own and in a variety of 'cold and flu' remedies. It is also frequently prescribed in combined preparations, such as co-codamol (paracetamol and codeine) and co-dydramol (paracetamol and dihydrocodeine). Although the quantity of paracetamol sold over the counter on any single occasion is controlled (16 tablets to a packet, one packet per customer), this does not prevent the purchase of large quantities of the drug.

Clinical effects of paracetamol overdose

Paracetamol is the most common agent used in deliberate self-poisoning in the UK. It is also associated with some inadvertent unintentional ('accidental') poisonings, particularly if taken in combination with preparations containing paracetamol. There are usually few acute clinical effects of paracetamol overdose—patients may be asymptomatic or simply experience nausea during the first 24h, but in severe overdose, liver damage may result and cause later deterioration. Some patients progress to fulminant (fatal) liver failure, combined in a minority with renal failure (from acute tubular necrosis).

Co-proxamol

Until recently, this combination of paracetamol and dextropropoxyphene was in widespread use as a painkiller for the long-term treatment of moderately severe pain. However, due to concerns about its role in overdose, it is no longer licensed in the UK. Deaths were attributed to the dextropropoxyphene component in overdose (particularly when taken with alcohol), as a result of cardiotoxicity/respiratory depression.

Mechanism of toxicity

Under normal (therapeutic) circumstances, paracetamol is metabolized in the liver, being conjugated to give the glucuronide or sulphate. In overdose, these mechanisms are saturated and instead paracetamol is metabolized to a toxic metabolite (N-acetyl-p-benzoquinoneimine), which itself can usually be inactivated by glutathione in the liver, but once the store of glutathione is used up, damage to liver cells (hepatocytes) ensues. The fatal dose varies between individuals, but may be as little as 10g, particularly in high-risk groups (e.g. alcoholics, malnourished).

Treatment

N-acetylcysteine is an effective antidote to paracetamol. It acts principally by replenishing glutathione stores. It is given intravenously and to be most effective, needs to be given within the first 8h after overdose. Treatment depends upon the amount taken, the time of ingestion, the weight of the patient, and the paracetamol blood level and is described in detail in the *British National Formulary* (see ♒ http://www.bnf.org).

Aspirin and non-steroidal poisoning

Aspirin (acetyl-salicylic acid)

Aspirin is implicated in far fewer attempted and completed suicides than paracetamol. The clinical effects vary according to the individual and the amount taken, but include hyperventilation, epigastric pain, tinnitus, deafness, and in severe cases, coma and convulsions. Aspirin acts as a stimulant upon the respiratory centre in the brain which is responsible for the characteristic hyperventilation.

Non-steroidal anti-inflammatory drugs (NSAIDs)

These drugs include ibuprofen and diclofenac. Gastrointestinal upset may result from poisoning, but serious effects are uncommon. Mefenamic acid poisoning is particularly associated with convulsions.

Harold Shipman

Crimes

Harold Shipman was a GP based in the northwest of England. Despite earlier suspicions when doctors had told police of their concerns about the number of cremation forms he had requested them to countersign, it was a forged will which eventually provoked extensive investigation. Following the death of his patient Kathleen Grundy, her daughter suspected that her will had been forged and this was traced to a typewriter in Shipman's surgery. The exhumed body of Mrs Grundy revealed traces of opioid. His victims were all women, mostly living alone and elderly, whom he injected with diamorphine. He was convicted on 15 counts of murder in 2000, although the number of deaths for which he was responsible is thought to number 200 or more.

Shipman inquiry

The government convened the Shipman Inquiry which published its final report in 2005. The Third Report (14/7/03, Command Paper Cm 5854) considered the system for death and cremation certification and for the investigation of deaths by coroners and stated that '(C)ertification of the cause of death by a single doctor is no longer acceptable'.

Protecting the public

The Shipman case demonstrated the inherent potential risks when a GP works—and certifies death—alone. This is no longer possible in the UK, following the introduction of primary care groups with responsibility for clinical governance. However, in this context, it is interesting to speculate as to whether, had the cases been referred for autopsy, the crimes would have been detected earlier. It is likely that the elderly victims would have exhibited at least some macroscopic abnormality or pathology which may, in the absence of suspicious circumstances or toxicology, have been deemed sufficient to have caused death.

Noting that toxicological analysis would have revealed the true cause of death, it is worth asking whether toxicology is now being instructed in similar, apparently routine 'sudden natural' death cases?

Shipman's death

Shipman hanged himself in Wakefield Prison in January 2004 and left no information relating to other deaths. The underlying motives for his actions remain unclear.

Public health

Although the primary concern of the forensic investigation is to establish a cause of death and collect evidence for any subsequent criminal proceedings in an individual case, the investigation of deaths associated with drugs should include an important public health remit.

Death certification

Public health policy and preventative strategies almost invariably rely on published mortality data. It is imperative that such data are as accurate as possible, which means, in practice, that death certificates should include a comprehensive statement of the role of drugs in the death.

- Avoid vague and ambiguous terminology such as 'mixed drug intoxication/overdose' or 'inhalation of gastic contents/vomit'.
- Name all drugs found at postmortem toxicology which are relevant to the death (taking advice from the toxicologist especially regarding the significance of metabolites).
- Ensure that information is communicated to local drug action teams, primary care specialists, and other relevant agencies. If necessary, open new channels of communication to facilitate this.

A *drug-related death* is a death in which the medical cause of death is related to the action of the drug or drug toxicity.

A *drug-unrelated death* is a death which was not directly caused by the drug but in which a drug was a contributing factor—e.g. a motor vehicle collision whilst under the influence.

Note that the death of a drug user does not necessarily make the death drug-related nor, indeed, even associated with drug use.

Drugs in sport

The World Anti-Doping Agency (see ✍ http://www.wada-ama.org) is the body responsible for publishing the list of substances which are prohibited in various sports. The 'Prohibited List' is updated annually and published at the start of the year. It provides a comprehensive list of all banned substances.

The 2009 list includes:
- Anabolic agents.
- Hormones and related substances—e.g. growth hormone (GH), insulin-like growth factors (IGF-1), erythropoiesis-stimulating agents (EPO), chorionic gonadotrophins (CG), insulins, corticotrophins).
- Beta-2 agonists (NB asthma medication such as salbutamol requires a Therapeutic Use Exemption).
- Hormone antagonists and modulators—e.g. aromatase inhibitors, selective oestrogen receptor modulators, agents modifying myostatin function.
- Diuretics and other masking agents.

Some substances are only prohibited during competition, including:
- Stimulants
- Narcotics
- Cannabinoids
- Glucocorticosteroids.

Others are only prohibited in particular sports
- Alcohol—e.g. aeronautics, archery, automobile, karate, powerboating.
- Beta-blockers—e.g. bobsleigh, bridge, golf, gymnastics, sailing, snooker, skiing.

Approach to drugs by athletes

Professional athletes are advised to take extreme care when taking any medication which has not been specifically approved by their doctor or medical adviser. The case of Alain Baxter (Winter Olympics, 2002) who unknowingly took methamphetamine (in the North American version of a commonly available nasal spray) illustrates this point.

Deaths

Although cases are rare, deaths as a result of the misuse of these prohibited substances are encountered. The extent to which the misuse of other 'performance enhancing' drugs such as sildenafil citrate (Viagra®) are associated with sudden death is not yet known. A full toxicological analysis should be carried out in all deaths associated with sport as even in amateur or low-level sport an individual may misuse a variety of substances. The presence of drugs may also be a coincidental finding.

Drugs and substance dependence

Opioid dependence

- Buprenorphine (Subutex®, Suboxone® (with naloxone))
- Methadone (Methadose®)
- Dihydrocodeine (DF118®) (sometimes preferred by users as it comes in tablet form).

National Institute for Health and Clinical Excellence (NICE) Guidance

'Methadone and buprenorphine (given as a tablet or a liquid) are recommended as treatment options for people who are opioid dependent.

A decision about which is the better treatment should be made on an individual basis, in consultation with the person, taking into account the possible benefits and risks of each treatment for that particular person. If both drugs are likely to have the same benefits and risks, methadone should be given as the first choice.

Different people will need different doses of methadone or buprenorphine. People should take methadone or buprenorphine daily in the presence of their doctor, nurse or community pharmacist for at least the first 3 months of treatment and until they are able to continue their treatment correctly without supervision.

Treatment with methadone or buprenorphine should be given as part of a support programme to help the person manage their opioid dependence.'[1]

Alcohol dependence

Disulfiram (Antabuse®).

Reference

1 NICE (2007). *Drug misuse – Methadone and buprenorphine.* Available at ℘ http://guidance.nice. org.uk/TA114

Further reading

Department of Health (England) and the devolved administrations (2007). *Drug misuse and dependence. UK guidelines on clinical management.* London: Department of Health (England), the Scottish Government, Welsh Assembly Government and Northern Ireland Executive.

Glossary of drug terminology

The following vocabulary may be useful when taking or reading witness statements regarding the use or misuse of illicit and/or prescribed medication. It must be emphasized that this vocabulary is both local and transient in nature and the use of the terms (particularly by witnesses) does not necessarily bear any relation to the actual substances taken.

- **2CB** (4-bromo-2,5-dimethoxyphenethylamine)—(spectrum, venus, erox, cloud 9s, etc.), hallucinogenic drug analogous to ecstasy.
- **4-MTA** (methylthioamphetamine)—a derivative of amphetamine with effects similar to MDMA (ecstasy).
- **Amphetamine (and methamphetamine)**—stimulants (speed, upper, sulph, whiz, base, etc.). Also used to treat attention deficient hyperactivity disorder (ADHD).
- **Barbiturates**—(barbies, goof balls, nembies, gorillas, red/pink/blue ladies/devils) recreational drug leading to mild euphoria (cf. alcohol).
- **Base**—(basing, freebasing) usually referring to crack cocaine.
- **Benzodiazepine**—(benzos), psychoactive drugs including diazepam (Valium®), chlordiazepoxide (Librium®), nitrazepam (Mogadon®), flunitrazepam (Rohypnol®) and temazepam (eggs, ruggers, rugbies, Edinburgh Es, vitamin T, beans, mazzies, tems—but also Temgesic®—etc.).
- **Buprenorphine**—(Subutex®, Suboxone®), an opiate substitute used as an alternative to methadone. Temgesic® is licensed for analgesia only.
- **Cannabis**—(grass, herb, hash, hashish, dope, weed, puff, draw, ganga, joint, skunk, blow, black, marijuana, THC, etc.), the active ingredient is tetrahydrocannabinol (THC). Smoked, eaten, or infused.
- **Chasing the dragon**—to smoke heroin—usually by placing powdered heroin on foil and heating from below.
- **Cocaine**—(C, Charlie, coke, dust, lady, snow, Percy, toot, white, aunt, etc.) crystalline alkaloid obtained from coca plant. Usually snorted or sniffed.
- **Crack**—(rock, stones, pebbles, base, etc.) a freebase form of cocaine usually using sodium bicarbonate as the base. Typically smoked.
- **Crystal meth**—(methamphetamine, meth, ice, crystal, zip, speed, chalk, glass, crazy, yaba, go-fast, amping, etc.). Usually smoked with long lasting effects (4–10h).
- **Dihydrocodeine**—(DHC, diffs, Dfs), an opioid substitute used as an alternative to methadone (also a prescribed analgesic).
- **DMT**—dimethyltryptamine is a naturally occurring tryptamine structurally analogous to psilocin and with hallucinogenic properties.
- **Delirium tremens (DTs)**—a medical emergency associated with significant mortality caused by alcohol withdrawal (see 🕮 p.256).
- **DTTO** (Drug Treatment and Testing Order)—intended to give offenders the opportunity to reduce their drug use and related crime.
- **Dual diagnosis** (or comorbidity)—coexisting psychiatric condition and substance use.
- **Ecstasy** (3,4 methylenedioxymethamphetamine)—(MDMA, E, eckies, love doves, sweeties, XTC, etc.), a synthetic substance which promotes increased energy, euphoria and empathy.
- **Flashback** (see HPPD)—a temporary state associated with hallucinogenic drugs in which the user re-experiences the episode.
- **GHB** (gammahydroxybutrate)—(liquid ecstasy, liquid X, get her to bed).

- **Heroin**—(brown, dragon, china white, H, horse, junk, skag, shit, smack etc.), opiate drug synthesized from morphine.
- **HPPD** (see flashback)—hallucinogen persisting perception disorder is a DSM-IV condition in which a user of hallucinogenic drugs (particularly LSD) continues to persistently experience an altered reality.
- **IV or i.v.** (intravenous)—(i.e. injection directly into a vein) or 'mainlining'.
- **Ketamine**—(special K, super K, vitamin K etc.), powerful anaesthetic with hallucinogenic properties.
- **LSD** (lysergic acid diethylamide)—(acid, blotter, dots, drop, flash, liquid acid, rainbow, flash, paper magic, etc.).
- **Magic mushrooms**—(liberties, magics mushies, psilocybin, shrooms, etc.).
- **Methadone**—a frequently used heroin substitute for treatment of opioid dependence ('methadone maintenance therapy'). An alternative to abstinence and promoted as an effective harm-reduction intervention.
- **Naloxone**—an opioid antagonist used to treat opioid overdose (blocks the actions of the opioid and reverses respiratory depression, although it has a shorter half-life than some of the drugs it is used to reverse). There is some controversy as to whether opioid-dependent patients should be issued with 'take home' naloxone for use in emergency situations.
- **Nitrates**—(amyl-, butyl-, hardware, liquid gold, poppers, ram, stag, stud, thrust, TNT, etc.)
- **Opiate**—a drug derived from poppy plant (e.g. opium, morphine, heroin).
- **Opioid**—refers to the whole group of natural, synthetic and semi-synthetic compounds that act on opioid receptors.
- **OTC** (over-the-counter medication)—drugs which are legally available from a pharmacy, but the quantity may be controlled (e.g. paracetamol).
- **Overdose**—use of any drug in a quantity high enough that acute adverse physical or mental effects occur. A dose higher than the prescribed therapeutic dose. Some drug users frequently deliberately 'overdose' in order to maximize the drug's effect—this does not imply suicidal ideation.
- **PCP** (phencyclidine)—(angel dust, monkey dust etc.).
- **Psilocin** (4-hydroxy-dimethyltryptamine (4-HO-DMT))—a hallucinogenic alkaloid found in 'magic mushrooms' (with psilocybin).
- **Rohypnol®**—(roofies, rope, R2, etc.) A benzodiazepine associated with 'date-rape' (drug facilitated sexual assault—DFSA).
- **Skin-pop**—inject subcutaneously (typically when veins difficult to find).
- **Solvents**—substances commonly found at home (e.g. hair spray, glue, cleaning substances, and gas fuel canisters) used as volatile solvent abuse.
- **Speedball (snowball)**—cocaine mixed with heroin.
- **Steroids (anabolic)**—(pumping, juice, weights, etc.), facilitate the development of skeletal muscle.
- **Street** (or 'diverted')—often used to refer to a prescribed drug which has been sold illegally.
- **Sublingual**—administration of a drug by placing it under the tongue (utilizing the abundance of blood vessels to achieve effective absorption).
- **Viagra®**—sildenafil (poke, V), prescribed for the treatment of erectile dysfunction, but with recreational value and use.

Antidepressant drugs

An alphabetical list of some of antidepressant drugs which may be encountered in forensic medical reports is shown here. For further information and a complete list of drugs licensed for use within the UK, consult the *British National Formulary.*[1] Non-medics are advised that this list is presented for the primary purpose of assisting name identification and reporting —it is intended neither as a guide to their use nor their appropriateness in a given clinical situation.

- Amitriptyline (TCA)
- Citalopram (Cipramil®) (SSRI)
- Clomipramine (Anafranil®) (TCA)
- Dosulepin (dothiepin, Prothiaden®) (TCA)
- Dothiepin (Dosulepin)
- Doxepin (Sinepin®) (TCA)
- Duloxetine (Cymbalta®, Yentreve®) (SNRI)
- Escitalopram (Cipralex®) (SSRI)
- Fluoxetine (Prozac®) (SSRI)
- Fluvoxamine (Faverin®) (SSRI)
- Imipramine (TCA)
- Isocarboxazid (MAOI)
- Lofepramine (TCA)
- Nortriptyline (Allegron®) (TCA)
- Paroxetine (Seroxat®) (SSRI)
- Phenelzine (Nardil®) (MAOI)
- Sertraline (Lustral®) (SSRI)
- Tranylcypromine (MAOI)
- Trimipramine (Surmontil®) (TCA)
- Venlafaxine (Efexor®) (SNRI).

Key to abbreviations

- MAOI: monoamine-oxidase inhibitor
- SNRI: serotonin and noradrenaline re-uptake inhibitor
- SSRI: selective serotonin re-uptake inhibitor
- TCA: tricyclic antidepressant.

Reference

1 Joint Formulary Committee. *British National Formulary.* London: British Medical Association and Royal Pharmaceutical Society of Great Britain. Latest edition avilable at ℘ http://bnf.org

Analgesic drugs

An alphabetical list of some of analgesic drugs which may be encountered in forensic medical reports is shown here. For further information and a complete list of drugs licensed for use within the UK, consult the *British National Formulary*.[1] Non-medics are advised that this list is presented for the primary purpose of assisting name identification and reporting—it is intended neither as a guide to their use nor their appropriateness in a given clinical situation.

Opioid analgesics

- Buprenorphine (Temgesic®)
- Codeine
- Diamorphine (heroin)
- Dihydrocodeine (DF118®)
- Dipipanone (Diconal®)
- Meptazinol
- Methadone
- Morphine (Oramorph®, Sevredol®)
- Oxycodone
- Papaveretum
- Pentazocine
- Pethidine
- Tramadol (Zamadol®, Zydol®).

Other analgesics and non-steroidal anti-inflammatory (NSAI) drugs

- Aspirin
- Aspav® (aspirin and papaveretum)
- Co-codaprin (aspirin and codeine)
- Paracetamol (acetaminophen)
- Co-codamol (paracetamol and codeine)
- Co-dydramol (paracetamol and dihydrocodeine)
- Ibuprofen (Brufen®
- Nefopam (Acupan®).

Note

Co-proxamol—an analgesic highly toxic in overdose containing dextro-propoxyphene and paracetamol. UK Licences for all products containing co-proxamol were cancelled by the Medicines and Healthcare Products Regulatory Authority (MHRA) at the end of 2007 (although doctors could prescribe the unlicensed product to existing patients on a 'prescriber has responsibility' basis).

Reference

1 Joint Formulary Committee. *British National Formulary*. London: British Medical Association and Royal Pharmaceutical Society of Great Britain. Latest edition avilable at ℘ http://bnf.org

Forensic science

Introduction to forensic science

Context

It is not the purpose of this book to provide instruction in the forensic sciences. However, it cannot be over-emphasized that forensic investigation is a multidisciplinary team effort and it is imperative that individual members of the team have at least an elementary understanding of the roles of experts in other disciplines. Not only does this ensure that evidence gathering, analysis, and interpretation is carried out efficiently and effectively, but it also goes some way to ensuring that expert witnesses in a court setting are, indeed, experts in the subjects to which they speak.

Definition

What is meant by the term 'forensic science'? Arguably, there is no such thing, if the term is intended to refer to a separate and clearly defined discipline. Forensic science is really an umbrella description relating to the practice of *any* science within a legal context. It is worth emphasizing that good forensic science is, therefore, nothing other than good science applied to a forensic context.

Why then include a chapter which purports to cover the 'forensic sciences'? This chapter simply presents an overview of the scientific disciplines which to a greater-or-lesser extent are often called upon in forensic practice. It is not claimed to be inclusive of all the forensic sciences, nor suggested that it describes any of them in any depth.

Key features

In general terms, forensic science means the application of rigorous scientific methodology and validated laboratory practices and techniques in order to generate results which can be used as evidence.

Key concepts relating to evidence include:
• Protection
• Recording
• Collecting/recovery
• Preserving (especially avoiding contamination)
• Analysing
• Interpreting
• Evaluation
• Presenting.

It should be noted that errors at any stage of this process may cause an otherwise strong case to collapse. Not only does this lead to a miscarriage of justice in that individual instance, it also results in an erosion of the public's confidence in the forensic sciences.

The importance of adhering strictly to the SOPs and operating guidelines in forensic laboratories cannot be over-estimated.

Forensic science and the court

How scientific evidence is presented in the court room is an oft neglected part of this chain. It should be clear that no matter how good the science, if it is poorly presented to a lay audience (i.e. the jury) it will fail to convince. Yet just as the scientist or other expert witness has an obligation to present their evidence clearly with precision and accuracy, this book is also intended to assist the lawyer in his or her ability to question and cross-examine such evidence.

Forensic science agencies and organizations

- Forensic Science Society
- American Academy of Forensic Sciences (AAFS)
- The Australian and New Zealand Forensic Science Society (ANZFSS)
- European Network of Forensic Science Institutes (ENFSI)
- Scottish Police Services Authority (SPSA) Forensic Services.

Crime scene management

What is a crime scene?

Although this might seem obvious, it is in fact one of the most important questions to be asked. A crime scene is defined whenever an illegal act is suspected to have taken place. The crucial issue is to define the physical limits of the crime scene—this is important as it should contain the maximum possible quantity (and quality) of evidence, whilst occupying a volume in which it is practical to search. Depending on the type of offence alleged to have been committed, this might be a room, a house, or even a whole street. It should be obvious that the wider the crime scene is defined, the greater the disruption to the public and this has to be balanced against the need to secure 'all' the evidence. The crime scene can also include areas in which evidence relating to the alleged offence might be located, even if this is not where the offence occurred. There are also circumstances in which the decision as to *when* a situation becomes a 'crime scene' is important. If a child has been reported to be late home from school, when (and where) does this become a 'crime scene'? It is important that law enforcement officers are able to refer to clear guidelines and policies when confronted by such circumstances.

Priorities at a crime scene

These are:
• Preservation of life (of victims, the public, and investigators)
• Preservation of the scene
• Gathering of evidence.

Law enforcement officers arriving at an incident are often confronted by a confusion of events and should always treat a scene as a scene of crime until confirmed otherwise. This should include calling out a forensic pathologist if a death is considered to be suspicious.

It is advisable to err on the side of caution and assume that a scene is a crime scene in order to protect evidence. Downgrading a scene (e.g. to an 'accident' or 'sudden natural death') is straightforward and costs nothing other than minor inconvenience. It is likely that evidence will be lost if it is not treated as a crime scene initially—with significant negative consequences both for the investigation and the reputation of the law enforcement agencies.

A certain amount of 'common sense' must be exercised in the case of large-scale, 'public' crime scenes. For example, in the case of the Lockerbie air disaster (21 December 1988), bodies were removed from public view at the earliest opportunity.

Some crime scenes are difficult to define in physical or geographical terms—notably, Internet-based crime such as child pornography or fraudulent (financial or identity) activity.

Health and safety

All crime scenes are potentially hazardous. Risk cannot be removed entirely, but efforts must be made to carry out a rigorous risk assessment and implement appropriate precautions. Advice from other agencies (such as fire or maritime rescue services) should be sought if relevant.

Approach to the crime scene

Crime scenes are rarely static and the quality of evidence deteriorates with time. Steps should be implemented to reduce the rate and extent of deterioration including:

- Cordons
- Common approach paths
- Control of scene.

Typically, a crime scene requires an inner cordon, an outer cordon with a single entry point to both, and a single pathway to the focus of the incident. Although the primary concern at this stage should be the preservation of evidence, consideration to unauthorized viewing (particularly if outdoors) should be made and, if necessary, a tent or screen erected. Press interest in serious incidents is significant and although visual access must be limited, it important to handle this with sensitivity (especially as relatives, friends, and neighbours of victims may be present). A Scene Entry Log should be maintained as quickly as possible and any possible sources of contamination (e.g. blankets which may have been put over a deceased) kept for examination at a later date.

Modern practice requires that whenever there is a crime scene, there should be a crime scene manager (CSM, who may be the Senior Investigating Officer, SIO). This CSM takes charge of the scene, including controlling and recording access of other experts. Forensic pathologists and forensic scientists, no matter how experienced, must act in accordance with the crime scene manager. The *only* exceptions are emergency medical staff treating injured people who remain at the scene.

If the crime involves several scenes, then a crime scene coordinator is appointed. Crucial to this role is to ensure there no cross contamination between scenes (which may, of course, involve the same experts).

Recovery of evidence

Recovering evidence from a crime scene is the responsibility of a wide range of experts. In certain types of incident it is likely that law enforcement officers will work in close collaboration with other statutory agencies such as aviation, marine, customs, fire, and environmental (pollution) investigators or organizations such as those with a remit to protect wildlife:

- Civil Aviation Authority (CAA)
- Air Accidents Investigation Branch (AAIB)
- Marine Accident Investigation Branch (MAIB)
- HM Revenue and Customs (HRRC)
- Department for Environment Food and Rural Affairs (DEFRA)
- Royal Society for the Prevention of Cruelty to Animals (RSPCA)
- Royal Society for the Protection of Birds (RSPB).

Crime scene investigation

Background

Crime scene investigation should attempt to address each of the following issues:

- Has a crime been committed?
- How/when/where was it committed?
- What is the identity of the perpetrator?

Note that a scene or incident might involve one or more designations. For example, a scene of a sudden death might prove to be drug-related and as such would have potential implications for a prosecution for supply of drugs or even manslaughter/culpable homicide.

   If in doubt, it is important to treat a scene as a crime scene to avoid the risk of losing vital evidence. A scene can always be downgraded at a later stage, once investigators are confident that no crime has been committed.

Accident or crime scene?

Lockerbie

Although initially clearly a scene having all the characteristics of a major *accident*, investigation into the Lockerbie air disaster (21 December 1988) revealed that it resulted from a criminal act. More recently, railway 'accidents', have resulted in criminal prosecutions on the basis of corporate manslaughter legislation.

Corporate manslaughter

The first UK case of corporate manslaughter involved OLL Ltd. Peter Kite, the Managing Director was jailed for 2 years (after appeal) in 1994 following the deaths of four teenagers in a canoeing incident at an outdoor activity centre at Lyme Regis, Dorset.

Crime scene recording

It is important that crime scene investigation includes crime scene recording. This should involve the use of traditional techniques, such as photography (always employing a scale for reference) and scale drawings (using computer software), but should also make use of crime scene management and reconstruction software. The ability to create a virtual scene is a valuable tool to assist interpretation and evaluation of evidence and/or events at a later date.

Crime scene evidence

The question of whether the evidence is believed and 'proves' the case as presented by the prosecution is, of course, a matter for the jury or judge to decide. Prior to that consideration, it is imperative that the integrity of the prosecution's evidence is preserved and can be demonstrated to the court. A chain of continuity should exist for each item of evidence, providing a complete audit trail accounting for all movement, handling, storage, and analysis from the scene to the mortuary/laboratory and, if appropriate, presentation in court. It should be possible to scrutinize the chain at any point to eliminate the possibility of contamination, damage, or deterioration having occurred which might be prejudicial to the case. All Health and Safety procedures associated with the handling, storage, and analysis of the item or material should also be documented so any adverse effects are known and can be described to the court.

Locard's principle

Edmond Locard (1877–1966) is often regarded as the father of modern evidence-based forensic science. The famous dictum summarizing his work:

'Every contact leaves a trace'

is axiomatic with the basic principle of forensic science. In purely practical terms, this simply means that it is always worth looking for evidence wherever a 'contact' is suspected. Remember that although this necessitates thorough and comprehensive police work at every crime scene, it says very little about the evidential significance of whatever might be found.

Significance of evidence

Note that in order to acquire evidential significance the contact does not need to be directly between two people. Suppose 'A' is alleged to have committed a crime against 'B'. If there has been physical contact between A and B then it is possible that there has been a direct transfer between the two: for example, semen, blood, hair, or DNA from one individual is transferred to the other (perpetrator to victim *and/or* victim to perpetrator). Matching the transferred sample to the source establishes contact. However, evidence of contact does not establish a reason for the contact and does not, therefore, 'prove' the prosecution's case. The defence might argue that there is an alternative and innocent explanation, that the sample has been transferred by an alternative mechanism (such as third-party contact), or that the sample has been contaminated by poor collecting, handling, storage, or analysis.

Alternatively, there might be a transfer from a common source which establishes indirect contact between individuals 'A' and 'B': the presence of a particular pollen, dust particles, fragments of a particular glass or fibres can provide evidence that 'A' and 'B' were 'at the same place' or, more generally, exposed to the same source of the sample. Again, note that this does not necessarily say anything about when this exposure occurred or why.

Applications in alleged sexual assault

Both the profound power and limitations of Locard's principle are manifest in allegations of rape. If semen is identified in a sample obtained from the complainant, then the science can prove (subject to the usual arguments about transfer, contamination, etc.) that sexual intercourse occurred. If, however, the suspect does not deny that sexual intercourse occurred, then the evidential significance of the science is minimal (the issue being whether there was consent to the act, not whether the act took place). Even if there is conclusive scientific evidence of contact, an 'alternative explanation' may render this evidence irrelevant to the case.

DNA from mosquitoes

Spitaleri and colleagues[1] report a case in which DNA matching that of a homicide victim was recovered from the blood meal stain of a mosquito found in the suspect's house. Although the technical aspects of this case are worthy of note, in this context the focus is the importance of the scene investigation and how an apparently innocuous finding (a squashed mosquito) actually held crucial evidence: scientific advances do not replace thorough and comprehensive police work:

- Note that if no evidence of contact is found, this does not establish that no contact took place.
- Evidence of contact does not establish guilt and the absence of evidence of contact does not establish innocence.

Reference

1 Spitaleri S, Roman C, Di Luise E, *et al.* (2006). Genotyping of human DNA recovered from mosquitoes found on a crime scene. *International Congress Series* **1288**:574–6. (Progress in Forensic Genetics 11: Proceedings of the 21st International ISFG Congress, Ponta Delgada, September 2005.)

Identification: matching and uniqueness

Basic concepts

In forensic investigation, there is another concept which is just as important as Locard's principle, namely the concept of identification—matching and uniqueness. A forensic sample which is obtained from a crime scene (for example, DNA, a fingerprint, a fibre, a fragment of paint, or a hair) only acquires evidential significance once it can be identified with, or matched to, a reference sample recovered elsewhere or from a suspect.

Unique match

The concept of a unique match is of particular importance in a court room. If a particular witness reports seeing a 'red car with a white stripe' leaving a crime scene, it is not sufficient to locate *any* white striped red car. A successful prosecution requires that the unique vehicle be identified (and proved to be such to the required standard of proof). In this example, a fragment of paint recovered from the scene can (by comparing chemical composition of the fragment to various paint manufacturers' databases) be matched to a particular batch and/or series of vehicles: it is unlikely that it can be matched to a unique vehicle unless a 'physical fit' can be achieved. Note that although chemical analysis of the paint fragment may enable investigators to focus on a particular class of car, it is only once a suspect vehicle is identified that a unique physical fit match is possible.

Matching

The extent to which 'item A matches item B' is often a question of magnification. Tearing a piece of paper into two pieces well illustrates this point. At a distance, the detail of the tear may be insufficient to distinguish unique features: the visible detail is not specific enough to enable a unique match to be made. As the torn edges are examined at higher magnifications, the required level of detail is exhibited and a match can be made with confidence. But note that at even higher resolutions, the 'perfect match' will be lost as minute tags and fragments are displaced and lost and the pattern is distorted. The skill of the forensic scientist is not only to know where and when to *start* looking but also to know when and where to *stop*. Irrelevant detail can be as misleading as insufficient information.

In a court of law, the expert should be cautious about matching an injury with a unique weapon. In most cases, the correct terminology to use is that an injury 'is consistent with' a type of weapon.

Knife injuries

For the forensic pathologist, it is important to appreciate that injuries can rarely be matched to a unique weapon such as a knife. The best that can usually be achieved is that the medical expert who examines the injury is able to state that the findings are 'consistent with' a particular type of weapon. This may include, for example, a knife produced as evidence in court. To state that the injury was caused by one particular knife requires more—an obvious example being if the tip breaks off during an attack and remains in the body. The tip can then be matched uniquely to the knife by a 'physical fit' procedure.

Gunshot injuries

Although it might be possible to state that a bullet recovered from an injury was fired from one particular gun, the injury itself can usually only be matched to a class or type of weapon.

Certain injuries are more likely to reveal information about the type of weapon (see p.164).

The Ruxton case

Double murder

The Ruxton case was an early demonstration of the success of forensic science and led to an increased professional and public trust in the technological advances being employed in the court room. Ruxton was an Indian-born doctor living near the border between England and Scotland. On 14 September 1935, he murdered his wife, Isabella, and her maid, Mary Rogerson, mutilating their bodies and scattering the remains in an attempt to render them unidentifiable.

Pioneering techniques

The discovery of human remains under a bridge in Scotland was the chance event which initiated the investigation. A forensic team led by forensic pathologist John Glaister and the anatomist James Couper Brash used pioneering techniques of photographic superimposition and managed to identify the bodies and produced the key evidence in the successful prosecution.[1] Whether this level of 'match' would be accepted by a court today is open to debate.

Trial

Dr Ruxton's trial took place in March 1936 and lasted 11 days. He was found guilty and sentenced to be hanged to death. He admitted guilt before his execution.

Reference

1 Glaister J and Couper Brash J (1937). *Medico-Legal Aspects of the Ruxton Case*. Edinburgh: Livingstone.

Daubert

The Daubert test

The so-called 'Daubert' test was introduced in the US courts as a way of regulating the admissibility of scientific evidence. The test requires that the two conditions of relevance and reliability are satisfied before expert scientific evidence can be admitted.

Relevancy test

The relevancy test simply requires that the evidence to be submitted is relevant to the issues of the case. This prevents irrelevant science being produced which, no matter how rigorous or persuasive it is, is simply irrelevant to the questions before the Court. This prevents juries being misled by irrelevant science.

Reliability test

The reliability test requires that scientific evidence and techniques:
- Are tested in actual conditions not only in the controlled environment of the laboratory;
- Have been subject to peer review, publication, and general acceptance within the relevant scientific community;
- Have a known error rate (which should be close to zero); and,
- Have standard procedures so they can be reproduced and tested by other experts in different settings.

The Daubert standard has particular relevance to the admissibility of evidence based on low copy number DNA analysis. Note that pseudo-scientific techniques would generally be excluded on the basis of Daubert (although whether they have an investigative role is open to further debate).

Further reading

Daubert v. Merrell Dow Pharmaceuticals, 509 US 579 (1993).
Huber P (1991). *Galileo's Revenge: Junk Science in the Courtroom*. New York: Basic Books.

Trace evidence: background

The nature of trace evidence

Trace evidence denotes any type of evidence which may be recovered from a scene in small amounts. The presence of trace evidence at a scene depends on at least three factors: how easily it separates from the source; the nature of the contact; and the nature of the surfaces involved. Any material which is capable of being transferred in small amounts from one object or place to another has the potential to be of trace evidential value. For example, soil, pollen, vegetable matter, gunshot residue, explosives, fire accelerants, body fluids, and illegal drugs. Analysis leading to a match with a reference sample may be more informative and discriminatory in some cases than others.

Interpretation

It should be obvious that although the techniques used to analyse trace evidence may produce a match between a sample from a crime scene and a reference sample (e.g. one taken from a suspect) they provide no explanation (exculpatory or otherwise) of *how* or *why* that sample was at that location.

Case of Ross Rebagliati

Ross Rebagliati was a Canadian snowboarder who tested positive for tetrahydrocannabinol (THC) following his gold medal winning performance at the Nagano Winter Olympic games in 1998. Rebagliati did not deny the scientific evidence of his sample, accepting that he had inhaled cannabis smoke. His successful defence, however, was that the cannabis smoke was the result of his friends smoking cannabis and that he had inhaled it coincidentally because of his proximity.

The case is a good example of detecting trace evidence which was sufficient to prove that an event took place (i.e. inhalation of cannabis smoke), but insufficient to prove that an offence had occurred.

Trace evidence: glass

The main property used to compare pieces of glass is the refractive index (RI). When light passes from one material to another with a different RI, the light path is bent. Conversely, if the two materials have the same RI, the light travels straight: this lack of bending is exploited in the most common technique used to assess the RI.

Glass refractive index measurer (GRIM)

This involves placing a small piece of the glass sample in a depression containing a transparent oil on a microscope slide. The RI of the oil can be changed as its temperature changes. At one temperature, the RI of the oil will equal the RI of the glass. Since there is now no bending of the light at the interface between the glass and the oil at this temperature, the light travelling through the whole assembly is unaffected. Knowing the RI of the oil at all temperatures gives the RI of the glass, which can then be identified from reference databases.

Density of glass is also a useful property in identifying the type or source of a sample of glass.

Physical fit matching of fragments of glass can be useful in, for example, a 'hit and run' incident. Fragments recovered at the scene may be matched to those remaining in a headlight on a suspected vehicle. In order to have evidential significance; however, the prosecution should be confident about the 'uniqueness' of the claimed match.

Trace evidence: paint

The nature of paint

The features of paint are physical (colour, texture, layers) and chemical (ingredients). Tiny fragments (<1mm) of paint from multilayered sources, such as car bodywork, can be embedded in a resin and sliced through to show the layers of primer, undercoats, and top coats. As with many items that may look the same colour under normal lighting, some items may look very different in other lighting conditions such as UV or monochromatic sources.

Spectrophotometry

This is also used in paint examination, except that in contrast to fibre analysis, which uses measurement of the light transmitted through the fibre, paint analysis uses reflected light (reflectance spectrophotometry). Paint analysis is similar to other organic chemistry, as most of the pigments used in paints are organic compounds. However, some additives give paints specific qualities such as waterproofing, antifungal, fire, or heat proofing, insulating, or flow modifiers. Many of these are metals, or metal compounds which can be detected using scanning electron microscopy (SEM). An electron beam is used to bump electrons within atoms of the sample right out of the atom. This leaves a gap that other electrons in the atom fill, so they drop into the gap left by the ejected electron. As they do so, they emit energy as X-rays. The amount of energy is characteristic of the jump that the electron makes going from its high orbit around the atom to its new low orbit. The jump is different in different elements and can be used to detect, for example, gunshot residue.

If a suspect source is identified (e.g. a vehicle) it might be possible to achieve a physical fit with a paint fragment.

Case of Malcolm Fairley (1985)

One of the most notable cases in which fragments of paint were of evidential significance was the 1980s case of 'The Fox' (Malcolm Fairley). Paint fragments found at a scene were matched to a British Leyland 'Austin Allegro' produced during 1973–1975. A vehicle which matched this colour was later identified at a suspect's home address. This evidence was crucial in focusing the investigation—it would not have been sufficient to secure a conviction. Fairley was subsequently convicted of a series of violent sexual assaults and rapes and sentenced to six life terms.

Trace evidence: hairs and fibres

Hairs and fibres can be described by colour and shape. The fibre can be natural (e.g. wool) or man-made (e.g. nylon). The shape (morphology) of a fibre can be established by microscopic analysis. Examining morphology can differentiate human and animal hairs due to species-to-species variations; the scale pattern; the ratio of the width of the central region of the hair to the width of the hair, etc.

Hairs from different body sites have characteristic cross-sections:
• Head: Caucasian (elliptical), African (oval), and Asian (round).
• Beard, pubic, eyelash: oval.

There may be considerable variations in hair morphology, even in hairs from one individual.

Colour represents the chemical and physical make-up of the fibre. Colour can be natural (i.e. introduced as the fibre is being made) or as a result of artificial dyeing (note that a person's 'hair colour' *in vivo*, may not be the hair colour as determined by chemical analysis).

Microspectrophotometry

This exploits the different absorption and transmission characteristics of light of different materials, due to their component atoms, elements, and ions. Light of different and known wavelengths in the visible spectrum is shone through the fibre and an absorption pattern or wavelength scan produced. Scans produced from a sample fibre can be compared with those of reference fibres of known characteristics. Using these techniques, dyes that appear the same colour to the naked eye can be distinguished because they are made up of different components.

Man-made fibres are usually made from long chains of carbon atoms with various atoms and chemical groups added, giving particular properties. Chemical bonds between carbon and these other atoms (and also itself) each absorb light of a different wavelength in the infrared (IR) region of the electromagnetic spectrum. Each fibre and the textile made from that fibre, can be characterized by its absorption spectrum in the IR region of the electromagnetic spectrum. The most common technique to do this is the Fourier transform infrared spectroscopy ('FTIR').

Fibres may also be characterized by **Ramen spectroscopy** (which looks at vibrational energy of the molecules of the fibres) and their birefringence (which is a function of the fibre's refractive indices).

These techniques have, for the most part, replaced destructive methods of analysing the dye components in fibres, which would have been extracted from the fibre and separated by thin layer chromatography.

Determining the melting point of a fibre as well as pyrolysis-gas chromatography (which thermally breaks samples down in to smaller molecules which are then analysed by gas chromatography and mass spectrometry) may be of relevance in differentiating between man-made fibres. Hairs are also a source of DNA. A complete nuclear cellular DNA profile is potentially available from the cells that comprise the root and mitochondrial DNA can be recovered from hairs that have no roots.

Fingerprints

Types of fingerprints

Visible prints—fingerprints made by touching glass or, for example, with an ink-covered finger are clearly visible to the naked eye.

Latent prints—a fingerprint not visible without treatment (e.g. application of powder) is termed a latent print. These consist primarily of perspiration from sweat pores.

Plastic prints—when the finger is pressed into a soft material (e.g. chocolate, clay, fresh paint, etc.) a print is made by creating a negative ridge impression.

History

In the journal *Nature* (1880), Henry Faulds (1843–1930) published a paper entitled 'On the Skin-Furrows of the Hand'. He wrote that 'when bloody finger-marks or impressions on clay, glass etc., exist, they may lead to the scientific identification of criminals ... the pattern was unique'. These recognizable patterns form the basis of the classification system which has been adopted in most English-speaking countries. Sir Edward Henry (1850–1931) based his system on three basic types of fingerprint patterns which had been recognized by Sir Francis Galton (1850–1911), namely loops, arches, and whorls. There are also subtypes of the types, but generally speaking, loops are defined where at least one ridge enters from one side, curves round, and exits at the entry side. Arches have ridges flowing from one side to another, rising in the centre in a wave-like pattern. Whorl classification is complex, due to the subtypes, the most simple of which encompass spiral, circular, and oval ridge patterns. As well as the basic pattern type, ridge characteristics including ridge endings and bifurcations may be seen and used for comparison and identification.

Two axioms form the basis for fingerprint identification:
• Fingerprints are unique.
• Fingerprints do not change through life.

Print comparisons

The process of comparing a print obtained from a scene with the comparison print can reach one of the following conclusions:
• The investigated print is identified as coming from the same donor as the comparison print.
• The investigated print has insufficient information to enable a conclusion about origin.
• The investigated print is unfit for identification, but exhibits detail sufficient to exclude specific donors.
• The investigated print enables the expert to state that the investigated person cannot be excluded as the donor.
• The comparison print is of insufficient quality (the procedure should be halted and a new comparison print may be obtained).

Minimum point rules

Historically, a match was confirmed on the basis of the minimum number of points rule (or an empirical standard approach). However, there is no scientific or statistical basis for the assertion that a match requires a certain (e.g. 12 or 16) number of 'identical' points. Generally, a minimum points rule has now been replaced by a more integrated approach in which the court hears evidence from an expert witness who uses a qualitative and quantitative approach to reach a conclusion.

Human error

In addition to the question marks over the scientific status of fingerprint evidence, the techniques and methods employed are particularly prone to human error. One of the most notable cases in recent years is that of Shirley McKie, a police officer with Strathclyde Police. Experts at the Scottish Criminal Records Office mistakenly identified her fingerprints at a crime scene. She was subsequently charged with perjury and although being found not guilty, the case has become an internationally important landmark in the role of fingerprint evidence in modern forensic investigation. A further example of human error was seen after the Madrid bombings (March 2004), in which the US Federal Bureau of Investigation erroneously matched digital images of latent prints to an Oregon lawyer, Brandon Mayfield.

Although there are many documented cases of a wrong 'match', unverified techniques used to obtain ('lift') the print and the continuing debate over the 'uniqueness' of patterns, the use of fingerprints remains a potentially quick and cheap method of identifying bodies.

Prints from a body

When an unknown body is discovered, consideration should always be given to obtaining fingerprints. These are fragile and should be taken before remains are moved. If the epidermis is 'de-gloved' (bodies in water), it is possible to take the print from the 'glove'. In some circumstances (e.g. extensive burning, mummification) it might be desirable to submit the whole hand to a fingerprint expert for examination and with specialist techniques, retrieval of prints. Prints obtained from a deceased individual should be compared with those stored on databases or with fingerprints taken from personal property once an identity is suspected.

Forensic analysis of DNA

DNA and individuality

Our apparent individuality (e.g. hair and eye colour or predisposition to diseases such as cystic fibrosis) arises because of differences in our *genes* (regions or **loci** of DNA which control hereditary characteristics *exhibiting genetic variation known as alleles*). The combination of the two genes (one inherited from each parent in the form of **chromosomes**) is the **genotype** and a person's **phenotype** is the observable result of the genotype. In a forensic context, these differences are relatively tiny (the variations are limited by the need to maintain the functional ability to code proteins) and are of limited use.

DNA profiling

The basis of DNA (deoxyribonucleic acid) profiling in forensic science is in the areas of non-coding DNA lying between the genes (sometimes referred to as 'junk' DNA) which comprises about 98.5% of the **genome** (the complement of the 46 chromosomes normally present). As these regions have no coding function, the variation is unlimited and the possible combinations are such that individuals are (at least to the order of 1 in billions) unique. The only exception is identical twins in whom both the genotype and the 'junk' DNA is identical.

Short tandem repeats

Forensic analysis examines regions of the genome called short tandem repeats which are repeated sequences of DNA (typically 4–6 base pairs in length). The variation (and conversely the uniqueness of the individual) arises because the number of repeats is highly variable (polymorphic) across the population (e.g. the locus known as D18S51 [with the sequence AGAA] has been found to be repeated between 7 and 27 times in different individuals). A heterozygotic individual will have different versions of each loci inheriting one from each parent. A homozygotic individual inherits the same version from both parents.

Polymerase chain reaction (PCR)

PCR is a method of increasing (amplifying) the quantity of a DNA sequence obtained from a sample exponentially. Typically a PCR involves 28 cycles, which increases the original sample by a factor of approximately 270 million. In the UK, current forensic practice is to amplify 10 loci (in the US 13 loci are routinely examined), plus a determination of the sex of the individual from a locus known as amelogenin (based on XX chromosomes for females and XY for males).

Electrophoretogram

The process of 'typing' or 'profiling' is managed by a computer which produces a graphical representation (an electrophoretogram or electropherogram) usually showing peaks along three colour-coded horizontal axes. The position of the peak along the axis indicates the size (number of repeats). Note that the form of this graphical output is dependent on the software used and more sophisticated packages also provide interpretative analysis.

Alongside each peak the number of repeats found at that locus will usually be stated. Note that although the height of each peak in a heterozygous person should be the same as it represents the quantity of DNA, there is significant variation because of the chemistry and dynamics of the amplification process. The height of peaks can also be useful in determining which allele comes from which source in a mixed sample.

Paternity disputes

Paternity disputes can be resolved using DNA analysis. If the alleles of the disputed parent are inconsistent with those inherited by the child, then that individual can be excluded as a biological parent. If the alleles are consistent with the child's alleles then the individual is possibly a biological parent. It is important that reference samples are available from all the potential parents.

Mitochondrial DNA

Mitochondrial DNA is inherited from the mother, so is a useful method of tracing the maternal line. In a forensic context, this genetic material is important because it is more resilient to degradation than nuclear DNA. It mutates at a faster rate than nuclear DNA and has less discriminatory power, because all female members of the family will share the same mitochondrial DNA (ignoring mutation). It can be a useful tool when identifying victims of mass disasters. Analysis of mitochondrial DNA requires the sequencing of two hypervariable regions.

Familial DNA

Familial DNA is based on the theory that family members are more likely to have similar DNA. In 2004, Craig Harman was convicted of manslaughter following a close (but not exact) match between a sample obtained at a crime scene and a family member on the DNA database. In the James Lloyd case (2006), a DNA match was made following the close match of a DNA sample obtained from Lloyd's sister after a driving offence. He had committed rapes and sexual offences in the 1980s.

Low copy number

Low copy number DNA analysis remains controversial. The technique is used when only a very tiny quantity of DNA is recovered—such as from a fingerprint. In order to generate sufficient DNA for analysis, this requires more PCR cycles with the consequence that contaminants and other residual DNA will also be amplified. As techniques to recover more minute quantities of DNA develop, the amount of DNA transferred via innocent contact also increases. This potentially results in a greater number of 'matches'—but 'matches' with little or no evidential significance.

Further reading

Low copy number DNA testing in the Criminal Justice system. Available at ⧉ http://www.cps.gov.uk/publications/prosecution/lcn_testing.html
Omagh Bombing Trial: *R v Hoey* [2007] NICC 49.

Interpretation of DNA analysis

Importance of interpretation

*The **interpretation** of* DNA analysis is at least as important as the science which underlies it. If two profiles (e.g. one from a crime scene, the other from a suspect or a database) have the same alleles at all of the profiled loci, then the samples 'match'—this means that both samples could have originated from the same source. The random match probability is the probability of obtaining that match if the samples did not come from the same source. This is not the same as the probability that the suspect is innocent.

If the two profiles do not match, then the two samples do not come from the same source—a suspect can, therefore, be absolutely excluded (ignoring the possibility of human error or sample contamination).

Random match probability

This is derived from multiplying the probabilities for the individual loci (derived from frequencies observed in tested samples of specific populations) together—for 10 loci this is in the order of 1 in billions.

Stutters

These are artificially generated small peaks which appear due to the chemistry of the PCR process—the problem with a 'stutter' is knowing whether it is indeed a 'stutter', or a small peak representing another source of DNA such as a mixed sample. This is a subjective decision made by the reporting scientist—a peak will usually be considered a stutter if <15% of the size of the main peak.

Mixed samples

These are those obtained from more than one source. In some cases, it might be straightforward to subtract a known source (e.g. the female in a case of alleged rape), but if DNA from multiple sexual partners is present, the result might be inconclusive. A number of markers on the Y chromosome have been identified. These can be valuable to discriminate between multiple male contributors in a mixed biological sample.

Partial profiles

These arise when it is not possible to analyse 10 loci—either due to the quantity or quality of DNA recovered from the sample. A random match probability can still be calculated, but this will have less discriminatory power and will carry less evidential value.

Interpretation of profiles

Conclusions and statements are made from interpretation of the profile as a whole, rather than a single locus, and this is particularly relevant when making conclusions as to the number of contributors to a sample. While two peaks indicates *at least* one contributor, if every locus of the profile had one or two peaks the profile would be taken as originating from a single source sample. The examples shown in Figs. 15.1–15.4 are illustrative of the possible results at a single locus.

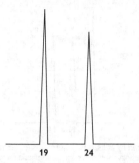

Fig. 15.1 Peaks produced most likely by one heterozygous individual. Examination of further loci might indicate more than one contributor to the sample in which case a) at least one heterozygous individual, or b) at least two homozygous individuals, or c) a combination of homozygous and heterozygous individuals who share one allele.

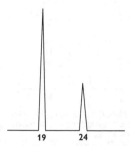

Fig. 15.2 Peaks produced by a) (at least) two homozygous individuals—note that the smaller peak is <50% of the larger peak and is unlikely therefore to have come from a single heterozygous individual or b) one heterozygous individual and one homozygous (for allele 19) individual.

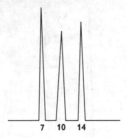

Fig. 15.3 Peaks produced by at least two individuals (potentially a combination of heterozygous and homozygous). This usually implies a mixed sample; however, individuals with chromosomal abnormalities (e.g. Down syndrome with trisomy 21) could produce a similar pattern depending on the loci tested.

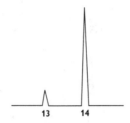

Fig. 15.4 Peaks produced by either a) a stutter and at least one homozygous individual, or b) a heterozygous individual and a homozygous individual (for allele 14), or c) two homozygous individuals.

National DNA database

The UK database
The UK has the world's largest DNA database, with profiles from >5% of the population stored. In the USA, the comparable figure is <1%. Legislation governing samples obtained for and retained on the national DNA database is in a state of flux. The Crime and Security Bill 2009–2010 (England and Wales, Northern Ireland) proposes new time limits for the retention of DNA samples, DNA profiles, and fingerprints and extends the circumstances in which such samples can be collected. The Bill responds to a European Court of Human Rights judgement and represents a scaling-down of earlier proposals to enable indefinite storage of some profiles.

Controversy
DNA databases are the subject of controversy, particularly regarding the potential uses of the data out of the criminal justice area (e.g. health-related information and insurance). Furthermore, as the number of profiles stored on the national DNA database increases, the likelihood of a coincidental or adventitious match also inevitably increases. The risk of a chance match would be significantly reduced if the number of loci tested was increased.

Alternatives to DNA analysis
Although DNA analysis has certainly taken over from a lot of other methods in becoming the technique of choice for forensic 'identification' purposes, it should be noted that other methods retain usefulness in certain circumstances:
- Blood groups—a quick and easy method of elimination.
- Anthropology—able to narrow a search on the basis of age and sex.
- Fingerprints—may identify an individual not on a DNA database.
- Cheaper techniques are likely to retain a role within the developing world.

DNA analysis in perspective
It must be remembered that without a reference sample, profiling a sample recovered from a crime scene will not result in a positive identification. DNA analysis is based on achieving a comparison between two samples, one of which has a known source. From the perspective of the criminal justice system, a national DNA database (with appropriate international communication) provides an important reference source—the civil liberty and ethical issues arising from calls to make it a universal database are issues still to be resolved.

Further reading
Gill P, Jeffreys AJ, and Werrett DJ (1985). Forensic applications of DNA 'fingerprints'. *Nature* **318**:577–9.

Exonerating the innocent

Almost invariably, techniques of forensic science and medicine are thought of as being used to convict the guilty. However, one of the earliest uses of DNA evidence was arguably even more important—to exonerate the innocent.

The Colin Pitchfork case

In 1983, Lynda Mann was raped and murdered in the Leicestershire town of Narborough. A semen sample identified a type A blood group and an enzyme profile matching 10% of the male population. In 1986, Dawn Ashworth was sexually assaulted and murdered in the same town—evidence from her body indicated the same attacker had committed both murders. Police had a suspect who confessed to the second killing, but denied involvement in Lynda Mann's death. Convinced the suspect was responsible for both deaths, the police approached Jeffreys who, with Gill and Werrett, had described the potential for using DNA profiling in forensic cases. Semen samples obtained from the two murder victims were compared against a suspect's blood sample. Analysis conclusively proved that both girls were killed by the same man. However, crucially, DNA evidence proved that this was not the suspect. Given that the police had a confession relating to the killing of one victim, it is probable that if the case had proceeded to trial, the suspect would have been convicted and the case closed. In addition to the miscarriage of justice that would have entailed, it would also have left the guilty man at liberty.

In order to identify the man responsible for the murders it was, therefore, simply a task of finding the individual who matched the two existing samples. Thus the world's first intelligence-led DNA screen took place involving 5000 men from three local villages who were asked to provide blood or saliva samples. Blood grouping was used to identify the 10% of men with the killer's known blood group and DNA profiling was subsequently carried out on these individuals.

The guilty man almost escaped justice by getting a friend to give a blood sample using his name. Fortunately, a conversation relating to the switch was overheard and a local man, Colin Pitchfork, was arrested and later convicted. This demonstrates that even with the best scientific methods available human factors are just as important.

Sean Hodgson case

In 2009, Sean Hodgson was freed after spending 27 years in jail for a murder which he initially confessed to, but DNA techniques indicated that he did not commit. This period of imprisonment is one of the longest terms served following a miscarriage of justice in the UK.

Further reading

Gill P, Jeffreys AJ, and Werrett DJ (1985). Forensic applications of DNA 'fingerprints'. *Nature* **318**:577–9.

Forensic biology

The advent of DNA profiling has had a huge impact on the importance of biological evidence, making the latter seem less relevant, particularly in relation to the identification of individuals involved in a crime scene. However, the older techniques are still important in determining the type of biological fluid or sample that has been found, even if being less discriminatory for personal identification.

Blood identification

Blood is the body fluid most often deposited and most easily identified at a violent crime scene—it is red and visible to the naked eye. Indeed, the simple presence of blood can provide information about events at a scene due to its location and distribution on surfaces such as floors, walls, clothing, and moveable objects. Whether the blood is still wet or has discoloured with age, may provide some information regarding the time it was placed where it was found. However, blood is not always easy to find at a scene, so screening techniques should be used. It is noted that the presence of blood at a scene does not necessarily imply a crime—a sudden natural death from ruptured oesophageal varices, for example, may be often accompanied by copious quantities of blood.

Presumptive luminal test

A crime scene can be screened for the presence of blood by spraying the area with a solution of luminal and looking for and photographing the chemiluminescent glow produced by blood. The chemistry of the reaction involves an oxidization of the luminol compound by the haem component of red blood cells, including a release of pale blue or yellow-green light (depending on the reagent preparation). Luminol is very sensitive and thus, very useful, but it can give a false positive by reacting with other oxidizing chemicals.

Presumptive tests are useful in indicating the presence of a substance quickly and cheaply. They can be used at the scene. They provide qualitative, not quantitative, information and are not definitive. Other tests should be carried out at the laboratory. In practice, some scenes 'obviously' contain large amounts of blood, in which case such tests are unlikely to be carried out.

Stain collection and transportation

The way a stain is collected, packaged, and transported will depend on its location and whether it is wet or dry. If the stain is on a moveable object and has dried, it is possible to transport the whole stain, by putting the stained article (or sample if the article is too bulky) in a paper bag or envelope. Representative unstained areas of the stained item should also be collected and packaged separately from the stained samples, to act as a negative control. In some cases, a *dried stain* may be swabbed with a moistened cotton swab and transported on the swab in its protective container placed in paper packaging. The containers may be ventilated to assist drying of the swab.

Damp environments

Prolonged exposure to damp environments accelerates decomposition and growth of micro-organisms, which can compromise the sample, so samples should be dried as soon as possible. A scraping of dried material may be collected and transported in paper packaging, rather than swabbing the sample.

Wet articles which cannot be dried on site should be transported in plastic bags and dried out at the laboratory for subsequent storage in paper.

Further tests

Further tests carried out at the laboratory on the collected samples include chemical reactions that produce a colour change in the presence of the oxidizing haem component of red blood cells. Two commonly used tests are the KM (Kastle–Meyer) and LMG (leucomalachite green) tests.

Source of blood

The advent of DNA profiling technology has largely superseded the previously used identifying tests, which fell in to the discipline of serology.

Species identification

This is particularly relevant in the area of forensic wildlife or animal cases (e.g. illegal importation). Tests involve immunological components that give a visible precipitation stain when blood of a particular species is present. The precipitate results when antibodies, which are immunological molecules that have specific recognition characteristics such that they only bind other molecules of a particular shape and structure (which are species specific), encounter such molecules. The molecules to which antibodies bind are known as antigens and when the species-specific sets of antibodies and antigens that are used in the tests interact, a precipitate of the bound antibody–antigen complexes forms enabling the species of a sample to be identified.

ABO typing

Prior to DNA analysis, the science of immunology provided the methods to distinguish individuals on the basis of the presence or absence of specific antigens. The most common tests have been to determine the ABO blood group and phosphoglucomutase (PGM) type of a sample. Karl Landsteiner was awarded the Nobel Prize for Medicine in 1930 for his classification of the ABO blood system and determining compatibility/incompatibility for blood transfusions on the basis of this system.

ABO typing is useful and well established, although its power of discrimination is limited. There are three possible antigens of the ABO group which are present on red blood cells, namely A, B, and O and the combination of these results in four possible blood groups, A, B, AB, and O, which can be detected immunologically. Each individual inherits two of the antigenic variants, one from each parent, which may be the same or different (Table 15.1).

Table 15.1

Parent 1	Parent 2	Offspring
A	A	A
B	B	B
O	O	O
A	B	AB
A	O	A
B	O	B

The frequencies of the different ABO blood groups vary from population to population.

Testing

When blood of an individual who is of the A blood group is mixed with antisera containing anti-A antibodies, the red blood cells and the antibodies will agglutinate, clumping together to form a precipitate. If antisera containing anti-B antibodies is added to red blood cells from an individual who is of the A blood group there will be no antigen–antibody reaction and the red blood cells will not precipitate. Red blood cells from an individual who is of the AB blood group will agglutinate with both anti-A and anti-B anti sera.

While it is possible to exclude an individual as being the source of an unknown sample if the blood types are not the same, one can only conclude that an individual who does have the same blood type as a sample could be included in the population of possible donors, along with others who also share the blood group type in question.

ABO and paternity testing

Blood group typing has also been useful in paternity dispute cases. An individual's blood group is a combination of the variants they inherit from their parents; each parent donating one variant to the child. If the blood group of a child could not result from the possible combinations of the blood groups of the known parent and the parent in dispute, then the parent in dispute would be excluded as the parent.

Phosphoglucomutase (PGM)

PGM is an enzyme involved in the metabolism of carbohydrate. PGM typing has a greater power of discrimination than ABO typing because there are 10 different forms that can be detected. PGM is especially useful because the enzyme can be detected in body fluids other than blood, for example, semen, saliva, and vaginal fluid.

One method of identifying the polymorphic variants uses a technique called isoelectric focusing (IEF). The four different PGM variants are identified as 2+, 2−, 1+, and 1− and each individual will have two variants, making up their genotype. The two variants making up an individual's genotype may be the same or they may be different, giving 10 possible combinations that can be differentiated by IEF.

While the prevalence of PGM in a number of body fluids is widespread, the finding of ABO type in non-blood body fluids depends on the secretor status of a person. 80% of humans are secretors and are a source of ABO-typeable material other than blood.

Blood pattern analysis

Whilst blood analysis may provide evidence of the source of a sample, it may also reveal important information as to the events that occurred at a scene of crime. The pattern of blood spatters, distribution, apparent age, and amount can help determine the sequence of events, including, for example, relative and absolute motion, position of the victim/assailant, and a time frame. Blood is a viscous fluid (about 6x as viscous as water) with a predictable behaviour. To form a blood spatter, the surface tension of the blood must be overcome.

Role of blood pattern evidence

Blood pattern evidence can be used to establish:
- Direction of travel of the blood droplets and source.
- Distance from source to impact surface.
- Angle of impact.
- A sequence of events (incident reconstruction).

It is important to understand the limitations of this type of analysis. Patterns are formed as a result of the relative motions between the source and the impact plane—these may not be easily or directly translated into absolute motions or pathways.

Blood drops

A blood drop which impacts at an angle of 90° will usually form a circular shape. The extent of satellite drops gives an indication of the velocity of impact (or if vertical, the distance fallen). A smooth non-porous surface such as a bathroom tile or glass is likely to produce less satellites (i.e. a smoother circle) than a rough surface such as a piece of wood. Arterial pressure and/or movement means that blood can be transferred in an upwards direction in addition to falling as a result of gravity.

The length (L) and width (W) of the drop are measured. The approximate angle of impact (Ai) is given by:

$$L/W=\sin(Ai)$$

Distribution of blood

The largest quantities of blood are often located where the assault ended or, if the victim moved, at the place where they collapsed/died. This is because at the start of an attack, the victim is more likely to be mobile and blood will be distributed over a wider area. Furthermore, a continued attack will exacerbate existing and create new wounds. As the victim (and/or the assailant) become covered in blood, it is more likely that smears and staining will be present on walls and floors. If a body has been moved from the primary scene where an attack took place to a secondary site then blood may not be found: the absence of blood (in the presence of significant wounding) is an indication that a body has been moved.

Cast-off blood

Cast-off blood may be produced as a result of the centrifugal forces when weapons such as blunt instruments or sharp knives are swung in an arc. The blood marks along the arc will change shape reflecting the angle of impact. Cast-off should be distinguished from arterial spurt.

Wipe

A wipe occurs when a moving object comes into contact with a blood stain. The direction of motion is usually apparent. A *swipe* is created when a moving object covered in blood comes into contact with a surface. The direction of travel is less obvious in this case, although thinning or feathering of the stain means that the mark gradually disappears in the direction of travel. Occasionally, especially when the initial contact was gradual and light, feathering appears on both sides of a swipe in which case the direction of motion is very difficult to ascertain.

Flow patterns

Since blood is a fluid, it moves under the influence of gravity. A change of direction in an otherwise uninterrupted flow signals movement. This can be observed if a body is moved soon after death (i.e. whilst blood is still liquid and able to move under gravity).

Fingerprints in blood

Fingerprints (in addition to more obvious patterns such as footwear) may be found in blood—these can be significant as they establish that contact occurred after the blood was deposited. Insofar as footprints represent the direction of travel, they can be useful when reconstructing the incident.

Origin of blood

Determining the point of origin of a series of blood marks requires convergence analysis. By estimating the parabolic 'flight path' of a number of points the origin can be plotted. Lasers and computerized reconstructions have replaced the traditional string pathways. Convergence analysis invariably requires the assumption of a single stationary point of origin; however, this is not always the case in practice.

In practice, it is rare to find patterns not obfuscated by other stains—these complex scenes require careful interpretation.

Forensic identification of semen

Context

The identification of semen may be of relevance in a sexually motivated crime or allegation of rape. The presence of semen is not required to prove the crime of rape and the presence of semen at a scene does not prove that rape occurred.

Identification

Semen is not as visibly obvious to the naked eye as blood, although it will fluoresce when UV light is shone on it. However, urine will also fluoresce under UV light, hence, this is a presumptive test. An amount large enough to be seen by the naked eye will be a yellowish-white stain, but swabs will be taken for other presumptive and/or confirmatory tests to be done in the laboratory. Semen is comprised of sperm cells in seminal fluid. The most common presumptive test is for a constituent of seminal fluid called acid phosphatase (AP). The AP test involves the application of a cocktail of chemicals that will generate a purple colour when AP is present.

Microscopy

A commonly used confirmatory test is the microscopic observation of sperm cells. A smear is made on a microscope slide and stained with one of a selection of dyes (haematoxylin or Christmas tree stain) and then identified under a microscope (purple or red, respectively). The process is time consuming, especially the fewer the sperm cells there are and can be hard to interpret, depending on the amount of contaminating cellular material (e.g. vaginal or faecal matter). The number of sperm cells found is scored on an arbitrary scale of negative or 1–5 levels of positive. The presence of tails on the sperm cells is also noted as this is a certain identification for sperm; the problem being that the tails will degrade or separate from the sperm head very easily after ejaculation and depending on the conditions in which the semen is left or stored.

Prostate specific antigen

The assay for prostate specific antigen or p30 (prostate specific antigen, PSA) is an alternative confirmatory test that stains for another constituent of seminal fluid. It is a time-consuming immunological assay, but is proof positive for semen. It is especially useful in identification of semen with no or few sperm cells.

Location of semen

In suspected rape cases, the location of the semen within the body following vaginal or anal sex is very useful in determining whether penetration may have occurred at all and how long previously. Identification of an individual has been assisted by use of tissue types such as ABO group if secretor positive, or PGM testing.

Forensic identification of other fluids

Urine

Urine is generally not tested for in the laboratory as there is no good, specific assay. Being mainly a solution of salts in water with few cells, it is also not an optimal source for DNA testing. Its main use is in toxicological assays for alcohol and the presence of drugs.

Saliva

Saliva is almost entirely water, but contains other substances, the most important of which is amylase, an enzyme used to digest carbohydrates.

Presumptive test

The suspect material is mixed with a starch solution. Iodine is added and this turns the solution blue-black if the starch is still intact. If amylase is present, it digests some or all of the starch and the test solution will stay yellow-brown (colour of iodine). This procedure for this presumptive test is not optimal and has been modified into the Phadebas test.

Phadebas test

Starch molecules are attached in an insoluble dye complex and when digested by amylase, it releases dye that becomes visible and can be measured or photographed, depending on whether the assay is done in a test tube or using Phadebas-impregnated paper. Although the chemistry is not very sensitive and other body fluids (e.g. semen, vomit, vaginal secretions) contain amylase giving a positive reaction, the relative concentration of amylase in saliva means that it gives a stronger reaction than other fluids. Amylase is relatively stable so positive results can be found after many months. As with semen, identifying an individual has been assisted by use of tissue types (e.g. ABO group, if secretor positive).

Faeces

This is not a good source of evidence or identification, other than giving an idea of food intake. Faeces are mainly bacteria, undigested food residue, gut-lining cells, and blood pigment breakdown products. DNA profiling is inefficient because although many gut-lining cells are shed into the gut, these are usually dead and undergo bacterial degradation.

Bone

In addition to the anthropological information such as age, stature, and sex, carefully prepared bone samples can produce DNA for profiling. Best results are obtained with mitochondrial DNA profiling rather than standard profiling—much depends on the bone used and its condition.

Hair

Hairs and other fibres (whether natural or man-made) are usually considered trace evidence. Hairs and fibres are compared to reference samples using morphology and colour comparison. Plucked scalp hairs are likely to be healthy, alive, and intact, with a root of skin cells from the point of insertion in the scalp. These cells are sufficient to act as a source of DNA for profiling and can therefore be of evidential significance.

Forensic anthropology

The primary role of the forensic anthropologist is to identify and interpret human remains. In this task, there may be overlap with the forensic pathologist: neither should exclude the expert contribution of the other.

Identification

In addition to cases in which an unidentified human body is discovered, either by accident or as the result of a deliberate search, the discovery of skeletal remains is relatively common during building work and other excavations. Although the final and definitive identification of human remains may require DNA evidence, the forensic anthropologist provides a quick, inexpensive, and convenient way of narrowing down the focus of an investigation. Note that unless and until there is a reasonably small number of 'suspects', reference DNA samples are unlikely to be available. The preliminary questions to be addressed by an anthropologist should include:

- Are the remains human or non-human?
- Are the remains 'forensic' or archaeological?
- How many individuals are there?

All skeletal material should always be referred to a forensic anthropologist or forensic pathologist for advice on these questions. Erroneous assumptions made by an inexperienced investigator at this stage are likely to be prejudicial to a successful investigation in the longer term.

If the answers to the earlier listed questions indicate that the remains are human and are of an age to be of interest to the medicolegal authorities (usually less than 50–75 years), the key tasks are to determine the biological profile:

- Sex (sexual dimorphism, particularly the skull and pelvis).
- Age (development and epiphyseal fusion).
- Stature (derived from published formulae using the length of the long bones).
- Race (skull morphology—although controversial).

The techniques employed to determine these primary characteristics vary according to the condition and extent of the remains available, the likely age range (for example, epiphyseal fusion has limited application in the mature skeleton), and the context of the discovery.

It is important not to quote precise findings for the primary characteristics. Age and stature should always be quoted as ranges and sex as a probability. There is considerable debate as to whether racial origins can be usefully determined by an examination of remains and findings should be reported with caution. Remember that the purpose of this examination is not to provide an individual identification, but to focus and guide the investigation which will lead to a positive match (most obviously by reducing the number of potential matches from a missing persons list).

Disease
Skeletal evidence of disease can reveal information about the deceased's medical history. Unless these conditions had been diagnosed during life, this is unlikely to provide any assistance in making an identification.

Disarticulated bones
The forensic anthropologist is able to interpret disarticulated bones. This may provide crucial evidence of animal disruption and ante- and/or post-mortem dismemberment (including cannibalism). This evidence is likely to be critically compromised if the remains are not retrieved, stored, and transported by an experienced forensic anthropologist/archaeologist.

Trauma
Evidence of trauma either prior to or as the cause of death can sometimes be recognized on skeletal remains. In mass grave excavations, bodies frequently reveal evidence of gunshot injuries—the site and characteristics of the bony injury can be useful to distinguish between, for example, execution (which may be illegal) and injuries received during battle (which may not).

Mass disasters
Although in many major incidents, bodies are recovered almost immediately, this is not always the case. If remains are severely decomposed, mutilated, or otherwise unrecognizable, a forensic anthropologist can provide useful clues as to identity. These should be confirmed, if possible, by DNA techniques prior to repatriation and appropriate disposal, as mistakes in identification can be devastating to families and relatives (as well as to the reputation of forensic services and international agencies).

Human rights abuses
Particularly in conflict and ex-conflict countries, the forensic anthropologist investigates allegations of human rights abuses and war crimes and provides evidence for criminal proceedings (usually under the auspices of the United Nations). The work frequently involves the excavation and interpretation of bodies from mass graves and can identify injury types, use of child soldiers, postmortem mutilation, and provide evidence to identify and subsequently repatriate remains.

Body farms
Much information about the process of human decomposition has been gained from research performed at 'body farms' (see 📖 p.35).

Further reading
British Association for Human Identification: 🔗 http://www.bahid.org
Forensic Anthropology Society of Europe (FASE): 🔗 http://www.labanof.unimi.it/FASE.htm

Forensic archaeology

The primary task of the forensic archaeologist is to locate and/or retrieve concealed human remains and to do so in such a way that evidence is preserved. Whereas the activity of the forensic anthropologist takes place in the mortuary or laboratory, the forensic archaeologist works at the scene. In the USA, the terminology is ambiguous and the role of the archaeologist tends to be included under the term anthropologist.

It should be emphasized that forensic archaeologists do not search for 'dead bodies'. Rather they search for various anomalies, such as soil disturbances which are indicators that a body (or drugs, illegal weapons, money, etc.) may be buried. Trained dogs are also available to locate bodies (similar to the use of dogs in avalanche rescue situations). The majority of concealed (as opposed to buried) bodies are discovered by accident in which case the expert assists with the recovery and preservation of evidence from what is likely to be a disturbed and contaminated scene. A body buried by a perpetrator can remain undiscovered despite extensive searches (e.g. the body of one of Ian Brady's victims, Keith Bennett, has never been located on Saddleworth Moor), although other apparently unrelated events might provide the vital preliminary clue (e.g. following Peter Tobin's conviction for the rape and murder of Angelika Kluk in 2007, police searched a house where he had previously lived and discovered the body of Vicky Hamilton who had disappeared in 1991).

Tools for searching include:

- Aerial photography (preferably at dawn or dusk as angled sunlight casts shadows and highlights 3D features).
- Magnetometry (variations in magnetic fields).
- Ground penetrating radar (2D profiles of reflected radar pulses are plotted to generate a 3D image of the surveyed area).
- Resistivity (near-surface variations in electrical resistance).

A forensic botanist (or a botanist with the experience of acting on the instructions of a legal authority) will be able to interpret plant repopulation following soil disturbance.

The decision to use line-searching/walking should be a balance between using small numbers of trained experts and (often significantly) larger numbers of willing and enthusiastic volunteers. If volunteers are forthcoming, then searching is optimized by interspersing trained experts throughout the line and focusing expertise on areas identified as being likely locations. Those in charge of coordinating such a search should never forget that community resources might be extremely useful when appropriately managed, yet can often feel excluded if offers of assistance are dismissed without adequate explanation.

Excavation and retrieval

During excavation, which may involve horizontal or vertical trenches, the trained archaeologist must document and record all findings, including taking note of position (absolute and relative) using GPS (global positioning system) when appropriate. Subject to the burial matrix, it might be possible to recover toolmarks, footprints, and other impression evidence in addition to physical items such as bone. Particular care must be taken to identify and recover all the small bones (such as the phalanges). The absence of these bones at a burial site might be evidence that the body was moved from a previous location. The absence of these bones back at the mortuary should never be the result of inadequate excavation or recovery.

Examination and interpretation (either by the same individual or a forensic anthropologist and/or forensic pathologist) should, if possible, take place at a well-lit, fully serviced mortuary.

Forensic entomology

History

The association between flies and death (or dead bodies) has been known for a long time. The Ancient Egyptians appear to have understood the connection between the dead body, maggots and flies (*Book of the Dead*, Chapter 154), and Homer refers to swarms of flies around bodies on the battlefield (*The Iliad* XIX). The earliest reported use of insects to solve crime appears in the works of Sung Tz'u (1186–1249) who used the fact that flies swarmed to a murder weapon (a sickle) to elicit a confession from the guilty man. In the 16th century, the *Vanitas* school of Dutch artists often depicted the evanescent nature of human desire by placing a fly on a skull, whilst Emily Dickinson's (1830–1886) poem *Dying* focuses on a single fly in a room.

Body farms

There are several 'body farms' in the USA which are involved in the study of forensic entomology (see 📖 p.35).

Determining the postmortem interval

The most frequent role of the forensic entomologist is to estimate a post-mortem interval. However, it is important to be aware that it is only possible to quote a time that the body has been exposed to oviposition (egg laying). This is not necessarily the same as the time since death. This can be significantly different if, for example, the body has been moved or conditions have changed significantly in the interim.

There are two different methods of determining the time since oviposition, both based on the fact that insects are poikilothermic (their development rate fluctuates with temperature). This growth-rate/temperature relationship has been established in the laboratory for various species. It is essential to establish the identity of the species: this may be possible from larvae if they are at an advanced stage of development, otherwise rearing to adulthood (in the laboratory) is necessary. DNA profiling is likely to become useful in this area. Correct identification is essential, as different species have different developmental rates.

The comparative method compares the oldest specimen recovered from the crime scene to a development rate chart which gives the number of development hours (i.e. the time taken for the species to grow to the observed state of development) for various known temperatures. The temperature at the crime scene usually has to be estimated (even if the temperature is accurately measured after discovery, this only approximates to the temperature fluctuation during the period from the crime to the arrival of the law enforcement officers).

If the temperature at the scene (or, more likely, a nearby meteorological station) is known more precisely then the linear relationship between developmental rate and temperature can give a more accurate time since oviposition. A given species takes the same number of temperature units (known as accumulated degree hours, ADH) to develop to the same stage (within the upper and lower threshold limits for that species). For example, for *Calliphora vicina* (bluebottle blowfly), the development from egg to adult requires approximately 7200 ADH. It is possible, therefore, to sum the number of ADH and back-count on the development rate chart appropriate to the identified stage of larval development at the scene. An alternative to the ADH method is to use accumulated degree days (ADD), although if the temperature can be determined on an hour-by-hour basis, the ADH is more precise.

It is important to be aware that several variables affect the result and the postmortem interval should be regarded as an estimate, not an exact time. Variables include: location (the minimum developmental temperature varies significantly according to location), humidity, species mix, microclimate, maggot masses (which affect temperature), movement, and method of concealing the body.

The entomologist should attend at the scene if possible. Otherwise, specimens should be collected from the scene (flying insects—using an insect net) and body. Larvae should be collected according to a protocol agreed with the entomologist.

Other uses of entomology

These include identification of individual hosts by blood-meals (DNA analysis of haematophages), neglect (elderly or the young based on insects attracted to faeces), drug analysis (drugs can be detected in larvae feeding on a body), transportation, and smuggling (localized species found in shipments).

Accident investigation

Stings from bees and wasps can be a causal factor in accidents. Reactions to stings are classified into three degrees of severity:[1]

- *Hymenopterism vulgaris*—the majority of cases. Painful, but not serious or lethal although accidents can result from loss of concentration or panic.
- *Hymenopterism intermedia*—usually non-lethal, but caution is required when swelling of the tongue, neck, or throat results in impairment of swallowing and breathing.
- *Hymenopterism ultima*—lethal or near-lethal reactions to stings, usually as a result of anaphylactic shock.

Insects are a potentially significant threat as a result of bioterrorism, as they may be used as vectors to carry disease or other hazards. As weapons for military use, their significance depends on the extent to which their behaviour can be modified to achieve a particular objective.

Reference

1 Fluno JA (1961). Wasps as enemies of man. *Bull Ent Soc Amer* **7**:117–19.

Environmental forensics

Definition and scope

The techniques of forensic investigation have extensive application to the legal implications of human activity on the environment. The term was first used after the Exxon Valdez oil spill in Alaska (1989). The remit of 'environmental forensics' is wide-ranging, overlaps with other disciplines, and includes:

- Pollution (land, sea, noise).
- Chemical contamination (and decontamination procedures).
- Waste disposal and management.
- Wildlife crime (live animal smuggling, trade in animal products, endangered species).
- 'Conflict diamonds.'
- Fire behaviour in rural environments (particularly relevant to the investigation of bush and forest fires).

Methodology

Techniques include those derived from a number of different disciplines, including analytical chemistry, microbiology, biochemistry, geosciences, hydrogeology, and atmospheric physics, in addition to those routinely used by forensic scientists in other areas. Given the ever-increasing amount and scope of legislation relating to the environment, it is important that breaches are thoroughly investigated and that an evidence-base is established on which to prosecute offenders (often on the basis of corporate and strict liability).

Action

If law-enforcement officers suspect activity relating to any of these disciplines, it is imperative that advice from an appropriate expert or agency is sought as soon as possible.

Further reading

Convention on International Trade in Endangered Species of Wild Fauna and Flora:
 http://www.cites.org
Environment Agency: http://www.environment-agency.gov.uk
European Environment Agency: http://www.eea.europa.eu
Partnership for Action against Wildlife Crime http://www.defra.gov.uk/paw
Scottish Environment Protection Agency: http://www.sepa.org.uk
United States Environmental Protection Agency: http://www.epa.gov

Document analysis

The field of document analysis is wide-ranging and includes various scenarios in which questions are asked: forged handwriting and/or signatures (e.g. cheques, wills), identifying the author of handwritten material (e.g. blackmail letters), identity of printers, photocopiers, and other devices, timescale of entries (e.g. diaries, accounts), origin of paper, and tracking amendments and alterations.

Handwriting analysis

This includes authentication of a wide range of handwritten documents. Graphologists claim that handwriting reflects personal character traits—this is a different area entirely (and one with little forensic application). Letters are examined and compared on the basis of their shape and their construction (stroke order and direction) and also their relation to adjacent characters. Ideally, the comparison should be between the same text written in the same format—either capital letters (upper case), script (letters are not joined), or cursive (joined-up writing without lifting the writing instrument). This sample might be available from other handwritten documents or can be requested from a suspect. The latter approach has the advantage of being able to control the pen, paper, and text, but it also tends to emphasize variations resulting from stress and of course, introduces the risk of deliberate disguise. An expert opinion can state that the comparison is conclusive, supportive, or inconclusive as to whether the compared documents were written by the same or different individuals. Note that the assumption that an individual's handwriting is unique has little or no scientific or statistical basis.

Signatures

Although signatures are a form of handwriting, by their very nature they are highly specific. Forged signatures may be traced (so they lack natural flow) or practised (so they often lack accuracy). It is not possible to state that a signature is forged simply because it is dissimilar to another example, because of natural variation. Indeed, signatures which are too 'identical' should raise suspicion. When examined under a low power microscope, a forged signature may exhibit pauses and re-starts of strokes, jerky strokes (by writing very slowly) and evidence of tracing (pencil marks, indentations). These observations are objective. More subjectively, the expert may comment on morphological discrepancies (especially the proportions of characters) and such things as the position of the signature with respect to other content of a document.

Other document analysis

In addition to handwritten documents, inks, printing methods (e.g. laser, inkjet, dot-matrix), paper and other characteristics of printed documents can be analysed to establish date, source and potential falsification.

Further reading

Chip and pin card security: http://www.cardwatch.org.uk
Security features of Euro banknotes: http://www.ecb.int/euro/banknotes/security

Forensic miscellany

As indicated in the introduction to this chapter, any scientific discipline which finds itself involved in a case of legal significance can be regarded as a 'forensic science'. Some of those not previously discussed include branches of engineering, soil analysis, palynology (pollen analysis), ear identification (the European FEARID project), dendrochronology (used, famously, in the Lindbergh kidnapping case and also in several art and musical instrument fraud cases) and limnology (including the use of diatoms to diagnose freshwater drowning). All of these have some aspects which are considered controversial, but there are many examples of their use in successful prosecutions.

Soil analysis

The analysis of soil is particularly complex as it comprises inorganic and organic substances. Inorganic parts include particles of stones, sand, as well as chemicals such as salts. Organic constituents include dead and decaying vegetal matter, as well as pollen, microscopic insects, worms, and bacteria. Some attempts are being made to create databases of soil composition from different geographic regions and land uses. Potentially, the DNA profile of entire bacterial mixtures found in soil samples can be generated for identification purposes.

Pollen

Different plants produce pollen of different sizes, shapes, and quantities at different times of the year. Microscopic examination of clothing and other material or swabs of body surfaces, will often detect complex mixtures, and sometimes very specific types, of pollen. This may be used to identify the geographical source or location of origin of the pollen which may be useful in tracking the whereabouts of evidential material. The difficulty may not be so much in the ability to identify the pollen, but to evaluate its meaning under the circumstances.

Forensic accountancy

Although not covered by the usual meaning of the term 'science', it is worth also mentioning disciplines such as forensic accountancy. Crimes such as money laundering, fraud, and Internet or computer-related offences, often require extremely detailed analysis of financial transactions and electronic transfers of funds (almost invariably with no physical 'paper trail').

Other activities

Of greater controversy are those activities with little or no published or verified scientific basis, but are promoted by individuals as aids to investigation. These include various para-psychological or pseudo-scientific 'techniques' often promoted by charismatic individuals who target families or relatives of victims (whilst also claiming success with law enforcement agencies). It should be noted that if an individual 'predicts' the location of, for example, a murder victim often enough then they will, inevitably, get it correct eventually—this may well form the basis of the 'success' story. Whether or not such activities can assist an investigation is open to argument: what is less equivocal is the fact that they do not produce evidence which is likely to be accepted by a court of law (they would almost certainly fail the Daubert standard for admissibility of scientific evidence—see 🕮 p.507).

Note that there are various scientific disciplines, such as forensic psychology, which have an important role in informing an investigation, although they may provide little or no evidence which can aid conviction. A psychologist may, for example, interpret an incident to state that this-or-that scenario is more-or-less likely (often based on documented series of apparently analogous cases). This can often significantly benefit an investigation by providing an initial focus so that resources can be targeted appropriately. However, to suggest that an individual is, therefore 'guilty' on the basis of this type of analysis would be to commit a fallacy of induction.

Fire: background

Conditions for fire

Four conditions are required for a fire to ignite and continue to burn:

- Combustible material (fuel)
- Oxidizing agent (usually O_2)
- Energy (usually heat)
- A self-sustaining reaction.

Fuel and O_2 must be present in suitable proportions for combustion to occur. There are defined upper and lower limits out of which a fuel will not ignite. These are termed the 'flammability limits' of the fuel.

Energy may be generated by mechanical means, for example, friction as in the striking of a match; electrical means, for example, arcing or short-circuiting of electrical appliances; gaseous compression; and chemical or nuclear reactions.

Continuation of a fire

Once a fire starts, the heat produced from the exothermic reaction is usually sufficient for continuous re-ignition to occur and provided a supply of fuel and O_2 is maintained, the fire will continue. Removing one or more of these requirements, however, will result in the fire being extinguished—this provides the theoretical basis for fire-fighting.

Types of fire

Fires may be distinguished as flammable combustion or smouldering combustion, depending on whether flames are present or not.

Flammable combustion

Flames result from the burning of flammable gas. This gas may be the fuel itself causing the fire (e.g. natural gas); it may result from the pyrolysis (chemical breakdown due to heat) of solid fuels generating flammable gases; or from the vaporization of flammable gases from liquid fuels, such as petrol.

Smouldering combustion

In contrast, smouldering combustion, which is seen at the interface between solid fuels and air, is devoid of flames, generating only heat and light. Solid fuels, such as wood, which are based on carbon compounds, which pyrolyse to produce flammable gases, also produce char (impure carbon remains) and this char may continue to smoulder after the pyrolysis products have burnt (the basis of a charcoal barbecue).

Fire prevention and safety

Regulations

In the UK, various regulations (e.g. *The Furniture and Furnishings (Fire) (Safety) Regulations 1988* as amended) govern the ignition characteristics of materials used in furniture manufacture. These were introduced in response to concern about the number of fatalities arising from fires involving polyurethane foam. The regulations are out of the scope of this book, but they are relevant to investigators seeking to determine the cause of a fire and the cause of death in a fire-related fatality. Furniture made prior to 1950 is exempt from the regulations, but furniture of this era is still in widespread use. All furniture and furnishings to which the regulations apply should be appropriately labelled. Furniture donated free of charge (e.g. by a charity) or given away by an individual is not covered by the regulations. In most cases, landlords who rent homes as part of a business are obliged to ensure that any included furniture adheres to the regulations. The regulations in the UK are considered to be stricter than those in the EU or USA.

Toxicological analysis

Although CO is the most frequent killer in fatal domestic fires, the toxicologist should analyse postmortem samples for the highly toxic products of foam combustion (e.g. HCN) as this provides an audit of the effectiveness of this type of legislation.

Smoke detectors

The most significant fire safety improvement in the domestic setting has been the widespread installation of smoke detectors/alarms. These are required by building regulations to be fitted into new houses. Landlords letting property on a commercial basis must ensure adequate (as determined by the size of the house, for example) smoke alarms are fitted (including mains-powered alarms). Multiple occupancy properties (houses in multiple occupation, HMO) and commercial properties are covered by specific legislation which includes the use of fire doors and protected escape routes. Smoke detectors/alarms and fire doors are designed to increase the chance of escape once a fire has started: the regulations referred to here are intended to decrease the risk of fire starting.

Water sprinklers

Water sprinkler systems are relatively rare in domestic properties, but legislation requires the fitting of a sprinkler system in larger commercial properties. The Theatre Royal, Drury Lane, London, was fitted with a sprinkler system in 1812.

Behaviour of fire indoors

Observations of test fires in controlled laboratory environments, using defined settings and parameters, provide information regarding the course of a fire. Real fires may behave unpredictably because of unknown variables. Fires that burn indoors in a room can be described as going through a sequence of stages, namely:

• Ignition
• Growth
• Flashover
• Fully developed fire (post-flashover steady-state burning)
• Decay.

Ignition

A fire will ignite only if four conditions for ignition (see 📖 p.540) are present. Flame may be immediate or only after a smouldering fire has generated sufficient heat. A fire may smoulder for a period before self-extinguishing.

Growth

Fire may spread from the point of ignition (the 'seat'). The spread will depend on the availability of O_2 and position of fuel relative to the seat. Modern fabrics may contain substances that actively retard the fire development. Heat required for growth may be transferred by one of three mechanisms: thermal convection, thermal conduction, and radiation.

Thermal convection

Transmission of heat by the movement of gas or liquid molecules away from the source of heat. The flow of heated molecules set up by this mechanism creates convection currents and these currents of hot gas rise upwards from a fire due to the increased buoyancy of the heated gas molecules. In this way, a fire that starts at a lower level in a room will produce pyrolysis products that rise to form a layer of hot gas at the top of the room, below which the temperature of the air in the room will remain relatively cool. Convection is usually the most efficient mechanism of transferring heat from burning fuel and because of the upward currents, a fire in a solid framework will tend to burn upwards more readily than downwards or outwards.

Thermal conduction

This is the movement of heat through a medium as energy is transferred from molecule to molecule, without there being macroscopic movement of the medium (e.g. transfer of heat along a metal rod). The contribution that conduction plays in spreading heat in a room fire will depend on the thermal conductivity of the components and furnishings in the room.

Radiation

This is the transmission of heat in the form of electromagnetic radiation (largely responsible for causing flashover). Fuel above a flame may catch light and start to burn, which allows the fire to spread upwards. The extent of the flames depends on the availability of fuel and O_2.

A fire will usually burn in a conical shape, the narrowest part being at the bottom spreading outwards towards the upper regions of the affected area. This is provided the fire can spread outwards in all directions. If the fire is curtailed by a vertical surface (e.g. a wall), then a burn pattern in a shape approximating to a V will be formed on that surface.

Flameover

This is the ignition of the hot pyrolysis products that have risen to the ceiling by convection. It results in a rapid engulfment of the ceiling in flames and increased temperature of the affected area.

Dropdown

This occurs when items above the level of the fire, for example, curtains or larger structural components, fall to the ground and ignite. If dropdown is available in significant quantities, then this maintains a supply of fresh fuel to the fire. Ignited dropdown should not be confused with multiple fire seats (which have a high suspicion of being caused deliberately).

Flashover

This describes the instantaneous ignition of all the fuel (gas, solid, and liquid) in the room and occurs if the temperature in the room increases sufficiently (often following flameover). Flashover signals the end of effective search and rescue as it involves extremely high temperatures (>500°C). It is the transition from a content fire to a structural fire. Delaying flashover can create valuable search and rescue time and can be achieved by allowing the escape of heat, limiting the supply of O_2 and using fire fighting equipment to reduce the temperature in the room.

The investigator should have an understanding of flashover as it replicates the effects of, and can easily be mistaken for, an accelerated (arson) fire (e.g. wall charring from floor to ceiling). It also destroys more subtle evidence which might have pointed to a seat of ignition and evidence of criminality.

Fully developed fire (post-flashover steady state burning)

Following flashover, the heat release rate in the burning room will be at its maximum level as all of the available fuel in the room is involved. The rate at which the fuel burns is limited by the air supply: the fire is said to be ventilation controlled. It is likely that the rate at which pyrolysis products are produced will exceed the rate at which the O_2 required to burn these gases is supplied. Partial combustion and pyrolysis products that have built up, and which are present in hot smoke leaving the burning room may result in flameover.

Decay

The limiting factors to an indoor fire are availability of fuel and O_2. The source of energy (heat) is usually provided by the fire itself and is only limited if fire fighting occurs. If an indoor fire is limited by O_2, sufficient levels of pyrolysis products may still be produced so that, if the room is suddenly ventilated, rapid flaming combustion may again be supported. This is termed 'flashback'.

Behaviour of fire outdoors

Background

Outdoor fires can be naturally occurring phenomena or result from human activity. Fires which are of human origin may be started with deliberate and malicious intent ('arson') or inadvertently. The latter includes those fires which were started with a specific purpose (e.g. barbecue, bonfire), but which later spread out of control.

Development and spread

Outdoor fires follow a less complex sequence of events than indoor fires. A fire in an open area of horizontal ground will generate convection currents as the hot gases rise from the seat of the fire. At the same time, air will flow towards the base of the fire, so O_2 will not be in short supply, but whether the fire will spread will be dependent on fuel being adjacent to the base of the fire and the rate at which the fuel can be heated. Because of the flow of convection currents, hot gases will be carried up, so heating of the ground level fuel will be dependent on conduction and radiation. The fire will spread in a shape and course dependent on the characteristics of the surrounding fuel (type, size, distribution, and moisture), the weather, and environmental conditions (the topography). Fire will travel up-slope more rapidly than down-slope, as the flames preheat the fuel and make the process of ignition more rapid.

Fire barriers

Fire barriers are areas which contain no fuel. They are used to limit the spread of fire. If wind conditions are favourable, fire has the potential to 'jump' across these breaks. Thermal convection heats material across the barrier and particularly if the wind is sufficiently strong to transfer hot embers, fuel can ignite at remote locations. When used to protect property, fire barriers are known as 'Asset Protection Zones'. They comprise part of the design of developments which lie in proximity to high-risk fire areas.

Fire: investigation

The investigation of a fire scene should follow the procedures applicable to more general crime scene investigation. Fires starting accidentally may have public safety and legal implications (tort/negligence, Health and Safety), whilst deliberate ignition can give rise to various criminal charges (including murder).

Preserving life or evidence?

Perhaps more than in any other scene, there is often an inevitable conflict between the task of preserving life (and property) and the preservation of evidence. Before any evidence gathering can be allowed to take place, the fire must be extinguished (itself a process which is likely to compromise evidence) and the scene must be declared safe by an appropriately qualified person.

It is crucial that all investigators work together as a team and adhere to a single and consistent line of command. It is usual for the Fire and Rescue Service to lead the investigation of a fire, although other specialists will be called upon when relevant (e.g. the forensic pathologist will investigate fatalities).

Origin of fire

The primary questions in any fire investigation are to determine the seat and the cause of the fire. The detection of accelerants is a major part in the determination that a fire has been started deliberately, although this information must always be interpreted in conjunction with the circumstances of the scene and other evidence (witness statements regarding spread, forced entry, etc.).

Multiple seats

The presence of multiple seats tends to indicate that a fire was started deliberately, but these must be distinguished from dropdown and other incidental findings.

Smell of vapours

The smell of vapours at a scene suggests that an accelerant has been used in a fire. Trained sniffer dogs are potentially useful aids to an investigation. In industrial settings, it is more likely that fire accelerants might have been present for other reasons, so it is important to ascertain what chemicals if any, were present before the fire started.

Collected samples

Samples which are collected should be stored and transported in nylon bags. These are suitable because the level of hydrocarbon leakage through the bags is low (though they are permeable to alcohol and water). Other materials (for example, polythene) allow leakage of the typical accelerants that may be used at a fire, resulting in loss of evidence and the potential for contamination with other samples. Contamination is a significant problem with fire scene samples.

Analysis

Samples are typically analysed by GC–MS (gas chromatography–mass spectrometry) using samples from the head-space of the test sample. This process allows the components of the sample to be separated, giving a characteristic fingerprint of different fuels. The sensitivity of GC–MS allows trace as well as bulk samples to be analysed, and its ability to separate different components in mixtures enables the different components of mixtures to be isolated, from which identification may follow.

Interpretation of the analysis of samples taken from a fire scene can be difficult because of the confusion between the chemical profiles of samples and the other products of combustion or the breakdown products of hydrocarbons. Whilst fuels such as petrol and diesel have a characteristic fingerprint, components within these fuels and their breakdown products may correspond with those of furnishing and carpet pyrolysis products, making it different to tell if the analysis has detected the presence of an accelerant or the effect of fire from combustion of products normally present during a fire. Reconstruction of fire scenes is an important part of determining what happened to cause a fire and can aid interpretation of the results of the scientific analysis.

Arson

Arson is the deliberate and malicious setting on fire of property either owned by the individual (usually a fraudulent insurance claim) or by another person. Motives for arson are various and include revenge, fraud, vandalism, pyromania, 'enjoyment' (particularly the power and control over the emergency services), and the concealment of crime (including murder). Schools are frequently targeted by pupils/ex-pupils. Deliberate fire-setting is not limited to buildings, but can also involve waste ground and bush or forest areas.

Explosions and explosives

Physics

An explosion results when pressure in a space increases at a rate greater than can be dispersed or exceeds the ability of a containing vessel to hold it. There is a rapid release of energy, causing a violent effect. The explosive process can be mechanical, thermal, electrical, nuclear (fusion or fission), or as is the case in the majority of deliberate explosions, chemical.

Chemical process

The explosive process is initiated by supplying sufficient energy to the oxidizing agent component and the fuel component. A primary explosive may be used to initiate the secondary explosive. Firearms' cartridges work along these lines with the primer (primary explosive) triggering the propellant. The fuel component and oxidizing agent part of an explosive may be combined by physically mixing the components together or they may be part of the same compound—for example, nitroglycerine (glyceryl trinitrate) and TNT (2,4,6-trinitrotoluene). Inert substances may be added to make the explosive safer to handle (e.g. dynamite, which is based on nitroglycerine). Explosives which rely on physically mixing separate fuel and oxidizing agents together may use fuels such as sugars or other carbohydrates, carbon or hydrocarbons, powdered metals or sulphur, and common oxidizing agents including inorganic nitrates, chlorates, and percholates. Gunpowder is a mixture of carbon, sulphur, and potassium nitrate.

Detonating explosives

Otherwise known as 'high explosives', these do not usually need to be contained in order to explode. High explosives that are contained (e.g. military applications such as shells, grenades, bombs, mines), not only produce the powerful blast of the explosion, but also send fragments of the casing at high speed. In a detonating explosion, the reaction travels through the explosive medium at a speed in excessive of the speed of sound.

Low (deflagrating) explosives

In contrast to high explosives, these need to be contained in a vessel in order to explode. The direction of the subsequent blast can be controlled by having a deliberately constructed path of least resistance. The propellant of firearms is an example of a deflagrating explosive, as are flammable dusts such as flour, and mixtures of air and natural gas.

Condensed and dispersed explosives

Condensed explosives (solid or liquid) and dispersed explosives (gas or an aerosol, i.e. a fine dispersion of solid or liquid in a gas) may detonate or deflagrate, but detonations of dispersed explosives are rare.

Effects of the explosive blast

The destruction or effects of the explosive blast may indicate the type of explosive involved. In a condensed explosion, the maximum damage tends to coincide with the explosion centre (which may form a crater). The pressure of the detonation decreases away from the explosion centre. Detonation of a dispersed explosion, however, results in an increase of pressure away from the point of origin. There is a less clear relationship between pressure and distance from the explosion centre in deflagration of a dispersed explosive.

Detonations of condensed explosives cause maximal damage, often with a shattering or pulverizing effect. Deflagrations of condensed explosives tend to cause less blast damage, bending being the typical damage (often accompanied by extensive heat damage at the site of the explosive). In a dispersed deflagration, objects are often displaced, rather than shattered (walls may be pushed outwards) and objects within the actual explosion may be relatively unscathed. While craters may form when a condensed explosive is detonated on a surface, they are not produced by deflagration of a dispersed explosive. Explosions may also lead to fires.

Explosion investigation

The investigation of a scene of an explosion follows the principles as outlined for any scene of crime investigation. Whenever an explosive substance is suspected (either from observation of damage or from intelligence-led investigation) an appropriate explosives expert should be on scene. The possibility of similar unexploded devices (or 'booby-traps' if placed deliberately) should be assumed until the area has been declared safe. If fire starts as a result of an explosion, the priority is to extinguish this and ensure the scene is safe before proceeding.

Casualties

The fact that casualties may need to be attended to close to the scene of the explosion is an additional complication. Officers in charge should prioritize the need to maintain order amongst the likely chaos and panic resulting from such events.

Scene control

The scene of an explosion can cover a considerable area. As far as is practicable, the cordon should include all this area. Note that as distance from the explosion centre increases, the fragments of evidence are likely to get smaller, so a search must be thorough and comprehensive. Items outside a cordon are liable to be collected by the public (including 'souvenir hunters') and important information may be lost (including information which may be helpful in identifying victims). Debris may include parts of the explosive device (detonator, timer, container if used, remote control, etc.) which need to be collected and examined. Such material may lead to laboratory identification of remains of an explosive, origin of the components, how the device was constructed, triggered, and potentially the individual(s) or organization involved. It is not uncommon for terrorist or criminal organizations to claim responsibility for large explosions and although certain authentication procedures may be in place, this should not replace thorough investigation.

Unintentional explosions

In addition to the obvious criminal implications of deliberate incidents, explosions (such as gas explosions), resulting from poor maintenance of infrastructure and/or illegal installation, whilst not being deliberate, may lead to prosecution under tort/negligence and/or Health and Safety legislation.

Analysis

A number of techniques are used to analyse suspected chemical explosives. If a sample is suspected of containing a volatile explosive compound (e.g. nitroglycerine), then GC–MS may be used. Other chromatography methods, such as HPLC (high performance liquid chromatography), TLC (thin layer chromatography), or IC (ion chromatography, which separates ionic or polar species) are also used. SEM-EDX can identify which elements are present in a sample and IR spectroscopy can provide information regarding the chemical species or functional groups of the sample. Atomic absorption and emission spectroscopies may also be employed to analyse suspected explosives.

The context effect and scientific evidence

In forensic medicine and science, as in most areas of life, the context in which one looks at something changes how we perceive and interpret what we 'see'. Optical illusions and 'magic' tricks work on this principle—the natural tendency to interpret what we 'see' according to what we expect, given previous experience and other contemporaneous information including what we are told.

In a forensic context, one key question is how much should an expert know about the case before they carry out their examination? This is a balance between having sufficient knowledge of the circumstances of the event in order to make the appropriate investigations, on one hand, and relying too heavily on assumptions and 'context' on the other. It needs to be remembered that a complainant does not necessarily admit to all aspects of the alleged offence immediately and the expert should never miss finding evidence simply because there was no reported reason to look. This is particularly important when examining a child.

In a case of a sudden death of a young known drug user, toxicological tests are likely to be instructed routinely. But what about the apparently natural death of an elderly person? One need look no further than the Shipman case (see 📖 p.486) to see an example of how easy it is to accept an expert's opinion simply because it seems to fit what we assume happened.

To admit bias in the scientific process is not to admit dishonesty or lack of integrity. It is simply to accept that individuals use direct experience and interactions in different ways. The good investigator will be aware of these and take them into account when analysing scientific results and evaluating and interpreting evidence.

Further reading

Dror I, Charlton D, Péron A (2006). Contextual information renders experts vulnerable to making erroneous identifications. *Forensic Sci Int* **156**:74–8.
Saks MJ, Risinger DM, Rosenthal R, *et al.* (2003). Context effects in forensic science: A review and application of the science of science to crime laboratory practice in the United States. *Sci Justice* **43**(2):77–90.

Forensic statistics

Why are statistics relevant to forensic medicine? Expressions such as 'beyond reasonable doubt' and more obviously, 'on the balance of probabilities' are probabilistic statements. When dealing with complex scientific evidence, experts should be fully aware of statistical implications. Dangers associated with statistical and probabilistic evidence are more than adequately illustrated by the paediatrician Professor Roy Meadow.

'Meadow's law'

The aphorism, 'one sudden infant death is a tragedy, two is suspicious and three is murder until proved otherwise' became embodied in forensic orthodoxy during the latter part of the 20th century.[1,2] Sally Clark was convicted of murder in 1999 and released on appeal in 2003. The evidence of Meadow was crucial to Clark's conviction (and also in the similar Anthony, Cannings, and Patel cases).

Meadow's evidence was flawed because of a misunderstanding of statistics—he treated each death as an independent event, an assumption which if valid, justified multiplying the accepted probability for one event (approximately 1 in 8500) to give a figure which made it appear extremely unlikely that deaths were natural (1 in 73 million). Assumption of independence is erroneous, because there may well be genetic and/or environmental factors which predispose a family to sudden infant death ('cot death'), thus making a second death more (not less) likely.

Managing statistics in a forensic context

- Statistical or probabilistic evidence in court should be presented by a statistician or expert with an appropriate knowledge of the subject (more generally, illustrating the danger of an expert speaking outside the area of their expertise).
- Statistical or probabilistic evidence should never be quoted in isolation.

Sample size determination

Whenever law enforcement agencies recover suspected drugs (or, for example, DVDs containing pornographic images) it is necessary to know how many should be sampled to prove the offence. An appropriate statistical expert should be consulted for sub-sampling advice.[3]

Bayesian reasoning

This involves relating the probability before an observation (a priori) to that after the observation (a posteriori). Although increasingly used in forensic science, it has been criticized on the grounds that if one assumes guilt, it is easier to interpret evidence to support that assumption—the Prosecutor's fallacy (see 🕮 p.554). Bayesian thinking permits a pragmatic approach which permits investigators to focus on what are 'more likely' to be important pieces of evidence and disregard those less likely to be crucial.

References

1 Meadow R (1997). *ABC of Child Abuse*, 3rd edn. London: BMJ Books.
2 DiMaio DJ and DiMaio JM (1989). *Forensic Pathology*. St Louis: Elsevier.
3 Aitken C (1999). Sampling – How big a sample? *J Forensic Sci* **44**:750–60.

The prosecutor's fallacy

Forensic investigation is concerned with collecting evidence for presentation to a court if called upon by either the prosecution (or plaintiff/pursuer in a civil action) or the defence. As the techniques used to collect and analyse evidence become increasingly sophisticated, it is imperative that those who use and present the evidence—the scientific experts as well as the lawyers—are aware of the increased problems with the interpretation of evidence. This is a significant issue with evidence having a statistical basis.

The good prosecutor must avoid the fallacy of the transposed conditional.

Suppose that expert evidence indicates that the probability of finding the evidence on an innocent person is very small. This might be a sample of DNA or, indeed, any other type of evidence (such as a fragment of paint, pollen, or drug) which links the suspect with the crime. The fallacy is then to assert that the probability of the accused being innocent is, therefore, correspondingly small.

Example

The following example illustrates the fallacy. A witness to a robbery reports a man wearing a distinctive yellow jacket with a single red sleeve running from the crime scene. According to the manufacturer, only 4 jackets were manufactured like this out of a 10 000 production run. A suspect is identified and is found to own a jacket matching the description. The prosecutor's fallacy asserts there is a 4 in 10 000 chance of finding this jacket type and so the probability of innocence is only 4 in 10 000. But this transposition of probabilities is exposed as nonsense if we know that all 4 jackets with this distinctive pattern were sold from the same shop in the same town. Based on such a statistic, therefore, the probability of innocence is more like 3 in 4. Note that the prosecutor's fallacy tends to rely heavily on evidence where chance occurrence is unlikely and neglects evidence that has a higher probability of happening as being less useful, even if it may help establish that a suspect was not involved.

DNA evidence is particularly prone to statistical manipulation. Suppose a suspect has a DNA match to a crime scene with a probability of 1 in 50 000, that is $p=0.00002$. This is certainly useful evidence, but the prosecutor's fallacy is to claim that the probability of innocence is, therefore, also 1 in 50 000. Even if the population of the city is only half a million then 10 people from that geographical location could produce this DNA match. Thus, the probability of innocence, derived from this single item of evidence, is significantly larger (1 in 10).

How to avoid the fallacy

It is important to avoid either giving the impression, or the excuse, for a prosecutor to erroneously transpose the unlikeliness of an event to the unlikeliness of innocence.

It should be remembered that many strands of independent evidence properly used will reduce the likelihood of type 1 error.

It is equally important to bear in mind that the role of the medical or scientific expert is to disprove a null hypothesis, not to prove the prosecution's favoured theory.

Finding an unlikely coincidence of suspect sample and crime scene is not the same as proving guilt or establishing a lack of innocence.

The defence fallacy

In the earlier example, the defence argues that if the chance of match is 0.00002 then in a town with a population of 500 000 there are 10 possible matches. Therefore the DNA evidence is irrelevant since nine other people are also possible suspects. That is, the likelihood of guilt is only 1 in 10. The defender's fallacy is to only scrutinize the evidence piece by piece and ignore other relevant items of evidence before making a statement about the innocence of the suspect.

All the evidence should be considered, taken together. Individual pieces of evidence should never be treated in isolation.

Index